METHODS IN CELL BIOLOGY

VOLUME 26

Prenatal Diagnosis
Cell Biological Approaches

METHODS IN CELL BIOLOGY

Prepared under the Auspices of the American Society for Cell Biology

VOLUME 26
Prenatal Diagnosis
Cell Biological Approaches

Edited by

SAMUEL A. LATT

CHILDREN'S HOSPITAL MEDICAL CENTER
AND BRIGHAM AND WOMEN'S HOSPITAL
HARVARD MEDICAL SCHOOL
BOSTON, MASSACHUSETTS

and

GRETCHEN J. DARLINGTON

DIVISION OF HUMAN GENETICS
DEPARTMENT OF MEDICINE
CORNELL UNIVERSITY MEDICAL COLLEGE
NEW YORK, NEW YORK

1982

ACADEMIC PRESS
A Subsidiary of Harcourt Brace Jovanovich, Publishers

New York   London
Paris   San Diego   San Francisco   São Paulo   Sydney   Tokyo   Toronto

ACADEMIC PRESS, INC.
111 Fifth Avenue, New York, New York 10003

United Kingdom Edition published by
ACADEMIC PRESS, INC. (LONDON) LTD.
24/28 Oval Road, London NW1 7DX

LIBRARY OF CONGRESS CATALOG CARD NUMBER: 64-14220

ISBN: 0-12-564126-5

PRINTED IN THE UNITED STATES OF AMERICA

82 83 84 85   9 8 7 6 5 4 3 2 1

To our parents, spouses, and children

CONTENTS

vii

8. *Miniaturization of Biochemical Analysis of Cultured (Amniotic Fluid) Cells*
Hans Galjaard

9. *The Use of Growth Factors to Stimulate the Proliferation of Amniotic Fluid Cells*
Charles J. Epstein

10. *Fetal Cells from Maternal Blood: Their Selection and Prospects for Use in Prenatal Diagnosis*
David R. Parks and Leonard A. Herzenberg

CONTRIBUTORS

Numbers in parentheses indicate the pages on which the authors' contributions begin.

LINDSEY ALLAN, Department of Paediatric Cardiology, Guy's Hospital, London SE1, England (181)

MARY T. BEAUCHESNE, Division of Genetics (Obstetrics and Gynecology), Brigham and Women's Hospital, Harvard Medical School, Boston, Massachusetts 02115 (35)

STUART CAMPBELL, Department of Obstetrics and Gynaecology, King's College Hospital Medical School, London SE5 8RX, England (181)

GRETCHEN J. DARLINGTON, Division of Human Genetics, Department of Medicine, Cornell University Medical College, New York, New York 10021 (297)

ROBERT J. DESNICK, Division of Medical Genetics, Mount Sinai School of Medicine, New York, New York 10029 (95)

CHARLES J. EPSTEIN, Departments of Pediatrics and of Biochemistry and Biophysics, University of California, San Francisco, San Francisco, California 94143 (269)

HANS GALJAARD, Department of Cell Biology and Genetics, Erasmus University Rotterdam, Rotterdam, The Netherlands (241)

GREGORY A. GRABOWSKI, Division of Medical Genetics, Mount Sinai School of Medicine, New York, New York 10029 (95)

DAVID GRIFFIN, Department of Obstetrics and Gynaecology, King's College Hospital Medical School, London SE5 8RX, England (181)

KAREN M. GUSTASHAW, Division of Genetics (Obstetrics and Gynecology), Brigham and Women's Hospital, Harvard Medical School, Boston, Massachusetts 02115 (35)

JAMES E. HADDOW, Foundation for Blood Research, Scarborough, Maine 04074 (67)

LEONARD A. HERZENBERG, Department of Genetics, Stanford University School of Medicine, Stanford, California 94305 (277)

KURT HIRSCHHORN, Mount Sinai School of Medicine, New York, New York 10029 (1)

HOLGER HOEHN, Department of Human Genetics, University of Würzburg, Würzburg, Federal Republic of Germany (11)

DAVID KURNIT, Division of Clinical Genetics, Children's Hospital Medical Center, and Division of Genetics (Obstetrics and Gynecology), Brigham and Women's Hospital, Boston, Massachusetts 02115 (311)

SAMUEL A. LATT, Division of Genetics (Obstetrics and Gynecology), Brigham and Women's Hospital, and Division of Genetics, Children's Hospital Medical Center, and Department of Pediatrics, Harvard Medical School, Boston, Massachusetts 02115 (35)

D. LITTLE,[1] Department of Obstetrics and Gynaecology, King's College Hospital Medical School, London SE5 8RX, England (181)

MAURICE J. MAHONEY, Departments of Human Genetics, Pediatrics, and Obstetrics and Gynecology, Yale University School of Medicine, New Haven, Connecticut 06510 (229)

[1]*Present address:* Birmingham Maternity Hospital, Queen Elizabeth Medical Centre, Birmingham, England.

WAYNE A. MILLER, Prenatal Diagnostic Laboratory, Massachusetts General Hospital, Boston, Massachusetts 02114 (67)

STUART ORKIN, Division of Hematology–Oncology, Children's Hospital Medical Center, Boston, Massachusetts 02115 (311)

DAVID R. PARKS, Department of Genetics, Stanford University School of Medicine, Stanford, California 94305 (277)

DARRELL SALK, Division of Genetic Pathology, University of Washington, Seattle, Washington 98195 (11)

MARY McH. SANDSTROM, Division of Genetics (Obstetrics and Gynecology), Brigham and Women's Hospital, Harvard Medical School, Boston, Massachusetts 02115 (35)

RAY WHITE,[2] Department of Microbiology, University of Massachusetts Medical School, Worcester, Massachusetts 01605 (311)

[2]*Present address:* Department of Cellular, Viral, and Molecular Biology, Howard Hughes Medical Institute, University of Utah School of Medicine, Salt Lake City, Utah 84132.

PREFACE

Prenatal diagnosis is a rapidly growing field in which increasingly sophisticated analytical tests are used to obtain vital information about a patient, the fetus. The prenatal examination is, at best, a partial or indirect one, without communication from the patient. The volume of prenatal diagnostic tests has escalated dramatically over the past decade. Despite an increased use of antenatal diagnosis and an enhanced public awareness of the availability of the procedures, fewer than 20% of women for whom antenatal diagnosis might be indicated utilize the tests.

Subject, of course, to personal beliefs about the desirability of prenatal diagnosis, the frequency, scope, and complexity of diagnosis *in utero* could easily double over the next few years. This state of affairs has at least two implications for laboratory scientists. First, there will be an increased need for laboratory personnel who are highly competent with state-of-the-art techniques for performing prenatal diagnostic tests. Second, there will be an intense need and challenge for basic scientists to adapt current advances in biomedical instrumentation, molecular biology, and cell biology to the development of better diagnostic methodology.

This book addresses the needs anticipated both of active diagnostic laboratory staff, who wish information about current procedures and an indication of directions for future development, and of basic scientists, who wish to know not only what currently is being done in prenatal diagnosis, but also where opportunities exist for new applications of basic science to the field of prenatal diagnosis.

Following an overview and historical perspective by Hirschhorn, a series of chapters outlines basic information currently necessary to operate a prenatal diagnostic laboratory. These chapters hopefully will serve to increase standardization of techniques in an effort to improve the accuracy and success of antenatal studies. The chapter by Hoehn and Salk describes the types of cells expected in amniotic fluid samples, indicating current and anticipated studies of their biological features, while the chapter by Sandstrom, Beauchesne, Gustashaw, and Latt discusses methods of chromosome analysis as applied to these cells. Basic procedural detail is accompanied by an indication of directions for future development. Similarly, the chapter by Haddow and Miller discusses not only the methods for alpha-fetoprotein (AFP) analysis in the detection of open neural tube defects, but also the possible impact of widespread maternal serum AFP screening and the development of ancillary laboratory tests to reduce diagnostic ambiguity. At present, AFP analysis is performed primarily in a few central referral laboratories. However, with increased availability of diagnostic reagents, this situation might change, and the need for interlaboratory standardization will become more urgent. The chapter by Grabowski and Desnick details the types of biochemical tests currently available for prenatal diagnosis. These tests are typically spread over numerous specialty centers and will continue to grow in number with the development of new techniques and better definition of the biochemical basis of various inherited diseases.

Prenatal diagnosis typically utilizes ultrasound for both sample acquisition and ancillary examination of the fetus, and Campbell, Griffin, Little, and Allen have written an extensively illustrated chapter acquainting individuals involved with prenatal diagnosis with the types of information that might be forthcoming from ultrasound studies. Fetuses can also be examined by endoscopy and, as discussed in the chapter by Mahoney, direct sampling of fetal tissue can be done for diagnostic studies. The risk and complexity of fetoscopy limits its use, but in isolated situations, it can provide essential information not available by other techniques. Fetoscopy provides small samples that require miniaturized analytical techniques. As described in the chapter by Galjaard, miniaturization of amniotic fluid cell analyses is possible and can speed up the acquisition of diagnostic information. A reduction in the time required for analysis of amniotic fluid cells has long been a goal of the clinician and counselor who deal with expecting parents. As indicated in the chapter by Epstein, the speed and success of prenatal diagnostic studies can also be increased by stimulating cell growth. A burgeoning number of identified growth factors provides ample opportunity for attempts at increasing cellular growth rate.

In the diagnostic sequence, the process of amniotic fluid sample acquisition continues to be the source of greatest risk to the mother and fetus. The chapter by Parks and Herzenberg describes an exciting new approach to sample acquisition, based on the isolation in a cell sorter of fetal cells present in the maternal circulation. This approach requires complex instrumentation and thus far cannot provide cells capable of further division, as needed for metaphase chromosome analysis. However, improvements in both immunodiagnostic reagents and flow cytometric equipment can be expected, and further development in this area as it relates to prenatal diagnosis can be anticipated. Also, procedures for obtaining fetal tissue transcervically, very early in pregnancy, have recently been described, and those may well influence certain prenatal diagnostic strategies.

Finally, it is often desirable to obtain information about differentiated properties or genetic markers not typically expressed by amniocytes. The chapter by Darlington describes how amniocytes can be induced to produce liver-specific proteins by fusion with hepatocytes and indicates a broad area for applying somatic cell genetics to prenatal diagnosis. Similarly, the chapter by Kurnit, Orkin, and White describes how cloned nucleic acid probes provided by recombinant DNA techniques can be used to "read" the genetic information contained in amniocytes and other fetal cells. Ultimately, the presence of restriction endonuclease fragment length polymorphisms, to which mutant alleles can be linked, places virtually any genetic disease within range of DNA linkage analysis. An explosion in the scope of this approach can be expected as recombinant DNA techniques are applied to prenatal diagnosis.

The chapters included here were chosen to cover the major basic laboratory techniques of prenatal diagnosis presently available and other sources of relevant data utilized in making diagnoses (e.g., ultrasound), and to identify technologies that exploit new research advances. With time, it is anticipated that many of these new technologies will be incorporated into standard diagnostic protocols, while new methodology will continue to emerge. To further both practical and investigative developments in prenatal genetic diagnosis is a goal of this book.

The efforts of the authors of individual chapters, upon which the success of this volume depends, are greatly appreciated. Also, discussions with colleagues and students during the course of this work were extremely valuable. Perhaps the greatest debt of the Editors is to their families and their mentors. Gretchen Darlington remains grateful to Robert S. K. Krooth, Frank H. Ruddle, James V. Neel, and Alexander G. Bearn. Samuel A. Latt is indebted to his teachers, Herman W. Lewis, Elkan R. Blout, Herbert A. Sober, and Bert L. Vallee, to Park S. Gerald for providing him with an entry into human genetics, and to Mary Ellen Avery and Kenneth J. Ryan for encouragement and support essential for continued work in the field of prenatal genetic diagnosis.

SAMUEL A. LATT
GRETCHEN J. DARLINGTON

Chapter 1

Overview and Historical Perspective of Prenatal Diagnosis

KURT HIRSCHHORN

Department of Pediatrics
Mount Sinai School of Medicine
New York, New York

Of all the advances in human genetics made over the past few decades, the one with the greatest impact on the clinical application of this science has been the development of prenatal diagnosis. The nature of genetic counseling has changed from a recital of statistical risks for disease to the ability to predict accurately whether a fetus is normal or affected as to the abnormality for which it is at risk.

There is a story, which may be apocryphal, as to how prenatal diagnosis began. It is said that someone from the agricultural community in Israel was interested in discovering the sex of early bovine pregnancies because for a variety of economic reasons it is better to have female calves born and, if possible, to abort most male calves. One needs only one bull to fertilize many cows, but the cows give milk. When Barr and Bertram (1949) discovered that the X chromatin body could distinguish female from male cells, it was suggested to Sachs and Danon at the Weitzman Institute that it may be possible to determine the sex of the unborn calf by examining amniotic fluid cells for X chromatin. Apparently, attempts at amniocentesis in the cow frequently lead to spontaneous abortion. This project was therefore abandoned. However, Sachs and Danon maintained their interest in this problem and approached an obstetrician named Serr to try to predict the sex of human fetuses that were going to be aborted in any case for other reasons. In 1955, Serr, Sachs, and Danon described the feasibility of antenatal sex determination by the analysis of sex chromatin in freshly obtained amniotic cells (Serr *et al.*, 1955; Sachs *et al.*, 1956). Soon thereafter Fuchs in Denmark utilized this same technique for the first time for actual prenatal diagnosis of genetic disease (Riis and Fuchs, 1960). A number of women at risk for sons with X-linked recessive diseases, primarily hemophilia and Duchenne mus-

1

cular dystrophy, were subjected to amniocentesis and many of these women opted to abort male fetuses.

Since these first attempts, a new and revolutionary field of study of fetal cytogenetics, biochemical genetics, and other genetically related studies has evolved. In 1966, Steele and Breg published their successful technique for the culture and karyotyping of fetal cells obtained through amniocentesis (Steele and Breg, 1966). At about that time it also became possible to perform amniocenteses safely by the transabdominal route rather than by the riskier transvaginal route used in the early studies. The transabdominal approach had been developed for the purpose of third-trimester amniocentesis in the study of pregnancies at risk for Rh sensitization. The transabdominal route obviated the previously relatively common finding of amnionitis following transvaginal amniocentesis. Within a year of the report by Steele and Breg, Jacobson and Barter (1967) described the successful prenatal chromosome diagnosis of three pregnancies at high risk for chromosomal abnormalities. In that article they discussed a number of issues that have still not been completely resolved. These, of course, include a variety of ethical, moral, and legal questions that have been addressed in several publications (Littlefield *et al.*, 1973; Harris, 1974; Milunsky, 1976) and with which we are still struggling. An example of such problems relates back to prenatal sex determination, but for the simple selection of sex rather than in a pregnancy at risk for X-linked disease. Although it has been recommended (Powledge and Fletcher, 1979) that this not be done by reputable laboratories performing prenatal diagnosis, even here differences of opinion exist and have been stated rationally (Fletcher, 1979). Despite some unresolved issues, many thousands of prenatal diagnoses have been performed and the diagnosis of abnormalities has presumably helped many families with their decisions relating to high-risk pregnancies.

Several articles, and reports of large series have been published (Hsu and Hirschhorn, 1974; Galjaard, 1976; Hsu *et al.*, 1978; Golbus *et al.*, 1979; Milunsky, 1979) relating the world experience with cytogenetic and other prenatal diagnosis, and the reader is referred to these for a discussion of results, pitfalls, and problems.

Soon after the utilization of amniocentesis for cytogenetic diagnosis, it became clear that a number of inborn errors would be detectable by enzyme analysis of cultured amniotic fluid cells. Nadler, who was in the forefront of this development (Nadler, 1968), published a review of the early findings (Nadler, 1972), and some of the articles just listed provide compilations of those inborn errors that are currently diagnosable. It is almost impossible to keep up with the constant additions to these inborn errors, because new discoveries of enzyme defects are allowing an ever-increasing number of diseases to be diagnosed prenatally. Means for the detection of genetic diseases in which the specific defect is not known have also been suggested, such as the use of the nitroblue tetrazolium test

in cultured amniotic fluid cells for the prenatal diagnosis of chronic granulomatous disease (Fikrig *et al.*, 1980).

The question of the risks of amniocentesis was addressed in great detail in
studies in the United States (NICHD, 1976), Canada (Simpson *et al.*, 1976), and
Great Britain (Working Party on Amniocentesis, 1978). In general, the conclusions of these studies are that there is virtually no risk to the mother and that the
risk of inducing an unwanted abortion of the fetus may be as high as 0.5% or 1 in
200 attempts. It is likely that in competent hands the actual risk may be lower.
All these studies have reported 99% or better accuracy of results. The question of
the risk of ultrasound for the purpose of placental localization, determination of
gestational age, and the diagnosis of congenital defects has been raised, but until
now there is no short-term or long-term evidence of any real damage to the
unborn child from this technique.

A number of other methods have come into use for the purpose of prenatal
diagnosis. Amniography and fetography, popular in the early 1970s, have not
been widely used in recent years. Conventional X-rays have been of some use in
the detection of some bony abnormalities, but are not common in the general
armamentarium of prenatal diagnosis. The most important of the new techniques
in use for some years has been ultrasonography. Perhaps its most important
application is the determination of gestational age by the measurement of the
fetal biparietal diameter. This technique is crucial not only for studying the
growth of the fetus, but also for determining the exact gestational age of the
fetus, important for the interpretation of other studies, particularly the level of
alpha-fetoprotein in the amniotic fluid. Another common use of ultrasonography
is for the detection of multiple pregnancies, of critical importance for accurate
prenatal diagnosis because if there are twins, both sacs need to be tapped in order
for a correct answer to be given to the family. An important aspect of ultrasonography is the guidance of the obstetrician during amniocentesis. It becomes easy to
avoid puncturing the placenta or injuring the fetus, because in most cases it is
possible to locate and enter a window into the large pool of amniotic fluid under
the guidance of ultrasonography, when performed on the table on which amniocentesis is to be done. A reduction in bloody taps has been reported as a result
of this practice (Kerenyi and Walker, 1977). Finally, ultrasonography has been
extremely useful in the detection of a variety of congenital malformations, particularly anencephaly and meningomyelocele, as well as a variety of limb and
renal abnormalities (Kaffe *et al.*, 1977; Hobbins *et al.*, 1979). It has been
demonstrated that ultrasound is capable of diagnosing congenital heart disease
and, potentially, cardiac dysrhythmias (Kleinman *et al.*, 1980).

In addition to the biochemical studies of cultured amniotic fluid cells, the last
few years have seen advances in such studies of the amniotic fluid itself. The
most important advance has been the use of alpha-fetoprotein measurement in the
diagnosis of open neural tube defects (Brock and Sutcliffe, 1972). Elevation of

amniotic fluid alpha-fetoprotein is also associated with other anomalies, including omphalocele and intestinal atresia, as well as severe fetal distress or fetal death (Ainbender *et al.*, 1978). Of great interest and potentially wide application are the preliminary studies of Nadler's group (Walsh and Nadler, 1980; Nadler and Walsh, 1980) on the successful intrauterine detection of cystic fibrosis by a combination of enzymatic and separative studies of amniotic fluid.

A number of other innovative methods have led to further exciting advances. The development of narrow-bore fetoscopes has led to direct inspection of fetuses for certain types of anomalies (e.g., Laurence *et al.*, 1975). Much more useful, until now, has been the utilization of fetoscopy for fetal blood sampling (Hobbins and Mahoney, 1976). The application of biochemical techniques and those of molecular biology to such fetal blood specimens has already produced prenatal diagnoses of various hemoglobinopathies (Alter, 1979) and of hemophilia (Firshein *et al.*, 1979). The study of fetal white blood cells from these specimens is promising for the detection of certain immune-deficiency diseases and leukocyte abnormalities (e.g., Newberger *et al.*, 1979). If this technique is as safe as ordinary amniocentesis, prenatal chromosomal analysis may more commonly be performed on fetal blood, as already reported (Cordesius *et al.*, 1980), with answers obtained by 72 hours rather than the usual 2 to 3 weeks' wait, a terribly difficult period of time for the family.

Once a fetoscope is inserted, it is possible to obtain small samples of fetal skin. Utilizing this technique, followed by tissue culture or histopathological examination of the skin sample, a number of diagnoses have recently become possible. These include such primary skin diseases as epidermolysis bullosa letalis and other related diseases, such as several forms of ichthyosis (Elias *et al.*, 1980; Golbus *et al.*, 1980; Rodeck *et al.*, 1980). It has been suggested that such fetal skin fibroblast cultures may become useful for the diagnosis of diseases that show specific sensitivities of the DNA of the cultured cells to environmental agents. For example, it may be possible to diagnose ataxia telangiectasia prenatally by demonstrating the known increased cellular sensitivity to X-rays (Patterson *et al.*, 1979), and it has been suggested, although by no means proven, that fibroblasts from patients with Huntington's disease, and therefore perhaps fibroblasts from fetuses with Huntington's disease, may also be unusually radiosensitive (Moshell *et al.*, 1980). If the latter turns out to be true, it may at last become possible to approach rationally the counseling and prevention of this devastating entity. It has even been proposed that fetal muscle biopsy may be possible. If this is the case, a variety of primary genetic muscle diseases may become diagnosable, as has been suggested for Duchenne muscular dystrophy (Emery and Burt, 1980).

The techniques of modern molecular genetics have recently been applied to the DNA of amniotic fluid cells. With these highly sensitive methods, several forms of thalassemia and, in certain families, sickle cell anemia have become amenable to rapid diagnosis by the study of the uncultured amniotic fluid cells (Orkin *et al.*, 1978; Kan *et al.*, 1980). It is clear that the purification of many more probes for specific human genes, as well as the discovery of DNA polymorphisms linked to these, will allow a vast expansion of our ability for the rapid prenatal diagnosis of many genetic disorders.

Another approach to prenatal diagnosis is represented by the detection of a disease closely linked to a known polymorphic marker. The greatest success in this direction has been the use of HLA typing of cultured amniotic fluid cells in families where either the 21-hydroxylase deficiency type of the adrenogenital syndrome (Pollack *et al.*, 1979) or complement C4 deficiency (Pollack *et al.*, 1980) has shown appropriate segregation with an HLA haplotype.

There may be further advances on the horizon. One of the exciting findings that may have many applications is the ability to discover fetal cells in maternal blood. The use of the fluorescence-activated cell sorter is showing promise for the separation of the small number of circulating fetal cells from maternal blood (Herzenberg *et al.*, 1979). If this technique becomes satisfactorily accurate, a number of genetic diseases may be diagnosable prenatally without amniocentesis and at a much earlier time of pregnancy.

Another tool of the modern geneticist is the use of somatic cell hybrids. It may become possible in the not too distant future to utilize such hybrids, prepared from fusion of amniotic fluid cells derived from a pregnancy at risk to an appropriate rodent cell, for the purpose of turning on a human gene not ordinarily expressed in the cultured amniotic fluid cell. Such techniques may make it possible to detect diseases currently not amenable to prenatal diagnosis, such as alpha-1-antitrypsin deficiency, phenylketonuria, or other inborn errors ordinarily only detectable by liver biopsy.

It is probable that the prenatal discovery of disease will allow attempts at prenatal therapy. This has already succeeded in at least one inborn error, that of vitamin B$_{12}$-sensitive methylmalonicacidemia (Ampola *et al.*, 1975). It is hoped that early enough discovery of a variety of otherwise lethal or severely damaging inborn errors may become amenable to therapy not only by vitamins when applicable, but hopefully by the availability of newer therapeutic modalities of the future, such as enzyme replacement or even gene transfer.

I would like now to return to some of the ethical issues. As the ability to obtain a fetal karyotype becomes safer and more readily available (and, probably, less expensive), an ever-increasing segment of the population will be availing themselves of this service. Undoubtedly, the indications for the procedure will be liberalized and more "low-risk" patients will be studied. As already discussed, among them will be the couples who will request amniocentesis for the purpose of sex selection, choosing abortion if the unwanted sex is diagnosed. Individual medical centers may, for ethical reasons, choose to screen out these couples. However, eventually, as commercial laboratories expand their prenatal cytogenetic services, this issue may be determined by individual practitioners as part of their relationship with their patients. Since amniocentesis and midtrimester abortion are now legal in most areas, the only limitations on the availability of prenatal sex selection may be the physician's personal ethics and his or her medical judgment as to the safety of late abortions. Many now feel that to refuse amniocentesis and abortion for the trivial purpose of sex preference is not in harmony with the currently legal right to choose abortion, for whatever trivial reason.

The issue of the abortion of normal fetuses arises also in the case of multiple gestations. Refined ultransonic techniques and dye studies allow the localization of the separate sacs for amniocentesis and, therefore, the study of the individual fetuses. The decision to abort all the fetuses if one is abnormal, or to maintain the pregnancy for the preservation of the normal fetus, has already arisen on several occasions (Filkins *et al.*, 1978; Heller and Palmer, 1978). Aberg *et al.* (1978) reported a twin pregnancy at risk for Hurler disease. One fetus was found to be affected, the other normal. At 24 weeks' gestation, under real-time ultrasound, transabdominal intracardiac puncture was performed on the affected fetus, causing cessation of the fetal heartbeat. The other twin survived the procedure and was delivered at 33 weeks' gestation when spontaneous labor began. The dead fetus had been partially resorbed. Using this technique, it is possible to selectively preserve a normal fetus in a multiple gestation, as we have recently done at our institution in a pregnancy with one normal and one trisomy-21 twin (Kerenyi and Chitkara, 1981).

Some cytogenetic diagnoses may give rise to ambiguity in the minds of the genetic counselor and the patient. The unexpected finding of a 47, XYY, XXX, or even XXY fetus on amniocentesis presents significant problems. Certainly, for the patient who primarily fears the prenatal diagnosis for Down's syndrome, these abnormalities appear relatively minor. The information, along with emphasis that there is a spectrum of the clinical phenotypes, which include men and women of normal intellect, is presented to the patient as the state of our current understanding. The decision to maintain the pregnancy will depend on many factors particular to each situation: the pregnancy history; the presence or absence of normal children in the family; the age of the couple; religious convictions; and, possibly, the socioeconomic and educational level of the family. Similar issues pertain for decisions regarding 45, XO fetuses. Although the serious physical, particularly cardiovascular, abnormalities which these patients may have must be discussed, as well as the potential for difficult psychological adjustment to abnormalities of sexual development, the counseling should also include mention of the potential for a relatively normal life with normal life expectancy in most cases.

Problems of counseling stemming from the prenatal diagnosis of *de novo* balanced translocations or *de novo* pericentric inversions are difficult to resolve.

Jacobs (1974) has suggested, from analysis of newborn data and from studies of mentally subnormal populations, that the proportion of individuals with *de novo* translocations is significantly greater among the mentally subnormal. Jacobs reasoned that the observed abnormality might be caused by a small deletion or mutation at the breakpoint. In general, one can be reassuring in cases of familial translocation or familial pericentric inversion when no differences in morphology between the chromosomes of parent and fetus are observed with the appropriate banding studies. However, one must be cautious in the counseling of the parents of a fetus with an apparently balanced *de novo* translocation or inversion and advise them that the risk for congenital abnormalities and/or mental retardation may be greater than that in the normal population. The decision to terminate or maintain the pregnancy is, of course, left to the parents.

The rapid application of advancing technology from the basic sciences, clinical instrumentation, and other apparently unrelated research activities has already made a tremendous impact on our ability to diagnose genetic and congenital abnormalities in pregnancies at risk, and has given the clinical geneticist his most powerful tool in allowing families an important option in their reproductive decisions. It should be stressed that the availability of this option has induced many families to consider and to complete pregnancies, when previously they were unwilling to risk such a pregnancy or would have opted for an early termination if no answers were available. Since the results of most prenatal studies will indicate that the fetus is not affected with the condition for which it is at risk, prenatal diagnosis, in addition to being an accurate predictive measure for the prevention of the birth of children with anomalies, should be regarded as life-giving and lifesaving.

REFERENCES

Aberg, A., Mitelman, F., Cantz, M., and Gehler, J. (1978). *Lancet* **2**, 990–991.
Ainbender, E., Brown, E., Kierney, C., and Hirschhorn, K. (1978). *In* "Prevention of Neural Tube Defects" (B. F. Crandall and M. A. B. Frazier, eds.), pp. 169–178. Academic Press, New York.
Alter, B. P. (1979). *J. Pediatr.* **95**, 501–513.
Ampola, M. G., Mahoney, M. J., Nakamura, E., and Tanaka, K. (1975). *N. Engl. J. Med.* **293**, 313–317.
Barr, M. L., and Bertram, E. G. (1949). *Nature* **163**, 676–677.
Brock, D. J. H., and Sutcliffe, R. G. (1972). *Lancet* **2**, 197–199.
Cordesius, E., Gustavii, B., and Mitelman, F. (1980). *Br. Med. J.* **280**, 1107.
Elias, S., Mazur, M., Sabbagha, R., Esterly, N. B., and Simpson, J. L. (1980). *Clin. Genet.* **17**, 275–280.
Emergy, A. E. H., and Burt, D. (1980). *Br. Med. J.* **280**, 355–357.
Fikrig, S. M., Smithwick, E. M., Suntharalingam, K., and Good, R. A. (1980). *Lancet* **1**, 18–19.
Filkins, K., Kushnik, T., Diamond, N., Searle, B., and Desposito, F. (1978). *Am. J. Obstet. Gynecol.* **131**, 584–585.

Firshein, S. I., Hoyer, L. W., Lazarchick, J., Forget, B. G., Hobbins, J. C., Clyne, L. P., Pitlick, F. A., Muir, W. A., Merkatz, I. R., and Mahoney, M. J. (1979). *N. Engl. J. Med.* **300,** 937–941.

Fletcher, J. (1979). *N. Engl. J. Med.* **301,** 550–553.

Galjaard, H. (1976). *Cytogenet. Cell Genet.* **16,** 453–467.

Golbus, M. S., Loughman, W. D., Epstein, C. J., Halbasch, G., Stephens, J. D., and Hall, B. D. (1979). *N. Engl. J. Med.* **300,** 157–163.

Golbus, M. S., Sagebiel, R. W., Filly, R. A., Gindhart, T. D., and Hall, J. G. (1980). *N. Engl. J. Med.* **302,** 93–95.

Harris, H. (1974). "Prenatal Diagnosis and Selective Abortion," pp. 62–84. Nuffield Provincial Hospitals Trust, London.

Heller, R. H., and Palmer, L. S. (1978). *Pediatrics* **62,** 52–53.

Herzenberg, L. A., Bianchi, D. W., Schroder, J., Cann, H. M., and Iverson, A. M. (1979). *Proc. Natl. Acad. Sci. U.S.A.* **76,** 1453–1455.

Hobbins, J. C., and Mahoney, M. J. (1976). *Clin. Obstet. Gynecol.* **19,** 341–352.

Hobbins, J. C., Grannum, P. A., Berkowitz, R. L., Silverman, R., and Mahoney, M. J. (1979). *Am. J. Obstet. Gynecol.* **134,** 331–345.

Hsu, L. Y., and Hirschhorn, K. (1974). *Life Sci.* **14,** 2311–2336.

Hsu, L. Y. F., Kaffe, S., Yahr, F., Serotkin, A., Giordano, F., Godmilow, L., Kim, H. J., David, K., Kerenyi, T., and Hirschhorn, K. (1978). *Am. J. Med. Genet.* **2,** 365–383.

Jacobs, P. A. (1974). *Nature* **249,** 164–165.

Jacobson, C. B., and Barter, R. H. (1967). *Am. J. Obstet. Gynecol.* **99,** 796–807.

Kaffe, S., Rose, J., Godmilow, L., Walker, B., Kerenyi, T., Beratis, N. G., Reyes, P., and Hirschhorn, K. (1977). *Am. J. Med. Genet.* **1,** 241–251.

Kan, Y. W., Lee, K. Y., Furbetta, M., Angius, A., and Cao, A. (1980). *N. Engl. J. Med.* **302,** 185–188.

Kerenyi, T. D., and Chitkara, U. (1981). *N. Engl. J. Med.* **304,** 1525–1527.

Kerenyi, T. D., and Walker, B. (1977). *Obstet. Gynecol.* **50,** 61–64.

Kleinman, C. S., Hobbins, J. C., Jaffe, C. C., Lynch, D. C., and Talner, N. S. (1980). *Pediatrics* **65,** 1059–1067.

Laurence, K. M., Prosser, R., Rocker, I., Pearson, J. F., and Richards, C. (1975). *J. Med. Genet.* **12,** 334–338.

Littlefield, J. W., Milunsky, A., and Jacoby, L. B. (1973). *In* "Ethical Issues in Human Genetics" (B. Hilton, D. Callahan, M. Harris, P. Condliffe, and B. Berkley, eds.), pp. 43–51. Plenum, New York.

Milunsky, A. (1976). *In* "Genetics and the Law" (A. Milunsky and G. J. Annas, eds.), pp. 53–60. Plenum, New York.

Milunsky, A. (1979). "Genetic Disorders and the Fetus." Plenum, New York.

Moshell, A. N., Barrett, S. F., Tarone, R. E., and Robbins, J. H. (1980). *Lancet* **1,** 9–11.

Nadler, H. L. (1968). *Pediatrics* **42,** 912–918.

Nadler, H. L. (1972). *In* "Advances in Human Genetics" (H. Harris and K. Hirschhorn, eds.), Vol. 3, pp. 1–37. Plenum, New York.

Nadler, H. L., and Walsh, M. M. J. (1980). *Pediatrics* **66,** 690–692.

Newberger, P. E., Cohen, H. J., Rotchild, S. B., Hobbins, J. C., Malawista, S. E., and Mahoney, M. J. (1979). *N. Engl. J. Med.* **300,** 178–181.

NICHD National Registry for Amniocentesis Study Group (1976). *J.A.M.A.* **236,** 1471–1476.

Orkin, S. H., Alter, B. P., Altay, C., Mahoney, M. J., Lazarus, H., Hobbins, J. C., and Nathan, D. G. (1978). *N. Engl. J. Med.* **299,** 166–172.

Patterson, M. C., Anderson A. K., Smith, B. P., and Smith, P. J. (1979). *Cancer Res.* **39,** 3725–3734.

Pollack, M. S., Maurer, D., Levine, L. S., New, M. I., Pang, S., Duchon, M. A., Owens, R. P., Merkatz, I. R., Nitowsky, H. M., Sachs, G., and Dupont, B. (1979). *Lancet* **1**, 1107–1108.

Pollack, M. S., Ochs, H. D., and Dupont, B. (1980). *Clin. Genet.* **18**, 197–200.

Powledge, T. M., and Fletcher, J. (1979). *N. Engl. J. Med.* **300**, 168–172.

Riis, P., and Fuchs, F. (1960). *Lancet* **2**, 180–182.

Rodeck, C. H., Eady, R. A. J., and Gosden, C. M. (1980). *Lancet* **1**, 949–952.

Sachs, L., Serr, D. M., and Danon, M. (1956). *Br. Med. J.* **2**, 795–798.

Serr, D. M., Sachs, L., and Danon, M. (1955). *Bull. Res. Council Israel* **5B**, 137–138.

Simpson, N. E., Dallaire, L., Miller, J. R., Siminovitch, L., and Hamerton, J. (1976). *Can. Med. Assoc. J.* **115**, 739–748.

Steele, M. W., and Breg, W. R., Jr. (1966). *Lancet* **1**, 383–385.

Walsh, M. M. J., and Nadler, H. L. (1980). *Am. J. Obstet. Gynecol.* **137**, 978–982.

Working Party on Amniocentesis (1978). *Br. J. Obstet. Gynecol.* **85**, (Suppl. 2), 1–41.

Chapter 2

Morphological and Biochemical Heterogeneity of Amniotic Fluid Cells in Culture

HOLGER HOEHN

Department of Human Genetics
University of Würzburg
Würzburg, Federal Republic of Germany

DARRELL SALK

Department of Genetic Pathology
University of Washington
Seattle, Washington

METHODS IN CELL BIOLOGY, VOL. 26

I.   Introduction

In addition to their utility in the prenatal diagnosis of genetic disorders, midgestation amniotic fluid cells constitute a new and precious source of human cells for the purpose of cell biological investigation. Several properties contribute to the diagnostic and scientific value of these cells, the most important of which are (a) the presence in a single amniotic fluid specimen of multiple, morphologically and biochemically distinct cell types that are all derived from the fetus or from fetal membranes and thus are isogenic; (b) the feasibility of clonal expansion of these various cell types to obtain sufficient quantities of cellular materials for cell biological investigations of a single cell type; and (c) the distinctiveness of the predominant amniotic fluid cell type from the pre- and postnatal fibroblast cell types (WI-38 and skin fibroblasts) that have been virtually the only source material for studies of normal human cells in long-term culture. In this chapter we will review the morphologic and growth characteristics of these different amniotic fluid cell types and demonstrate their distinctiveness in terms of expression of various gene products. Finally, we will comment on their potential use in cell biological investigation.

II.   Cellular Content of Second-Trimester Amniotic Fluids

In addition to variable amounts of cellular debris and anucleate particles, second-trimester amniotic fluid contains between 10^3 and 10^5 nucleated cells per milliliter of fluid. There are several morphologic types present, but the greatest number are cells with small, densely staining, frequently pycnotic nuclei and with large, pale, often vacuolated cytoplasms. These squamous-like cells display ultrastructural characteristics of fetal epidermal cells at the same stages of pregnancy (Holbrook and Odland, 1975), and desquamation from the fetal epidermis is their most likely mode of origin. Individual amniotic fluids display great variability in the number of cells that are present. The reasons for this variability are not known with certainty, but development of the typical stratified epithelium from a simple two-layered structure (periderm and germinal zone) begins around the sixteenth week of gestation. Since this developmental change occurs with different velocities in different areas of the body, small differences in gestational age might have a comparatively large impact on the total amount of epithelial cornification and desquamation (Huisjes, 1978). The nonsquamous cell types suspended in second-trimester amniotic fluids range in their cytologic presentation from a variety of parabasal-like cells (occurring in isolation or as aggregates) to multiple forms of cuboid and columnar epithelial cells. A striking finding in many fluids is the presence of coherent sheets of epithelioid cells and/or syncytial aggregates comprising several dozen nuclei (Casadei *et al.*, 1973).

All epithelial surfaces in direct or indirect contact with the amniotic cavity are possible sites of origin of these cells: amniotic membranes, fetal epidermis, and the mucosa of the digestive, respiratory, and urogenital tracks (Herz *et al.*, 1979). Considering the widespread use of 16- to 20-week amniotic fluid specimens for clinical purposes, it is surprising that a systematic cytologic and histochemical investigation of this material has not yet been reported, whereas authoritative descriptions exist for amniotic fluids from the later stages of gestation (e.g., Huisjes, 1978). However, from the point of view of cell culture a satisfactory classification of the cellular components of second-trimester amniotic fluids emerges only after transfer and incubation of the native cell suspension in appropriate containers.

According to their behavior in the culture environment, nucleated amniotic fluid cells can be operationally divided into three separate categories. The first category includes cells that remain afloat even after prolonged periods of incubation (i.e., more than 72 hours); the majority of these cells consist of the squamous-like cells that originate from fetal epidermis. The second category includes cells that attach to the culture substrate (either shortly after plating or within a 3-day period) but do not grow sufficiently, if they divide at all, to form classical cell clones. In this category are the various types of "rapidly adhering" (RA) cells that were first described by Sutherland and others (1973, 1975). Gosden and Brock (1977, 1978) subsequently provided comprehensive information on the morphology, behavior, origin, and clinical significance of these cells that will be discussed in detail in the article by Haddow and Miller in the present volume. The third category of amniotic fluid cells includes those cells that attach to the culture surface and subsequently proliferate in a clonal fashion. These cells give rise to large, well-defined cell colonies of more than 100 (usually over 1000) cells per colony after 2–3 weeks of incubation. This chapter will deal primarily with the morphologic and biochemical characterization of the colony-forming cells.

III.   Clonal Morphology and Growth

According to their clonal characteristics, we have distinguished three principal classes of colony-forming amniotic fluid cells (Hoehn *et al.*, 1974, 1975a, 1978). The morphologic heterogeneity of the most distinctive cell types and their colonies are shown in Figs. 1–3, and their characteristics are described next. Figure 4 demonstrates that heterogeneity of clonal growth patterns is also demonstrated by cells derived from a variety of fetal tissues.

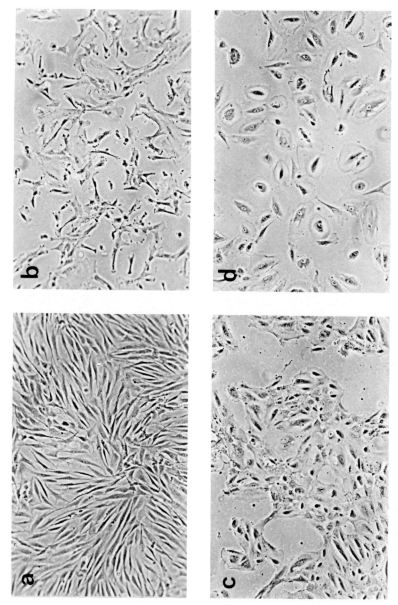

Fɪɢ. 1.   Living primary clones of amniotic fluid cells after approximately 1 week in culture (phase contrast). (a) F-type; (b) AF-type; (c,d) E-type.

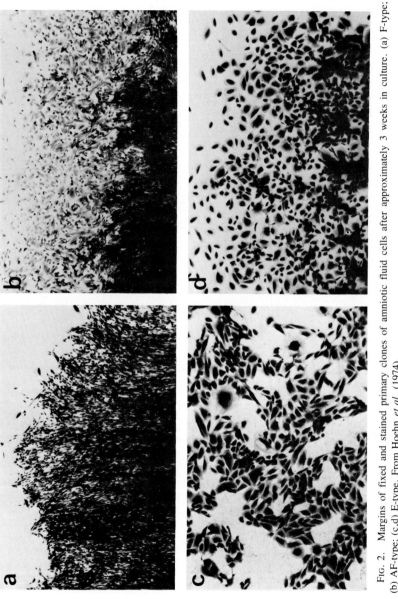

FIG. 2.   Margins of fixed and stained primary clones of amniotic fluid cells after approximately 3 weeks in culture. (a) F-type; (b) AF-type; (c,d) E-type. From Hoehn *et al.* (1974).

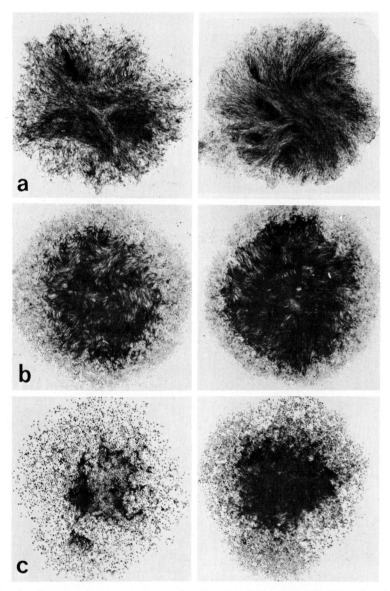

FIG. 3.   Examples of mature primary colonies of amniotic fluid cells after 14–16 days in culture. (a) F-type; (b) AF-type; (c) E-type.

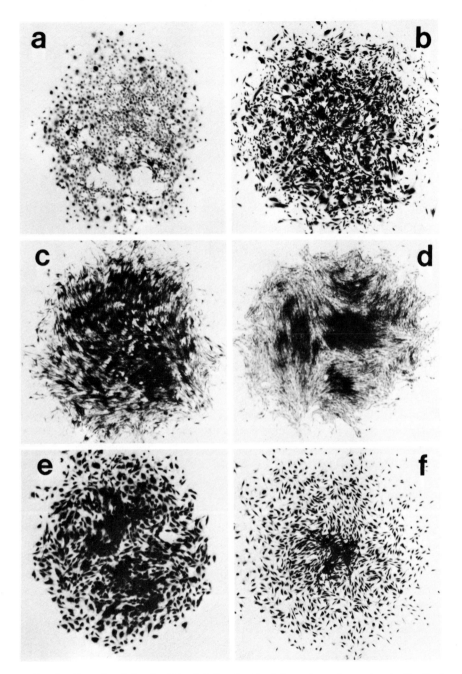

FIG. 4. Examples of clonal outgrowth in low-density platings of scrapings or trypsin digests of various tissues obtained from a 16-week-old fetus. Note the variability of cellular phenotypes and the lack of typical "fibroblast" morphology. (a) Amnion; (b) intestine; (c) oral cavity; (d) trachea; (e) kidney; (f) bladder.

TABLE I

In Vitro Growth Potentials of Colony-Forming Amniotic
Fluid Cell Types[a]

Colony type	Number of colonies[b]	Mean life span	
		CPD[c]	Standard deviation
F	15	52.8	14.5
AF	173	24.1	14.3
E	66	12.1	4.1

[a] Data summarized from Hoehn *et al.*, 1974.

[b] After 12–14 days in primary culture.

[c] Cumulative population doublings (CPD) achieved after initial isolation, transfer, and propagation to confluency of a single colony into a
25-cm² culture flask. CPD calculated on the basis of hemocytometer counts
at the time of weekly passage (Martin *et al.*, 1970).

A. F-Type Colonies

F-Type colonies consist of fibroblast-like cells that are indistinguishable from
cultured fibroblasts derived from skin. These F-type cells generate a characteristic ribbed and streaming pattern as they grow into mature colonies, as do skin
fibroblasts. Within these cell streams the individual spindle-shaped cells are in
close contact, overlap, and form multilayered sheets in areas of high cell den-
sities (the colony core). Amniotic fluid F-type cells have the greatest *in vitro*
growth potential of all colony-forming cells (Table I). If present in an amniotic
fluid specimen, they are likely to overgrow the culture at later stages of cultivation and/or during serial passage. However, not all 20-ml diagnostic amniotic
fluid specimens contain such F-type progenitor cells. In two series of experiments, fewer than half of the specimens gave rise to F-type colonies (Hoehn *et
al.*, 1974, 1975a). In rare instances (Schmid, 1977; Hoehn *et al.*, 1978) F-type
cells were shown to be of maternal rather than fetal origin, but the fetal derivation
of F-type cells cannot be doubted when they display male karyotypes consistent
with the sex of the fetus (Hoehn *et al.*, 1974). Iatrogenic introduction of maternal
fibroblast-like cells via needle puncture at the time of amniocentesis may have
embarrassing results (wrong sex diagnosis), and rarely may lead to other forms of
misdiagnosis.

B. AF-Type Colonies

AF-Type colonies are the most frequent that emerge from amniotic fluid cell
cultures. To the untrained eye, individual AF cells are only subtly distinct from

classical "fibroblasts" in that they tend to appear less polar and show greater marginal ruffling. They dramatically increase in size with serial passage and at later stages they resemble smooth muscle-type cells from human vasculature (Martin *et al.*, 1975). Mature (12- to 14-day-old) AF-type colonies have a dense core of multilayered nondividing cells surrounded by a loosely organized peripheral growth zone in which individual cells grow in all directions rather than in the parallel fashion characteristic of fibroblasts. This "bulls-eye" configuration of the mature AF colony is the most distinctive morphologic characteristic that differentiates F- and AF-type cells. This morphologic distinction at the level of clonal organization has been confirmed by a variety of biochemical parameters, as will be discussed (Sections IV–VI). Because of their prevalence in second-trimester amniotic fluids, this class of cells constitutes the principal cell source for cytogenetic and biochemical investigations for prenatal diagnosis. Although their average growth potential (Table I) is distinctly inferior to that of the F-type cell, the initial growth rates of AF colonies and their tolerance of passage by trypsinization make it possible to prepare large numbers of cells (up to 10^8) from 20 ml of fluid in less than 6 weeks of culture.

C.   E-Type Colonies

E-Type colonies consist of large polygonal cells with smooth margins. These cells grow in intimate contact with each other and their clonal appearance resembles that of AF clones except for the presence of a broader growth margin (Fig. 1). Virtually every 20-ml specimen of sixteenth-week amniotic fluid yields typical E-type colonies, but there are several morphologic variants of cells with these "epithelioid" characteristics. Some cultures display coherent sheets of E-type cells in which proliferation occurs centrally instead of in a marginal growth zone. Attempts at passage of such structures via trypsinization usually do not succeed, even though these cells can be cytogenetically analyzed by the *in situ* method of chromosome preparation (Schmid, 1975). Another example of variant epithelioid colonies are those that consist almost exclusively of large "potato chip"-like cells that have irregular nuclear morphologies ranging from simple lobulation to nuclear fragmentation and micronucleation. Such colonies are highly resistant to dispersion by trypsin, but even after successful trypsinization they will reattach but not proliferate; instead they secrete inordinate amounts of a PAS-positive extracellular matrix that covers the culture surface in a weblike fashion. The *in vitro* growth potential of all E-type cells is much less than that of either F or AF cells, and only occasional colonies give rise to mass cultures that can be propagated for more than two to three passages (Table I). Because they senesce *in vitro* so precipitously, chromosomal aberrations in colonies of E-type cells may reflect the somatic changes commonly observed in senescent cells (Salk *et al.*, 1981) rather than constitutional (zygotic) changes. Proper interpretation of aberrations in E-type cells therefore depends on simultaneous observations of F or AF colonies in the same culture.

IV.   Electrophoretic Profiles of Whole-Cell Homogenates

A.   One-Dimensional SDS–PAGE[1]

In our own laboratory, 14- to 16-day-old isogenic F-, AF-, and E-type amniotic fluid cell clones were isolated from primary amniotic fluid platings with stainless-steel cylinders and analyzed by one-dimensional SDS–PAGE (Johnston et al., 1981). Cell pellets obtained by trypsinization of second-passage clones (approximately 10^5 cells) were resuspended in 0.5-ml aliquots of Laemmli's buffer and loaded onto a continuous 6–15% polyacrylamide gradient gel 30 cm in length. After the run, the gels were stained with 0.25% Coomassie blue in a methanol–acetic acid solution.

Figure 5 shows the degree of separation achieved by this method. We were unable to find consistent qualitative differences among the 70–80 bands appearing on such gels. However, there were consistent quantitative differences among the three amniotic fluid cell types and between fetal and postnatal cells involving staining intensity of the four landmark protein bands designated 1–4 in Fig. 5. Even though Coomassie blue staining patterns cannot be evaluated stoichiometrically in areas of high protein concentration, the relationships among these landmark proteins were sufficiently consistent that clusters of cell types were evident in a two-dimensional plot of the ratios of the intensities of these bands (Fig. 6). The distinction based on the quantitative relationships among the four landmark proteins was clearest between fetal and nonfetal cells; it is most remarkable that fetal and postnatal cells of virtually identical in vivo morphologies (F-type amniotic fluid cells and skin fibroblasts) can be separated on the basis of the quantitative relationships among so few proteins. There was considerable variation and overlap among fetal cell types, although the E-type cells were the most heterogeneous in terms of electrophoretic profile, as they are morphologically.

B.   Two-Dimensional IEF–PAGE[2]

Because the separation of whole-cell homogenates on the basis of molecular weight and the analysis of total protein by Coomassie blue staining failed to show qualitative differences among the three classes of colony-forming amniotic fluid cells, the analysis was extended to newly synthesized proteins and the isoelectric

[1]See Laemmli, 1970.
[2]See O'Farrell, 1975.

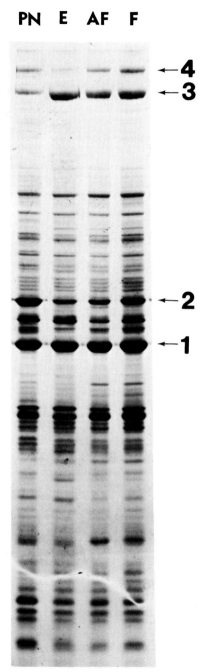

FIG. 5. One-dimensional electrophoresis in an SDS–polyacrylamide slab gel, stained with Coomassie blue. Shown are whole-cell homogenates of postnatal skin fibroblasts (PN) and amniotic fluid cell types E, AF, and F. Note the four landmark protein bands including (1) actin, (2) desmin, and (3) myosin. Adapted from Johnston *et al.* (1981).

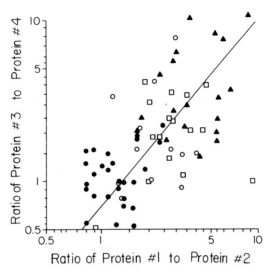

FIG. 6.   Quantitative relationships among the four landmark protein bands shown in Fig. 5 as a function of cell type. Solid circles, postnatal skin fibroblasts (PN); open circles, F-type; open squares, AF-type; solid triangles, E-type amniotic fluid cells. Adapted from Johnston *et al.* (1981).

point was added to the separation previously based solely on molecular weight (Johnston *et al.*, 1981). Cells were plated at a density of 0.5×10^5 per square centimeter in multiwell dishes and labeled with [^{35}S]methionine for periods of 2–3 hours. Approximately 10^6 counts were loaded for isoelectric focusing (IEF) in the first dimension, and a 12% polyacrylamide separating gel was used in the second dimension. The protein maps of the three cell types were compared by the "reference-constellation method" of Dewey and colleagues (1978): the entire gel area was divided into several domains demarcated by landmark protein spots.

Figure 7 illustrates three such domains for each of the respective amniotic fluid cell types. There are clear differences between the F-type cells and the AF- and E-type cells in each of these domains. For instance, the spots indicated by solid markings in the reference maps in Fig. 7 are absent from F-type cells but present in AF- and E-type cells. The spots indicated by the open circles with broken borders differ quantitatively: the amount is consistently reduced in F-type cells. There are surprisingly few qualitative differences in spot patterns between the

FIG. 7.   Selected landscapes from autoradiographs of two-dimensional gel electrophoresis of [^{35}S]methionine-labeled whole-cell homogenates. F-, AF-, and E-type amniotic fluid cells are shown in the columns as indicated, and consistent qualitative (solid) and quantitative (open) differences are indicated in the reference maps at the right (see text). Top row, pH 4–5 region; middle row, pH 5–6 region; bottom row, pH 6–7 region. Adapted from Johnston *et al.* (1981).

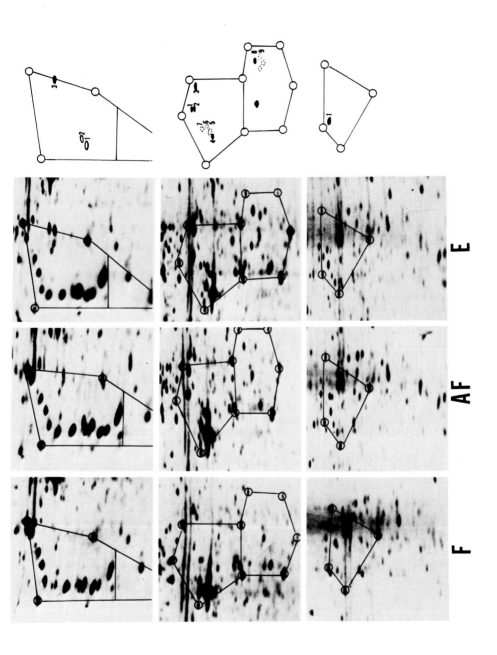

AF- and E-type cells. The open circles with solid borders in the acidic region (pH 4–5) indicate the area that most consistently differentiates the three cell types: both spots are apparent in AF-type cells, spot number 2 is less apparent in F-type cells, and both spots are greatly reduced in E-type cells. Because of minor variations in pattern between different electrophoretic runs, it is necessary to observe multiple runs to appreciate that other variations observed in Fig. 7 are not consistent.

In considering these findings one should keep in mind that the observed differences in the protein map cannot result from genotypic variation because all three cell types were derived from the same amniotic fluid specimen. Our preliminary studies with synchronized cultures and with aged cells suggest that the observed differences in the two-dimensional protein maps of F and AF/E cells are not due to differences in synthetic activity as a function of cell cycle state, culture age, or variations in the proportions of quiescent and cycling cells. The two-dimensional protein maps of primary amniotic fluid cell clones are consistent with the concept that F- and AF-type cells, in spite of their morphologic and growth-kinetic similarities, are derived from developmentally distinct cells that retain their differentiated patterns of gene expression during *in vitro* growth.

V.   Structural Matrix Proteins

A.   Procollagens

The production of collagen by cells derived from amniotic fluid was first suggested by the work of Macek *et al.* (1973), and the synthesis of type I collagen was subsequently demonstrated by Hurych *et al.* (1976). Priest *et al.* (1977) examined AF- and F-type cultures separately and recognized differences between their respective collagenous products: F-type cells synthesized a form of collagen indistinguishable from the ''interstitial'' collagen produced by cultured fetal skin fibroblasts, whereas AF-type cells produced a type of collagen that resembled ''basement membrane'' collagen.

Priest's group also demonstrated that AF (but not F) cells secrete a glycoprotein into the tissue culture medium that reacts with antibodies specific for epithelial basement membrane (Megaw *et al.*, 1977), and indirect fluorescent antibody studies indicated that this glycoprotein was associated with the extracellular matrix of both cultivated AF cells and a primary culture established from amniotic membranes of a human abortus specimen, whereas it was not identifiable in cultures of F-type amniotic fluid cells or fibroblasts derived from human skin.

Electron microscopy of the extracellular matrix of cultured F, AF, and skin fibroblast cells revealed findings consistent with the biochemical studies: extracellular type I collagen fibers could be visualized in F-type and skin fibroblast cultures, but not in AF cell cultures where fine filamentous material was observed admixed with amorphous material adjacent to cell membranes (Priest *et al.*, 1978). On the basis of all their findings, Priest *et al.* (1978) suggested that AF cells are derived from extra-embryonic, trophoblastic tissues.

In a later series of articles, Crouch and Bornstein (1978, 1979) characterized in great detail the spectrum of collagenous proteins produced by AF- and F-type amniotic fluid cells. According to their findings, F cells in culture synthesize predominantly type I and lesser amounts of type III procollagen. AF-Type cells, however, synthesize considerably less total collagen that consists principally of two types distinctly different from that produced by F-type cells. According to their respective positions in SDS–polyacrylamide gels, the smaller AF-type collagen was labeled AF2 and the somewhat larger molecule was labeled AF1 (Fig. 8). The amino acid composition of the AF1 molecule was found to be similar to that of basement membrane-type collagen (type IV), and its cyanogen bromide peptide patterns were distinct from those of types I, II, III, and A-B collagens when examined by SDS–PAGE (Crouch and Bornstein, 1979).

AF2, the second procollagen characteristic of AF cells, was found to be produced in different amounts by different clones and to contain three identical proα chains that are structurally and immunologically related to the proα1 chains of type I procollagen (Crouch and Bornstein, 1978). Despite differences in migration on SDS–PAGE and differences in solubility characteristics, there are marked similarities between the α1-chains derived from AF2 and from type I collagen; it appears that the differences between proα1 chains from AF2 and from type I collagens can be explained on the basis of increased posttranslational modifications (specifically hydroxylation) of the AF2 proα1 chains. Crouch and Bornstein concluded that the AF2 collagen has the chain composition $[\alpha1(I)]_3$ with higher degrees of hydroxylation of the prolyl and lysyl residues in the $\alpha1(I)$ chains than is found in type I collagen (chain composition: $[\alpha1(I)]_2\alpha2$).

Type I trimers ($[\alpha1(I)]_3$) similar to AF2 have been observed in non-amniotic fluid cell cultures treated with bromodeoxyuridine or embryo extract and in association with *in vitro* cellular senescence (Mayne *et al.*, 1975, 1976), in association with both inflammatory disease (Narayanan and Page, 1976) and virus-induced neoplasia (Little *et al.*, 1977), and in normally developing tissues in organ culture (Jimenez *et al.*, 1977; Munksgaard *et al.*, 1978). It is possible, as suggested by Little *et al.* (1977), that the type I trimer collagen represents an embryonic collagen type. The presence of this molecule in diseased tissues and tumors might reflect a process of "dedifferentiation" akin to the expression of the carcinoembryonal antigen or α-fetoprotein in some neoplasias (Crouch and Bornstein, 1978). Because F-type amniotic fluid cells do not synthesize this trimer, and because variable amounts of trimer and type I procollagen are synthesized by AF-type cells, it appears that production of the trimer is not a fixed

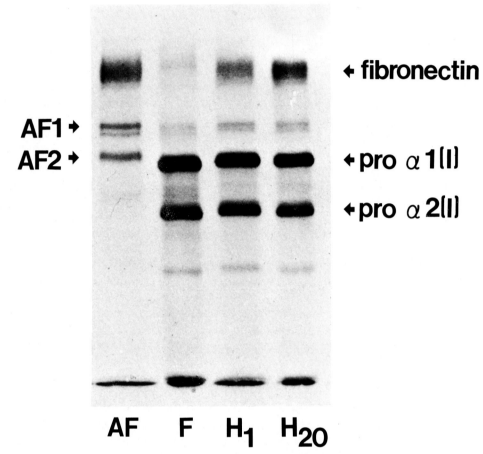

FIG. 8.   Fluorescence autoradiogram of reduced [³H]proline-labeled medium proteins of parental (AF and F) and hybrid cells (H₁ and H₂₀) on 5% SDS–PAGE. The arrows indicate the band representing fibronectin and the bands representing the four procollagen types characteristic of F-type (right) and AF- and E-type amniotic fluid cells (left). Adapted from Bryant *et al.* (1978).

characteristic of fetal cells, but rather that it reflects differences in the state of differentiation and/or embryologic derivation of AF- and F-type cells.

In addition to the increased amounts of hydroxylation of prolyl and lysyl residues in the α1(I) chains of AF2-, F- and AF-type cells appear to differ in the processing of their various procollagen molecules to intermediate p-collagens and collagen chains, in the time required for synthesis and secretion of procollagen molecules, and in the assembly or location of their disulfide bonds (Crouch and Bornstein, 1979). Whereas extensive F-cell procollagen processing occurs within several hours and a more limited amount of AF2-procollagen processing requires at least 12 hours, AF1 procollagen is not processed into procollagen intermediates in either the culture medium or the cell layer (Crouch and Bornstein, 1979). Compared with type I procollagen, the time required for synthesis and secretion of AF1 procollagen is prolonged, and type IV (AF1) procollagen secreted in the presence of α-α' dipyridyl lacks interchain disulfide bonds in contrast to type I procollagens.

B. Fibronectin

An additional structural matrix protein that has been examined in amniotic fluid cell cultures is fibronectin (Crouch *et al.*, 1978a,b). This glycoprotein, immunologically related to plasma cold-insoluble globulin (CIG), is enriched in amniotic fluid compared with plasma. It is secreted by both F and AF cells in culture and was shown to be associated with the pericellular and extracellular matrix by immunofluorescence. No qualitative difference was observed in the fibronectin secreted by these cell types although relatively more fibronectin was present in the secreted proteins of AF cells compared with F cells (Fig. 8).

It is evident from the work of Crouch and Bornstein (1978, 1979) and Crouch *et al.* (1978a,b) that the major constituents of the extracellular matrix of AF- and F-type cells are quite different. F-type cells produce principally type I collagen and lesser amounts of type III collagen. AF cells produce two less common forms of collagen: AF1 is similar to the type IV collagen associated with basement membranes and AF2 is a trimer of $\alpha 1(I)$ chains that are hydroxylated to a greater degree than the $\alpha 1(I)$ chains in type I collagen.

VI. Amniotic Fluid Cell Enzymes and Hormones

Because of their significance for the prenatal diagnosis of inborn errors of metabolism, many enzymatic proteins have been quantitatively determined in cultivated amniotic fluid cells (Gerbie *et al.*, 1972; Kabach and Leonard, 1972). In a critical review of such studies Burton *et al.* (1979) point out that there can be many factors that influence measured values of enzyme activity in such cells, such as the stage of gestation, amniotic fluid cell type, age of the culture, and tissue culture conditions. The influence of tissue culture conditions is well known to anyone involved with mammalian cell culture, and one of the first examples of enzyme activity variation in amniotic fluid cell cultures as a function of culture conditions was the fluctuation of lysosomal enzyme activities found by Sutherland *et al.* (1974) in 13 strains of amniotic fluid cells. In their own laboratory, Burton *et al.* (1979) observed that the type of medium, the timing of medium change, and the interval between plating and harvest or subculture affects activity measurements of the enzymes betaglucosidase and arylsulfatase.

One would expect that the morphologically distinct cell types that emerge in cultures of amniotic fluid would display differences in enzyme synthesis that reflect their respective states of differentiation and gene activity. Such cell type-specific expressions of enzymes was first recorded by Melancon *et al.* (1971), who found that the enzyme histidase was present in epithelioid, but not in fibroblastoid amniotic fluid cells. An example of quantitative variation in enzyme expression as a function of cell type is mentioned in the article by Burton *et al.* (1979): F-type cells display significantly higher cystathionine synthetase activities than E-type cells. There are comparatively few such examples of activity variation as a function of amniotic fluid cell type, possibly because enzymes tested can be grouped among the constitutive or "housekeeping" proteins universally present in cells during proliferation. A substantial change in the levels of such enzymes might be expected to occur only when cells switch from the replicative to the postreplicative state; during this period most mammalian cell types are subject to unbalanced growth with attendant changes in the size of protein pools and rates of protein turnover. An appropriate example for this situation is the increase in G-6-PD activity found in aging human skin fibroblasts (Fulder and Holliday, 1975).

With the possible exception of the histidase report (Melancon *et al.*, 1971), none of the enzyme determinations have yielded substantial clues as to the nature of the *in vivo* counterparts of cultivated amniotic fluid cell types. More promising leads have been obtained by the study of hormone synthesis in amniotic fluid cells. Priest and his colleagues (1979) examined AF- and F-type amniotic fluid cells and fibroblasts from fetal skin for the production of human chorionic gonadotropin (hCG), a peptide hormone normally produced by the placenta. AF-type cell cultures were found to produce this hormone, whereas F-type and fetal skin fibroblast cultures did not. The amounts of hCG produced by AF-type cell cultures declined progressively with subculture, and Priest *et al.* (1979) suggested that these cells gradually lose this differentiated function. The production of hCG by AF-type cells may imply that they originate from extra-embryonic trophoblastic tissues that are known to express this function *in vivo,* whereas F-type cells may be derived from fetal tissues proper, such as skin. Priest *et al.* (1979) point out that the morphology of AF-type cells is compatible with the morphology described by early reports of cultured abortus placenta, and they suggest that this interpretation is consistent with their measurements of hCG. The morphology of AF cells changes significantly as these cells age *in vitro,* however, and this fact has to be considered when comparing morphologic characteristics between published articles. Moreover, AF-type cells can definitely be cloned from midgestation fetal urines (Hoehn *et al.,* 1975b) and so a putative progenitor cell must also be represented within the urogenital system.

VII. Use of Amniotic Fluid Cells for Cell Biological Investigations

Methods for culturing cells obtained from amniotic fluids and the clinical applications of these techniques have been frequently summarized, most recently by Milunsky (1979). However, there are comparatively few articles on the experimental use of these cells. For the cell biologist, amniotic fluid from midtrimester human pregnancies constitutes a relatively novel source of normal human cells, but one that is becoming increasingly accessible and that provides some unique advantages. With the possible exception of human preputial epidermis (Sun and Green, 1977), amniotic fluid is the only source from which human epithelioid cells can be readily obtained and propagated without applying specialized culture techniques or growth factors. No other euploid human cell type is known that produces greater amounts of fibronectin in culture than AF-type amniotic fluid cells. Compared to fetal lung or postnatal skin fibroblast cultures, those initiated from amniotic fluid display extreme cellular heterogeneity at the morphologic as well as the biochemical level of analysis; this heterogeneity presumably is due to their origination from widely divergent *in vivo* tissues. Within a single specimen of amniotic fluid, however, this heterogeneous cell population shares the same genomic constitution, a fact that permits the assignment of apparent differences in gene expression of such cells to developmental differentiation rather than to differences in genotype. A very practical advantage of these cells for genetic studies is that their parental genomes are usually available for examination because parents rarely object to donating a blood sample or a skin biopsy for clinically necessary investigations at the time of amniocentesis. Moreover, follow-up studies with various additional cell types from the same individual (cord blood, umbilical cord, placenta, foreskin, etc.) may be readily available at the time of desired or natural termination of the pregnancy without recourse to unusual procedures.

In order to emphasize the more general cell biological importance of amniotic fluid cells, we will conclude this article reviewing their *in vitro* characteristics with two examples of research from our own laboratories. Other examples can be found in the published literature (e.g., Rankin and Darlington, 1979) and will be discussed in a later section of this volume.

A. Euploid Somatic Cell Hybridization with Amniotic Fluid Cells

The isolation of proliferating hybrid synkaryons from human diploid cultures has proved difficult because of the paucity of selective markers available. We have recovered actively proliferating hybrids from such strains using a nonselective technique employing dilute plating of fusogen-treated cell mixtures (Hoehn *et al.*, 1975c). The hybrid nature of the isolated clones was demonstrated by electrophoretic analysis of the G-6-PD phenotype and observation of DNA content by flow cytometry. These hybrid clones were found to be chromosomally stable (i.e., they remained pure tetraploids throughout their *in vitro* life span), and their growth potential was apparently determined in a co-dominant fashion by the proliferative potentials of the parental strains.

The question of gene regulation of ontogenetically divergent genomes was approached by fusing postnatal skin fibroblast-like cells to amniotic fluid E- and AF-type cultures (Bryant *et al.*, 1978). The phenotypic divergence between the parental strains in such heterotypic fusions facilitates the isolation of hybrids from dilute platings. Of a total of 202 isolates, 46 displayed G-6-PD type AB heteropolymeric enzyme; 19 of these 46 isolates proved to be pure hybrid clones on the basis of a stable tetraploid DNA content and chromosome complement. These 19 hybrids grew at a reduced rate compared to homotypic control (fibroblast) hybrids and tetraploids. However, the combination of a fibroblast with the epithelioid genome substantially improved the survival of the epithelioid genome during trypsinization and subculture. The production of extracellular matrix proteins in these hybrids appeared to be determined by the AF-type genome in the case of fibronectin and by the fibroblast genome in the case of procollagen synthesis (Fig. 8); technical considerations prevented a more detailed analysis of this interaction. Ribosomal gene activity was determined by the $AgNO_3$ histochemical procedure, and both parental genomes were present in the hybrids at the same level of activity as before the fusion. According to these results, genome regulation in heterotypic euploid hybrids appears to conform to the following rules: (1) the activity of household functions proceeds at the predetermined rate of each of the parental portions of the combined genomes; and (2) synthesis of luxury gene products may be dominated by the more specialized parental genome, even though there is no conclusive evidence for complete repression of either parental function.

B.   Flow Cytometry of Cultivated Amniotic Fluid Cells

For obvious reasons it would be desirable to abbreviate the interval between time of amniocentesis and time of final cytogenetic diagnosis. Many attempts have therefore been directed at speeding up the growth of prenatal cell cultures by various culture manipulations and addition of growth factors (Milunsky, 1979; see also the article by Epstein in the present volume). A completely different approach consists of high-resolution DNA content measurements of interphase amniotic fluid cells, either directly after amniocentesis or after a very brief period of culture. Because it has been shown that numerical chromosome aberrations may be recognized by flow-cytometric methods (Hoehn *et al.*, 1977), we decided to extend this approach to the cells suspended in midtrimester fluids. The results of these studies were discouraging. The DNA fluorescence histograms that were obtained were mostly of poor quality and, most disturbingly, were highly variable.

In order to determine the reasons for this variability we assayed isolated F-, AF-, and E-type amniotic fluid colonies. A series of five clones from each of these cell types was isolated from a single fluid and prepared and stained by the technique of Zante *et al.* (1976), as modified the Rabinovitch *et al.* (1981). This method yields high-quality DNA content histograms for a variety of mammalian cell types, including human diploid skin fibroblasts. Fixed samples are allowed to reach room temperature, centrifuged, and aliquots of 0.5×10^6 cells are resuspended in 0.8 ml of ethidium bromide (25 μg/ml in 0.1 M Tris with 0.6% NaCl). The sample is kept at room temperature for 10 minutes, and then 0.8 ml of mithramycin staining solution (50 μg/ml, 7.5 mM MgCl$_2$, and 12.5% ETOH) is added. RNase (0.1 ml of a 1% solution in saline) is added to the stained cell suspensions 30 minutes prior to flow analysis. Aliquots of internal standard particles (fluorescent polystyrene spheres, 9.7 μm approximate size; Duke Scientific, Palo Alto, CA) are diluted in the EB/MI dye combination (containing a 1% solution of NP-40) and added (in amounts depending on specimen concentration) to every experimental sample at the time of assay. Cellular fluorescence intensities are quantitated as fluorescence ratio (the mean value of the cellular fluorescence divided by the mean value of the fluorescence of the internal standard). The epi-illumination flow system is equipped with a multichannel analyzer for acquisition of up to four consecutive single-parameter fluorescence pulse height histograms. The excitation filters are BG38 and BG12, the dichroic mirror TK450, and the emission filter OG570.

Figure 9 shows the unexpected result of these experiments: the isogenic and karyotypically identical cell types fail to show uniform fluorescence values, and the relative fluorescence emission of the different classes of cells is inversely proportional to their respective cell sizes as determined by Coulter sizing (Rabinovitch *et al.*, unpublished). In apparent analogy to serum-deprived human skin fibroblasts, which lose cellular DNA fluorescence but increase their size (Rabinovitch *et al.*, 1981), variations in the degree of chromatin condensation must disturb the stoichiometric relationship between the amount of cellular DNA and binding of dye. The lesson from our initial studies with this system is that what is assayed with the chosen dye combination is not DNA per se, but the number of accessible binding sites and their distribution between donor and acceptor molecules that determines the extent to which energy-transfer phenomena enhance the total fluorescence. In recent studies we have used the nonintercalating dye DAPI (4',6-diamidino-2-phenylindole) to stain nuclei isolated by treatment with nonionic detergent (NP-40). In this system, there is a more predictable relationship between fluorescence and the expected DNA content of different amniotic fluid cell types. The fluorescence ratios of three

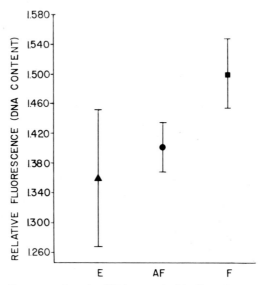

FIG. 9.   Relative fluorescence intensity (DNA content) of the G_1 peaks of isogenic E-, AF-, and F-type amniotic fluid cell clones assayed by flow-cytofluorometry and expressed as the sample to standard particle fluorescence ratio (vertical scale). The mean and standard deviation is shown for five clones each of E-, AF-, and F-type cells that were stained with ethidium bromide–mithramycin.

isogenic F-, AF-, and E-type amniotic fluid cell clones varied by only 0.6%. The average fluorescent ratios of ten male and eight female amniotic fluid cell clones differed by 1.76%, compared with the expected 1.72% difference in DNA content based on *in situ* cytophotometric data. The amniotic fluid cell system with its isogenic but variously differentiated cell types is an ideal system for the study of conformational changes of chromatin using appropriate fluorescent probes.

REFERENCES

Bryant, E. B., Crouch, E., Bornstein, P., Martin, G. M., Johnston, P., and Hoehn, H. (1978). *Am. J. Hum. Genet.* **30,** 392–405.

Burton, B. K., Gerbie, A. B., and Nadler, H. L. (1979). *In* "Genetic Disorders and The Fetus" (A. Milunsky, ed.), pp. 369–377. Plenum, New York.

Casadei, R., d'Ablaing, G., Kaplan, B., and Schwinn, C. (1973). *Acta Cytol.* (Baltimore) **17,** 289.

Crouch, E., and Bornstein, P. (1978). *Biochemistry* **17,** 5499–5509.

Crouch, E., and Bornstein, P. (1979). *J. Biol. Chem.* **254,** 4197–4204.

Crouch, E., Balian, G., Holbrook, K., Duskin, D., and Bornstein, P. (1978a). *J. Cell Biol.* **78,** 701–715.

Crouch, E., Balian, G., Holbrook, K., Hoehn, H., and Bornstein, P. (1978b). *Ann. N.Y. Acad. Sci.* **312,** 410–413.

Dewey, M. J., Filler, R., and Mintz, B. (1978). *Dev. Biol.* **65,** 171–182.

Fulder, S. J., and Holliday, R. (1975). *Cell* **6**, 67–73.

Gerbie, A. B., Melancon, S. B., Ryan, C. A., and Nadler, H. L. (1972). *Am. J. Obstet. Gynecol.* **114**, 314–320.

Gosden, C. M., and Brock, D. J. H. (1977). *Lancet* **1**, 919–922.

Gosden, C. M., and Brock, D. J. H. (1978). *Br. Med. J.* **2**, 1186–1189.

Herz, F., Schermer, A., and Koss, L. G. (1979). *Proc. Soc. Exp. Biol. Med.* **161**, 153–157.

Hoehn, H., Bryant, E. M., Karp, L. E., and Martin, G. M. (1974). *Pediatr. Res.* **8**, 746–754.

Hoehn, H., Bryant, E. M., Karp, L. E., and Martin, G. M. (1975a). *Clin. Genet.* **7**, 29–36.

Hoehn, H., Bryant, E. M., Fantel, A. G., and Martin, G. M. (1975b). *Humangenetik* **29**, 285–290.

Hoehn, H., Bryant, E. M., Johnston, P., Norwood, T. H., and Martin, G. M. (1975c). *Nature* **258**, 608–610.

Hoehn, H., Johnston, P., and Callis, J. (1977). *Cytogenet. Cell Genet.* **19**, 94–107.

Hoehn, H., Rodriguez, M. L., Norwood, T. H., and Maxwell, C. L. (1978). *Am. J. Med. Genet.* **2**, 253–266.

Holbrook, K. A., and Odland, G. F. (1975). *J. Invest. Dermatol.* **65**, 71–84.

Huisjes, H. J. (1978). *In* "Amniotic Fluid—Research and Clinical Application" (D. V. I. Fairweather and T. K. A. B. Eskes, eds.), 2nd Edition, pp. 93–129. Elsevier-North Holland, Amsterdam.

Hurych, J., Macek, M., Beniac, F., and Rezacova, D. (1976). *Hum. Genet.* **31**, 335–340.

Jimenez, S. A., Bashey, R. I., Benditt, M., and Yankowski, R. (1977). *Biochem. Biophys. Res. Commun.* **78**, 1354–1361.

Johnston, P., Salk, D., Martin, G. M., and Hoehn, H. (1981). *Prenatal Diagnosis* (in press).

Kaback, M. M., and Leonard, C. O. (1972). *In* "Antenatal Diagnosis" (A. Dorfman, ed.), pp. 81–94. Univ. of Chicago Press, Chicago.

Laemmli, U. K. (1970). *Nature* **227**, 680–685.

Little, C. D., Church, R. C., Miller, R. A., and Ruddle, F. H. (1977). *Cell* **10**, 287–295.

Macek, M., Hurych, J., and Rezacova, D. (1973). *Nature* **243**, 289–290.

Martin, G. M., Sprague, C. A., and Epstein, C. J. (1970). *Lab. Invest.* **23**, 86–91.

Martin, G. M., Ogburn, C., and Sprague, C. (1975). *Adv. Exp. Med. Biol.* **61**, 163–193.

Mayne, R., Vail, M. S., and Miller, E. J. (1975). *Proc. Natl. Acad. Sci. U.S.A.* **72**, 4511–4515.

Mayne, R., Vail, M. S., Mayne, P. M., and Miller, E. J. (1976). *Proc. Natl. Acad. Sci. U.S.A.* **73**, 1674–1678.

Megaw, J. M., Priest, J. H., Priest, R. E., and Johnson, L. D. (1977). *J. Med. Genet.* **14**, 163–167.

Melancon, S. B., Lee, S. Y., and Nadler, H. L. (1971). *Science* **173**, 627.

Milunsky, A., ed. (1979). "Genetic Disorders and The Fetus." Plenum, New York.

Munksgaard, E. C., Rhodes, M., Mayne, R., and Butler, W. T. (1978). *Eur. J. Biochem.* **82**, 609–617.

Narayanan, A. S., and Page, R. C. (1976). *J. Biol. Chem.* **251**, 5464–5471.

O'Farrell, P. H. (1975). *J. Biol. Chem.* **250**, 4007.

Priest, R. E., Priest, J. H., Moinuddin, J. F., and Keyser, A. J. (1977). *J. Med. Genet.* **14**, 157–162.

Priest, R. E., Marimuthu, K. M., and Priest, J. H. (1978). *Lab. Invest.* **39**, 106–109.

Priest, R. E., Priest, J. H., Moinuddin, J. F., and Sgoutas, D. S. (1979). *In Vitro* **15**, 142–147.

Rabinovitch, P. S., O'Brien, K., Simpson, M., Callis, J. B., and Hoehn, H. (1981). *Cytogenet. Cell Genet.* **29**, 65–76.

Rankin, J. K., and Darlington, G. J. (1979). *Somatic Cell Genet.* **5**, 1–10.

Salk, D., Au, K., Hoehn, H., and Martin, G. M. (1981). *Cytogenet. Cell Genet.* **30**, 92–107.

Schmid, W. (1975). *Humangenetik* **30**, 325–330.

Schmid, W. (1977). *Hereditas* **86**, 37–44.

Sun, T.-T., and Green, H. (1977). *Nature* **269**, 489–493.

Sutherland, G. R., Brock, D. J. H., and Scrimgeour, J. B. (1973). *Lancet* **2,** 1098–1099.
Sutherland, G. R., Butterworth, J., Broadhead, D. M., and Bain, A. D. (1974). *Clin. Chim. Acta* **52,** 211–217.
Sutherland, G. R., Brock, D. J. H., and Scrimgeour, J. B. (1975). *J. Med. Genet.* **12,** 135–137.
Zante, J., Schumann, J., Barlogie, B., Göhde, W., and Büchner, Th. (1976). *In* "Pulse Cytophotometry" (W. Göhde, J. Schumann, and Th. Büchner, eds.), Vol. II, pp. 97–106. European Press Medicon, Ghent, Belgium.

Chapter 3

Prenatal Cytogenetic Diagnosis

MARY McH. SANDSTROM, MARY T. BEAUCHESNE, KAREN M. GUSTASHAW, AND SAMUEL A. LATT

Division of Genetics, Department of Obstetrics and Gynecology
Brigham and Women's Hospital
Harvard Medical School
Boston, Massachusetts

I. Introduction

The overall problem currently addressed by prenatal cytogenetic analysis is the ascertainment of a fetal karyotype from information obtained on the cells present

Copyright © 1982 by Academic Press, Inc.

in an aspirate of the amniotic cavity. As outlined in the chapter by Hoehn and Salk, this aspirate can contain a mixture of cell types (Hoehn *et al.*, 1974; Megaw *et al.*, 1977; Priest *et al.*, 1977, 1978; Papp and Bell, 1979), most of fetal origin. However, in some cases, a few cells of maternal origin are also present. From this 10- to 20-ml sample, containing 10^3–10^5 cells per milliliter, not all of which are viable—based on dye exclusion (Gosden and Brock, 1978)—less than 0.1% actively incorporate ^{3}H-labeled thymidine, and 5 cells/ml proliferate in culture in a manner permitting metaphase chromosome analysis (Hoehn *et al.*, 1974). Moreover, during this proliferation, karyotypic abnormalities may arise *de novo*, and, even under optimal conditions, only a small fraction of proliferating cells will reach metaphase and be included in chromosome studies. The present chapter will describe methods for analyzing this highly selected subset of metaphase cells with the goal of making an accurate determination of the fetal karyotype. Factors that can confound this analysis, such as cellular heterogeneity and culture-induced chromosome changes, will also be discussed.

In view of the risks incurred during sample acquisition, as well as the concern for prompt analysis, emphasis on prenatal cytogenetic analysis is appropriately placed on strategies that minimize technical causes for the failure to obtain results. Thus multiple cultures should be established from a single sample, and manipulations of these cells should be staggered. Additional attention should be given to background information such as maternal age, parental karyotypes, fetal karyotype statistics, ultrasound results, in using the newly derived cytogenetic information to arrive at estimates of the relative likelihoods of particular fetal karyotypes. Other data, such as those from biochemical tests, should, when available, be incorporated into such estimates. Finally, existing strategies may well eventually be modified to incorporate newly evolving data on chromosome-specific gene markers (as summarized in periodic Human Gene Mapping conferences), as well as methods for detecting chromosome-specific DNA sequences (Gusella *et al.*, 1979; Lebo *et al.*, 1979; Scott *et al.*, 1979; Botstein *et al.*, 1980; Wolf *et al.*, 1980; Bruns *et al.*, 1981; Davies *et al.*, 1981; Davies, 1981), in developing approaches for resolving karyotypic ambiguities.

The primary indication for prenatal cytogenetic diagnosis is, at present, advanced maternal age. A commonly accepted cutoff is 35 years of age, at which the risk of autosomal trisomy is approximately 3/1000 (twice the level in the population as a whole). Beyond this age, the risk of such trisomy increases significantly (Siggers, 1978; Golbus *et al.*, 1979; Milunsky, 1979). Additional indications for prenatal cytogenetic diagnosis are a previous incidence of autosomal trisomy in a family, a balanced translocation in one parent, and fetal sex determination (to rule out X-linked recessive disease). The need for chromosome analysis on amniotic fluid samples obtained because of elevated serum alpha-fetoprotein levels is less clear. One study (Gosden *et al.*, 1981) suggests that the incidence of chromosomal abnormalities in this group of patients is not elevated (i.e., the test is probably not indicated). However, more data on this last category will be useful.

II.   Culture Initiation and Harvest

Approximately 10–20 ml of amniotic fluid, typically obtained between the sixteenth and eighteenth week of gestation, is used to carry out prenatal chromosome analysis. Samples, maintained at room temperature, can be transported to a cytogenetics laboratory in the syringe used in obtaining the amniotic fluid or in sterile nontoxic (e.g., Falcon #3033, 15-ml, white top) tubes. Use of appropriate sample containers increases the success rate of subsequent culturing. If a sample arrives in a syringe, it is transferred, under sterile laboratory conditions, to the Falcon tubes for centrifugation. Samples are divided in half and then treated separately, to reduce the ultimate impact of sporadic laboratory problems, such as culture contamination or equipment malfunction. Multiple samples arriving at a laboratory during any one day should be set up separately, to reduce the chance of a mixup in sample identity. The entire process of prenatal cytogenetic diagnosis, starting with sample receipt and followed by cell culture and chromosome analysis, should typically be accomplished within 3–4 weeks.

Samples are centrifuged (200 g, 600–800 rpm) for 10 minutes. The supernatant is decanted, leaving approximately 1 ml above the cell pellet. Five milliliters of this supernatant is saved for alpha-fetoprotein (AFP) analysis; the remainder is stored at $-20°C$ to be used for further study, such as measurement of hormone levels, if necessary. Each pellet is carefully examined macroscopically as to size and the presence of blood and/or coloration. Cell pellets can range from invisible to large. A clear sample might yield pellets tinged with blood. Pellets from grossly bloody or brown samples may contain small clots or tissue pieces. On the average, the pellet from a clear sample, obtained at 16–18 weeks, will be 4–5 mm in diameter (typical size), and a standard procedure can then be followed— that is, a total of six primary cultures and two monolayer cultures per case initiated. A seventh primary culture can be set up for harvest within 20 hours to check for rapidly adhering (RA) cells, an adjunct method for assessing the likelihood of a neural tube defect (Gosden and Brock, 1978; see chapter by Haddow and Miller). The number of primary cultures per case is reduced if the cell pellets are unusually small.

Primary cultures, obtained by inoculating cells directly onto a coverslip or a microscope slide inside a petri dish, yield discrete colonies, each presumably originating from a single cell (Schmid, 1975). Trypsinization prior to analysis is unnecessary. Monolayer cultures, in contrast, yield, with trypsinization, a mixture of cells from a number of colonies. Cell growth is sometimes better in these cultures—which are typically initiated with more cells—than in discrete colonies; and monolayer cultures can serve to provide backup material if other cultures fail. Specific procedures used to set up both types of cultures are summarized in the following paragraphs.

A.   Primary Cultures

Glass coverslips (e.g., 22 mm square, No. 1½) are presoaked in absolute ethanol and then flamed for sterilization. Sterile coverslips are placed in 35 × 10-mm petri plates, which have previously been labeled with the patient's code number. The amniotic fluid cell pellets are resuspended in 3–5 ml of media [e.g., Ham's F-10 + 20% fetal bovine serum + penicillin (50 units/ml), streptomycin (50 μg/ml), and L-glutamine (1 mM)]. An amount of 0.5 ml of the suspension is added onto each coverslip. The cultures are then incubated at 37°C in an atmosphere of 5% CO_2 and 95% air, without any disturbance (except, when relevant, for the single coverslip examined for RA cells) for 5–7 days. After this time, the media and most of the nonviable cells are removed by gentle aspiration and replaced with 2 ml of fresh media. This procedure is repeated twice weekly until the cell material is ready for harvesting.

B.   Monolayer Cultures

One-half to one ml of the original cell suspension is added directly to the surface of a culture dish or T-flask. Two to four ml of fresh media is added, and the mixture gently swirled to distribute the cells. Incubation then proceeds as described above for 5–7 days, after which the media is renewed twice weekly.

Low-volume samples are set up in fewer plates, maintaining enough to allow readings to be obtained from more than one culture. Bloody samples or samples less than 8 ml in volume can pose significant problems in obtaining sufficient cell growth. Evaluation of pellet size must include an allowance for erythrocytes. Special methodology for processing very bloody samples, using heparin, has been published (Felix and Doherty, 1979). However, this requires receipt of samples before clotting has occurred.

C.   Harvesting

1.   COVERSLIP PREPARATIONS

Primary cultures on coverslips are generally ready for harvesting 10 to 14 days after initiation. Samples acquired late in gestation (18 to 20 weeks and beyond) may be ready for harvest a few days sooner. A typical culture may contain three to five cell colonies of perhaps 2 mm in diameter. Mitotic activity can be judged by the number of "doublets" (i.e., rounded cells that appear refractile when observed under an inverted microscope). The existence of five or more such doublets, typically at the periphery of a colony, is a good indication that the culture is ready for harvesting (Fig. 1). Doublets are also seen in the center of a colony, but these will usually yield metaphases of unsatisfactory morphology. These are thus less useful as a guide for a decision to harvest.

Mitotic arrest is achieved by adding colcemid (0.25 μg/ml) for approximately 2 hours before harvest. Cultures are incubated during this period. Hypotonic treatment follows. The most common hypotonic solution used is 0.075 M KCl, either full strength or diluted as much as 1:1 with distilled water. Under warm, humid conditions, full-strength 0.075 M KCl is satisfactory. In cool, dry atmospheres, a diluted KCl solution works better. The hypotonic solution is added at room temperature. Approximately 10 drops from a Pasteur pipet are gently applied to the periphery of a culture containing 2 ml medium. Five minutes later, the medium plus hypotonic solution is removed by careful aspiration at the periphery of the culture dish. Fresh hypotonic solution (1½-2 ml) is then added slowly and allowed to stand for 15 minutes. Without removing the KCl, a fixative solution of 6:1 methanol–acetic acid is added dropwise, at the edge of the culture. After 5 minutes, the hypotonic–fixative mixture is removed and replaced by 1.5–2 ml of fresh 6:1 fixative. After a further 15 minutes, the fixative is removed by aspiration. This cycle is repeated twice more, using 3:1 methanol–acetic acid fixative, except that the coverslip is lifted out of the dish without removing the last fixative solution, and excess fixative is drained from the edge of the slip. One quick, gentle blow on the cell side of the coverslip aids in spreading the chromosomes. The coverslips are then supported upright and allowed to air-dry for at least 1 hour before proceeding with staining procedures. The coverslips are fragile and must be handled with care.

2. PREPARATIONS CULTURED DIRECTLY ON SURFACES OF PETRI DISHES OR FLASKS

Monolayer cultures, set up in dishes or flasks without cover glasses, are often subcultured before harvesting. Subculturing increases the number of cells and/or subsequent metaphase figures available for analysis.

The cells of monolayer cultures can be passed onto coverslips for chromosome analysis or into other plates or flasks. With this procedure coverslip cultures can then be harvested in 2–3 days. Subcultures without coverslips reach confluency in 3–5 days, depending on the number of cells introduced from the original monolayer. For routine work, a culture is usually split into two new cultures, one of which is kept in reserve, with the other used for harvesting.

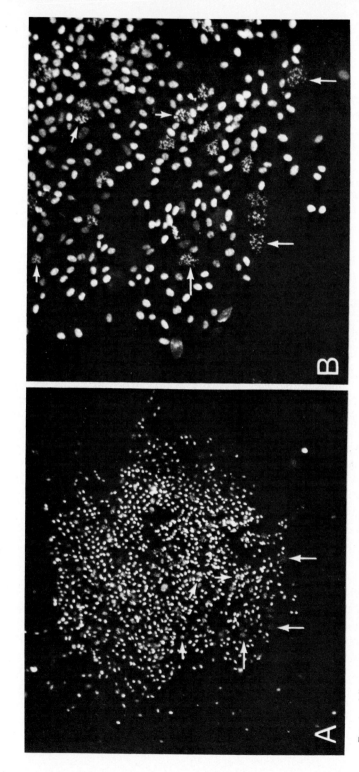

Fig. 1. Microscopic appearance of an amniotic fluid cell colony, grown on a coverslip. (A) The entire colony, stained with quinacrine (Table I). (B) A 2.5-fold further enlarged view of a sector of this colony. Large arrows point to well-spread metaphases (at the colony periphery) that are suitable for analysis. Smaller arrows point to poorly spread metaphases positioned toward the interior of the colony. By the morphological criteria of Hoehn and Salk (Chapter 2), this colony might be considered ''AF''-type, although, at this early stage of growth, identification is not absolutely certain.

Following mitotic arrest and trypsinization, cells are centrifuged, exposed 12–15 minutes to 0.075 M KCl hypotonic solution, and then fixed at least twice in 3:1 methanol:acetic acid before slide preparation.

III. Chromosome Identification

Approximately 2.5% of the amniocenteses performed because of advanced maternal age ($\geqslant$35 years) exhibit cytogenetic abnormalities (Milunsky, 1979). Though more than half of these abnormal diagnoses are trisomy 21, a wide variety of other abnormalities can occur. In addition to autosomal trisomies (with incidence increasing with maternal age) and X aneuploidy, various transmitted and spontaneous rearrangements can occur. One reason for the wide variety of abnormalities is the stage of gestation; not all abnormal karyotypes need be compatible with live birth (Boué et al., 1975, 1976, 1979; Carr and Gedeon, 1978). Many fetal chromosome changes require banding techniques for detection. Analysis of even normal or trisomic karyotypes can benefit from overdetermination from banding studies, even if most can be detected without banding (Fisher et al., 1980), primarily to assist in the differentiation between real chromosomal abnormalities and sporadic changes in chromosome scoring due to sample-preparation artifact. Thus banding analysis of at least a few cells is considered necessary (by the authors of this chapter) for prenatal cytogenetic diagnosis.

The authors' laboratory routinely utilizes two procedures, both of which yield positive (as opposed to reverse) banding patterns on all samples. The first, in which quinacrine (Caspersson et al., 1970, 1971, 1972; Czaker, 1973) is employed (Table I), affords moderate resolution, is highly reliable, and is especially

TABLE I

QUINACRINE BANDING[a]

---

1. Air-dry material (on a slide or a coverslip) for at least 1 hour before processing.
2. Immerse slides/coverslips in 100% methanol (5 minutes).
3. Stain with quinacrine dihydrochloride (20 mg/ml in H_2O) for 7 minutes.
4. Wash well with running water.
5. Immerse slide/coverslip in McIlvaine's buffer, pH 5.5 (0.043 M citrate–0.114 M sodium phosphate). A normal destaining time is 20 seconds; longer exposure to full-strength buffer reduces chromosome-staining intensity.
6. Wash well with running water. Air-dry. Store protected from light.
7. Mount for viewing in one part pH 5.5 McIlvaine's buffer diluted with four parts H_2O.
8. For fluorescence microscopy with incident illumination, use a 495-mm dichroic mirror (excitation) and a 510-nm barrier filter (emission).

---

[a] Modified from Czaker (1973).

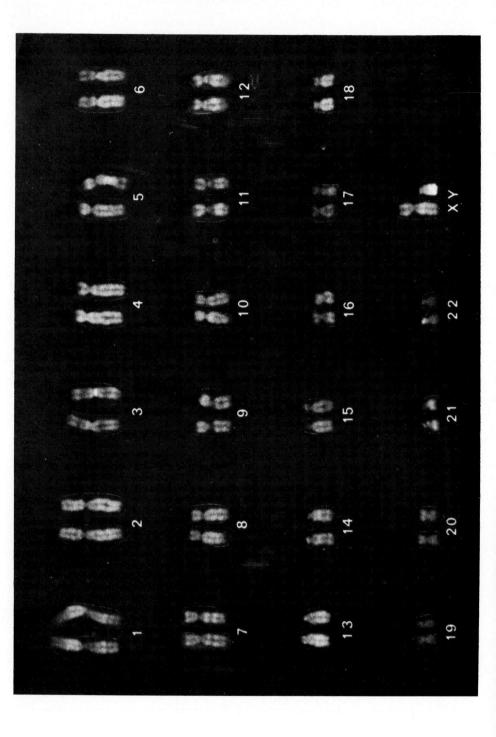

TABLE II

Giemsa–Trypsin Banding[a]

1. Use freshly prepared slides/coverslips.
2. Lay slides/coverslips flat in dish and flood with a 15% H_2O_2 (1:1 30% H_2O_2:H_2O) for 7 minutes.
3. Rinse slides thoroughly with distilled water.
4. Dry slides/coverslips on a hot plate (50°C) for approximately 1 hour.
5. Treat slides/coverslips in "working trypsin" solution in a Coplin jar for 3–30 seconds.[b]
   Stock trypsin—(GIBCO 5050) Stock trypsin is stored frozen in 4-ml aliquots.
   Working trypsin—4 ml stock + 46 ml Hanks' Balanced Salt Solution without Ca^{2+} and Mg^{2+} diluted just before use. The activity of this solution decreases rapidly with time, primarily because of enzyme autodigestion.
6. Rinse slides/coverslips in Hanks' Balanced Salt Solution (without Ca^{2+} and Mg^{2+}) with constant agitation.
7. Rinse slide/coverslip in distilled water for a few seconds.
8. Stain in 4% Giemsa (Gurr) made up in pH 6.8 buffer (one Gurr's buffer tablet per 100 ml; approximately 5 mM phosphate).
9. Rinse well in distilled water, then air-dry.

[a] From Seabright (1971, 1973).

[b] Trypsin is sensitive to pH, temperature, and age. To account for these factors (which may vary daily), as well as for variations between different slide preparations, it is usually necessary to test a range of exposure times.

useful for detection of certain polymorphic regions, including that in the distal part of the long arm of the human Y (Fig. 2). The second procedure utilizes Giemsa, after pretreatment of slides with trypsin (Table II) (Seabright, 1971, 1973). Success with this method is more variable than that with quinacrine, but the banding achieved is potentially of higher resolution, and the resulting preparations are permanent (Fig. 3). Giemsa–trypsin staining is also somewhat preferable to quinacrine for visualizing telomeric regions of chromosomes.

If detailed analysis of telomeres or Q-negative/G-negative bands is required, a reverse-banding procedure (Dutrillaux and LeJeune, 1971, 1975; Sehested, 1974; Verma and Lubs, 1975, Schweizer, 1976; Sahar and Latt, 1978, 1980; Latt et al., 1979a, 1980) can be very helpful. We have developed one procedure, which yields an essential R-band pattern, in which slides stained with chromomycin A_3 (a G-C specific dye) (Latt, 1977; Schnedl et al., 1977) are counterstained by methyl green (an A-T specific dye with an absorption spectrum overlapping the emission spectrum of chromomycin A_3) (Fig. 4; Table III). Energy transfer from chromomycin A_3 to methyl green is presumably extensive,

FIG. 2 (opposite). This karyotype is from a normal 46,XY male fetus. Cells were grown on coverslips, harvested in situ, stained with quinacrine, and photographed as described in the text (Table I).

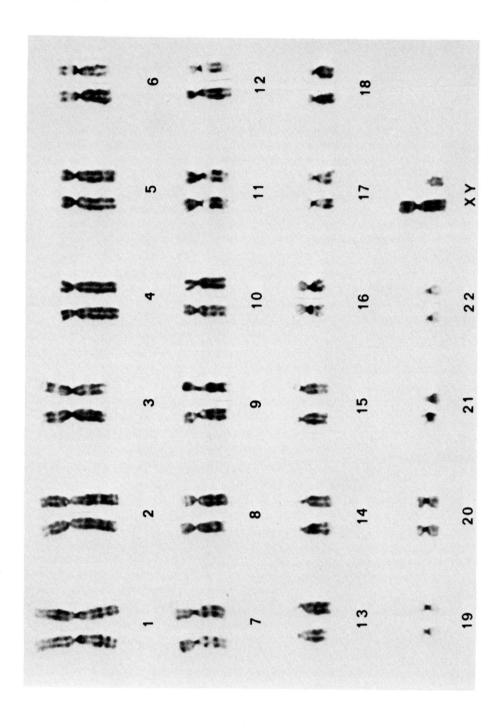

except where the interstain distance $\geqslant 50$ Å. The fluorescence of short clusters enriched for G-C base pairs would be relatively resistant to such quenching. Reverse bands thus seem to contain more of these clusters than do positive bands. Knowledge of the stain mechanism facilitates adjustment and optimization of staining conditions.

A variety of other stains are available for other specific indications. For example, C-banding (Arrighi and Hsu, 1971; Sumner, 1972; see Table IV) can be useful in identifying certain polymorphisms or delineating centromeric regions (e.g., to study chromosome fragments or, very rarely, to evaluate a pregnancy at risk for Roberts syndrome; Tompkins et al., 1979). Another double dye procedure (33258 Hoechst plus netropsin; Fig. 5, Table V; Sahar and Latt, 1980) or DAPI plus distamycin A (Schweizer et al., 1978; Schweizer, 1981) can further highlight certain polymorphisms, presumably by sequence-specific dye-binding competition.

A totally different approach for accentuating chromosome regions, according to their time of replication during S phase, utilizes BrdU incorporation during early or late S and 33258 Hoechst $\pm$ Giemsa staining (Latt, 1973, 1978) (Table V). Late-replication banding is particularly useful in examining the X, satellite DNA-containing secondary constrictions of #1, #9, and #16 (Fig. 6), and specific autosomal bands, such as those of 4q, 5p, and 13q (Latt, 1975). BrdU–dye methods depend on appropriate protocols of BrdU administration to cells prior to harvest (Table VI; Latt, 1976, 1978).

Additional staining procedures can assist the study of more limited chromosomal regions (Gagne and Laberge, 1972; Schnedl, 1978). Silver staining (Goodpasture and Bloom, 1975; Goodpasture et al., 1976) can be used to delineate 18S and 28S rDNA regions that are functionally active (Miller et al., 1976a,b). Immunofluorescent methods using antibodies (e.g., against 5-methylocytosine (Schreck et al., 1977) can highlight regions of #9, #15, #16, and the Y (Miller et al., 1974; Schnedl et al., 1975), which are also positive with 33258 Hoechst plus netropsin or DAPI plus distamycin A (Schweizer et al., 1978; Sahar and Latt, 1980).

Another class of cytogenetic methods addresses structural changes in chromosomes. Chromosome-breakage analysis can employ either nonspecific Giemsa or related staining, in which chromosome integrity can be determined but chromosome identification is unclear. Alternatively, banding stains can reveal aberrations (e.g., inversions, translocations), which might not change morphology. However, structural changes at telomeres may go unnoticed. Chromosome-breakage analysis has been employed for the prenatal diagnosis of Fanconi's

---

FIG. 3 (*opposite*). This karyotype is from a normal 46,XY male fetus. Cells were grown as a monolayer in a T-flask, harvested by trypsinization, processed by the Giemsa-trypsin banding procedure, and photographed as described in the text (Table II).

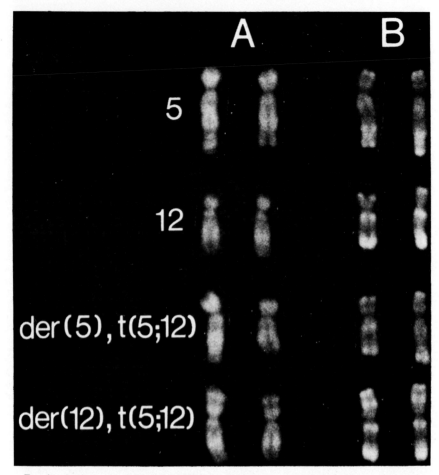

FIG. 4. Analysis of a reciprocal translocation by chromomycin A_3-methyl green fluorescence. This cell is from a fetus who had a parent with a reciprocal t(5q;12p) translocation. The chromosomes shown were stained with chromomycin A_3 plus methyl green as described in Table III. The translocation chromosomes (second and fourth columns) are apparent. The fetus had the translocation in a balanced form and was born phenotypically normal.

anemia (Auerbach *et al.*, 1979). More sensitive detection of chromosome fragility or the impact of mutagen-carcinogens on chromosomes is often possible with sister chromatid-exchange (SCE) analysis (Latt, 1974a,b; Perry and Evans, 1975; Wolff, 1977; Latt *et al.*, 1979b). Detection of SCEs requires halogenated nucleoside (e.g., BrdU) incorporation for at least the penultimate preharvest replication cycle. SCEs are markedly elevated in Bloom syndrome (Chaganti *et al.*, 1974), and SCE analysis may prove useful for prenatal diagnosis of fetuses at risk for this condition (Fig. 7).

TABLE III

CHROMOMYCIN A₃ PLUS METHYL GREEN REVERSE-FLUORESCENCE BANDING[a] —CHROMOMYCIN
A₃ STAINING[b]

1. Prepare chromomycin A₃ solution (0.5 mg/ml in 0.14 M phosphate buffer, 5×10^{-4} M Mg^{2+}) pH 6.8; cool to 0°C (ice bath) while mixing to dissolve. The chromomycin A₃ solution, kept at 4°C in the dark, is stable for at least 1 week.
2. To stain, cover the slide or coverslip surface with approximately four drops of dye solution and add a coverslip (stain for 20 minutes).
3. Rinse slides twice with pH 6.8 buffer (1 minute each time).
4. Slides stained with chromomycin A₃ can be stored for several days.

METHYL GREEN OVERSTAIN[a]

1. Prepare solution of methyl green (dye purified by thin-layer chromatography is optimal) 0.34 mg/ml in 0.01 M sodium acetate–0.01 M NaCl (pH 4.2). The optical density of this solution should be approximately 16 at 630 nm. This solution is stable for approximately a week when protected from light.
2. Just before using, dilute the stock methyl green 1:1 with 0.1 M NaCl–0.1 M HEPES (pH 7.0).
3. Flood the slides with the pH 7.0 methyl green solution and stain for 4 minutes.
4. Shake off the stain and wash with glycerin.
5. Mount in glycerin.
6. Use the same microscope settings as employed for quinacrine: 495-nm dichroic mirror (excitation primarily with 435-nm Hg line) and 510-nm barrier filter.

[a] From Sahar and Lalt (1978).
[b] From Jorgenson *et al.* (1978) and Van de Sande *et al.* (1977).

TABLE IV

C-BANDING[a]

1. Dry slides on a slide warmer at 50°C.
2. Heat distilled water, 5% BaOH,[b] and 2 × SSC (0.30 M NaCl–0.03 M sodium citrate, pH 7) to 60°C.
3. Soak slides in 0.2 M HCl (1 hour) and then rinse with distilled water.
4. Dip slides in a hot 1% Ba(OH)₂ solution[b] (50°C) for 15–20 seconds (exact time variable), and rinse vigorously in two changes of distilled H₂O (60°C).
5. Incubate slides in 2 × SSC at 60°C for 1 hour.
6. Rinse thoroughly with distilled water.
7. Stain with Gurr's Giemsa (2–4%) in pH 6.8 buffer.
8. Rinse with water.

[a] From Sumner (1972).
[b] Use a 5% Ba(OH)₂ stock solution, in H₂O, heated to 60°C. Just before use, dilute this 5% solution to 1% Ba(OH)₂ with H₂O (60°C), and cool to 50°C.

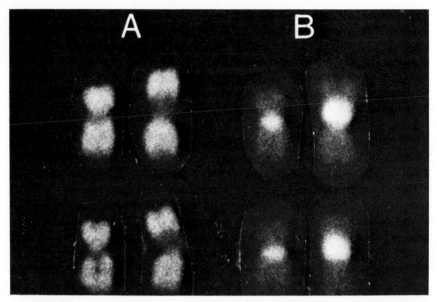

Fig. 5. The use of 33258 Hoechst plus netropsin to detect a pericentric inversion of chromosome #9. Amniotic fluid cells were grown as a monolayer and trypsinized during harvest. The chromosomes shown were stained with quinacrine (Table I) or with 33258 Hoechst, followed by 10^{-5} *M* netropsin (placed directly on the slide prior to photography) (Table V). The inv(9) is shown to the right of its homologue.

In experiments with animal model systems, SCE analysis has been used to detect transplacental exposure of fetal tissue to clastogens (Kram *et al.*, 1979). The applicability of this approach to examining human fetal exposure (e.g., via parental contact with environmental mutagens) is less clear, primarily because of the brief duration ($\leq$ 1 week) of the SCE elevation following exposure (Stetka and Wolff, 1976; Nevstad, 1978).

A number of new developments in the delineation of cytogenetic abnormalities may ultimately find application in prenatal diagnosis. These include the detection of very small chromosome deletions as well as the characterization of chromosome sites with an increased frequency of breakage (i.e., fragile sites).

Small deletions in chromosome #11 or #13 have been associated with increased risk for Wilm's tumor and aniridia (Riccardi *et al.*, 1978; Kolota, 1980a) or retinoblastoma (Knudson *et al.*, 1976; Kolota, 1980b). Other deletions may underlie conditions presenting with morphological abnormalities (Sanchez and Yunis, 1977).

Detection of deletions smaller than a standard metaphase chromosome band typically require special techniques for preparing highly extended chromosomes. Yunis (Yunis, 1976; Yunis *et al.*, 1978, 1979; Francke and Oliver, 1978) has

TABLE V

33258 HOECHST STAINING (FOR LATE-REPLICATION BANDING, SISTER CHROMATID-EXCHANGE ANALYSIS, AND TWO-DYE PROCEDURES)[a]

Primary staining
1. Soak slides in 0.14 M NaCl–0.004 M KCl–0.1 M phosphate buffer, pH 7.0 (PBS) for 5 minutes.
2. Stain for 10 minutes in 0.5 μg/ml 33258 Hoechst in PBS. Use 33258 Hoechst that has been freshly diluted from a 50-μg/ml solution in H_2O.
3. Rinse slide for 1 minute in PBS.
4. Rinse for 5 minutes in a second change of PBS.
5. Rinse with distilled water.

Fluorescence microscopy (for chromosomes from cells pulsed with BrdU/dT for late-replication banding)
1. Mount slide in pH 7.0–7.5 buffer—e.g., McIlvaine's citrate-phosphate buffer (0.01–0.02 M citrate, 0.16–0.18 M phosphate).
2. Excite with UG-1/TK400 dichroic mirror combination and view fluorescence through a 460-nm barrier filter.
Note: Chromosome fluorescence fades rapidly, but contrast is good. Fluorescence microscopy may also prove of use in monitoring BrdU incorporation, if troubleshooting of fluorescence plus Giemsa staining is necessary.

Fluorescence microscopy (for 33258 Hoechst plus netropsin procedure)[b]
1. Cover slide, previously stained with 33258 Hoechst, with approximately 1 ml of a 10^{-5} M solution of netropsin* in pH 7.5 McIlvaine's buffer (1–5 minutes).
2. Remove excess buffer and mount the slide in 1:1 pH 7.5 buffer: glycerin or pH 7.5 buffer.
3. Observe as mentioned before; reduce exposure to netropsin if suppression of 33258 Hoechst fluorescence is too great.

Fluorescence plus Giemsa staining (for SCE analysis)[c]
1. Follow the 33258 Hoechst primary staining procedure given already.
2. Place specimens on slides, cell side up, in a 4 × 4-in. clear plastic petri dish.
3. Cover each slide with a mixture of (one volume of PBS and two volumes of a 75 μg/ml solution of 33258 Hoechst in H_2O). Put a 24 × 50-mm coverslip on each slide.
4. Place the cover on the petri dish.
5. Expose the dish to a 20-watt fluorescent light, 3–4 in. from the surface of the dish, for 6–10 hours.
6. Rinse the coverslips off the slide under warm running tap water. Do not try to pry the coverslip off.
7. Place the slides in prewarmed (60–65°C) 2 × SSC for 15 minutes.
8. Rinse the slides well in running distilled water.
9. Stain in 4% Giemsa (7 minutes).

---

[a] From Latt (1973; in press).
[b] From Sahar and Latt (1980).
[c] Adapted from Perry and Wolff (1974).
*Distamycin A (4.2 × 10^{-6} M) can be substituted for netropsin at this step (Schreck et al., unpublished data).

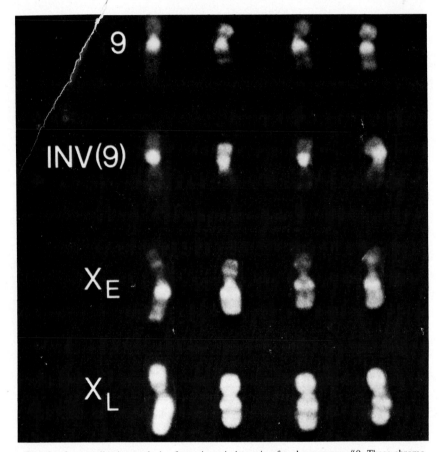

Fig. 6.   Late-replication analysis of a pericentric inversion for chromosome #9. These chromosomes are from amniotic fluid cells that were cultured in EMB (Eagle's Medium B) plus 15% fetal
bovine serum on coverslips, exposed to 10^{-4} M BrdU for 16 hours and then fresh medium containing
1.5×10^{-5} M dT for 7.5 hours. Colcemide, 0.25 μg/ml, was added 1 hour before harvest. The slides
were stained with 33258 Hoechst and analyzed by fluorescence microscopy (see Table V). Each
column in this figure contains #9 and X chromosomes from a single cell. The inv(9) (second row) is
apparent by the altered position of its late-replicating secondary constriction. The late X (bottom row)
is clearly distinguished from its homologue.

developed appropriate methodology, in which cells are blocked near the beginning of S phase with amethopterin, and then harvested at specific times (e.g.,
sufficient to reach prometaphase) after release from the block. Adaptation of this
approach to amniotic fluid cultures has been reported (Vogel *et al.*, 1978).

Recently, a form of X-linked mental retardation has been shown to be associated with a structural discontinuity near the terminus of the long arm of the X
(Howard-Peebles and Stoddard, 1979; Sutherland, 1979b). Though the

TABLE VI

BrdU Incorporation Protocols for Late-Replication Banding and SCE Analysis
(Amniotic Fluid Cells)

Late-replication banding
A. Highlight late-replicating regions.
1. Add 10^{-4} *M* BrdU to cells (16 hours is satisfactory for material cultured in EMB or Ham's F-10 plus 15% fetal bovine serum).
2. Change to medium without BrdU, add 1.5×10^{-5} *M* dT to fresh medium.
3. 6.5 hours later add colcemide (0.2 μg/ml).
4. Harvest for chromosome analysis 1 hour later.
B. Highlight early-replicating regions.
1. Add 10^{-4} *M* BrdU to cultures 6–7 hours before addition of colcemide.
2. Proceed as in steps 3, 4 under A. (e.g., 7.5 hours total terminal pulse time).[a]

SCE Analysis
1. Day 1: Initiate cultures with 3×10^5 cells per P-100 petri dish (proportionately fewer with a smaller container) in medium (e.g., Ham's F-10) plus serum (e.g., 15% fetal bovine serum).
2. Day 2: Change to fresh medium, add BrdU to 2.5×10^{-5} *M* dC to 10^{-4} *M*. From this point on, cells should be protected from light less than 350 nm.
3. Day 4: Add colcemide (0.45 μg/ml) 48 hours after addition of BrdU. Harvest 3–4 hours later.

[a] The exact time might be modified, depending on cell growth rate.

mechanism of this "fragility" is unknown, it might somehow involve folate metabolism, because the incidence of X-chromosome breakage is suppressed by exogenous thymidine and enhanced by addition of folate antagonists to cultures (Sutherland, 1979a). It is thus not surprising that subtle details of the culture medium composition (Sutherland, 1977; Keck and Emerit, 1979; Tommerup *et al.*, 1981) (e.g., pyrimidine content, dialyzable serum components) can influence the detection of this condition. Thus far, this methodology has been most successfully used with peripheral blood cultures (Sutherland, 1979b), although methods for its application to amniotic fluid cell culture have recently been published (Jenkins *et al.*, 1981; Shapiro *et al.*, 1982).

Small chromosomal fragments are occasionally seen in amniotic fluid cultures. Most are difficult to identify, whereas others can be assigned to segments of particular morphology, for which empirical clinical information on previous cases exists (Bernstein *et al.*, 1978; Brøndum-Nielsen *et al.*, 1978; Ramos *et al.*, 1979; Stetten *et al.*, 1981). In one condition, the "cat eye syndrome," variable numbers of unidentified chromosome fragments occur (Hsu and Hirschhorn, 1977). The importance of variations in the frequency of cells with fragments is not yet clear. One might anticipate that new approaches, (e.g., isolation of small chromosomes by centrifugation; Kaufman *et al.*, 1979), followed by analysis using recombinant DNA techniques, could permit clarification of the nature and significance of these fragments.

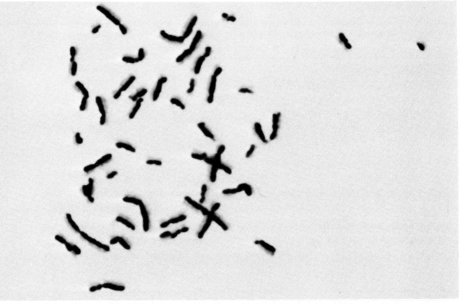

FIG. 7.   This metaphase is from a fetus whose parents' previous child had Bloom's syndrome. The cells were exposed to BrdU for 2 days (Table VI), and subjected to the 33258 Hoechst plus light plus Giemsa method (Table VI) for sister chromatid differentiation. This cell exhibits 9 SCEs, and the average for this fetus was 8 SCEs/cell (interpreted as normal). Fibroblasts from the previous sib exhibited an average of 53 SCEs/cell, compared with an average of 9 SCEs/cell for control fibroblasts.

IV.   Practical Problems in Amniotic Fluid Cytogenetic Studies

A.   Maternal Cell Contamination

Because transabdominal acquisition of an amniotic fluid sample can result in inclusion of maternal tissue, it is not surprising that maternal cells occasionally grow and are erroneously analyzed in "amniotic fluid" cultures. The frequency with which this occurs, estimated as twice the frequency of male fetuses erroneously identified as female prenatally (contamination of female cultures will typically be missed), is in the vicinity of 2 to 3 per 1000 (NICHD, 1976; Simpson *et al.*, 1976). Because, on the average, 1 in 50 of amniocenteses done for cytogenetic indications will involve a cytogenetically abnormal fetus (NICHD, 1976), maternal cell contamination could, in principle, result in one missed cytogenetic abnormality per 10,000–20,000 amniocenteses.

Comparison of parental chromosomal polymorphisms with those of the putative fetal cells, including examination of interphase nuclei for quinacrine–bright

Y chromatin, should permit identification of any maternal cells (Peakman *et al.*, 1977). At present, however, this is not practical to carry out on all cases with a 46,XX karyotype, and it is reserved for cases in which additional reasons for suspecting maternal contamination exist. Examples of such conditions include the extraordinarily rapid (< 10 days) outgrowth of a very large colony of 46,XX cells and observation of both 46,XX and non-46,XX (i.e., 45,X; 46,XY) cells, or 46,XX cells with different polymorphisms, in material derived from the same amniotic fluid sample. Routine use of multiple culture dishes can be highly informative, to the extent that maternal cell outgrowth is sporadic, as can hormone analyses (FSH, testosterone; Mennuti *et al.*, 1977) on amniotic fluid. Measurement of the latter might prove a cost-effective standard strategy for avoiding half of all inaccurate diagnoses due to maternal cell contamination. Another approach for identifying cell parentage, histocompatibility antigen testing (Niazi *et al.*, 1979), might ultimately prove practical, especially as improved immunological reagents become available and histocompatibility typing for other reasons (e.g., specific disease susceptibility; Rosenberg and Kidd, 1977) becomes more widespread.

B. Cytogenetic Findings of Questionable Significance

Unusual C-band or quinacrine–bright staining is typically attributed to polymorphisms, which are of negligible clinical significance (McKenzie and Lubs, 1975; Geraedts and Pearson, 1975; Buckton *et al.*, 1976; Magenis *et al.*, 1977; Matsuura *et al.*, 1978). When such adventitious findings occur in peripheral blood cultures, their significance can often be determined by examination of the patient. An analogous examination is not possible when an amniotic fluid sample is involved. Fortunately, one can usually obtain parental blood samples and, because inheritance of neutral chromosomal markers is straightforward, identify the heteromorphic marker in metaphase from one of the parents (Robinson *et al.*, 1976; Peakman *et al.*, 1977; Magenis *et al.*, 1977; Mayer *et al.*, 1978). In such studies, special staining techniques (e.g., involving dye pairs—Sahar and Latt, 1978, 1980; Latt *et al.*, 1979a, 1980) can often improve the sensitivity with which such polymorphisms can be detected.

Increased incidence of chromosomal breakage may be more difficult to interpret. Although baseline levels of chromosome aberrations are typically low (≤ 0.05 per cell) (Simoni *et al.*, 1979), the number of cells (≤ 100) suitable for analysis in most amniotic fluid cultures is not sufficient to detect with confidence any but markedly elevated breakage levels (e.g., ≥ 0.10–0.15 per cell). When chromosome breakage occurs throughout the genome, some type of infectious agent might be involved (e.g., Nichols, 1974). Though this is typically difficult to identify, it probably would not be evident in repeat cultures and it might not occur in duplicate cultures from the initial amniocentesis. Alternatively, if breakage, without any particular chromosome location, were consistently observed, a chromosome-fragility disease (German, 1972) might be suspected, and appropriate family historical information, together with special tests described in the previous section, might be considered. Another potential cause of chromosome breakage is maternal exposure to a chemical carcinogen or to high-energy radiation (Kram and Schneider, 1978). However, there is not yet an appropriate data base to permit evaluation of the contribution of this exposure route to fetal chromosomal abnormalities. Finally, in analogy with other data, breakage might be restricted to certain chromosomal loci, such as the previously mentioned, the structural discontinuity on the long arm of the X, associated with mental retardation (Sutherland, 1979a,b; Howard-Peebles *et al.*, 1979). Aberrations restricted to chromosome #17 have been associated with exposure to adenovirus-12 (McDougall, 1971), whereas breakage in the long arm of chromosome #16 corresponds to a heritable, clinically insignificant condition—manifest thus far only in lymphocytes (Magenis *et al.*, 1970). Hecht and McCaw (1979) have recently reviewed data on fragile sites in chromosomes.

C. *De Novo* Translocation

Approximately 2 in 1000 liveborns possess a *de novo* reciprocal translocation, that is, the parental karyotypes are apparently normal. For unknown reasons, *de novo* (but not transmitted) non-Robertsonian translocations appear to confer an increased risk for mental and physical abnormalities (Funderburk *et al.*, 1977; Aurias *et al.*, 1978; Evans *et al.*, 1978). The evidence for this derives from retrospective studies of malformed and/or mentally retarded individuals, a group with an approximately 5-fold increase in *de novo* translocations compared with the population as a whole. It is not known whether this reflects selection bias, an effect on genetic expression at the site of translocation, subtle nonreciprocity, an environmental insult causing many things in addition to the translocation, or a totally different reason. Very recently, it has been observed that an unusually high proportion of these *de novo* rearrangements seem to be of paternal origin (Chamberlin and Magenis, 1980).

In all cases in which the fetus shows a balanced translocation, analysis of parental karyotypes (including a check on polymorphisms) seems indicated. Management of those cases with normal parental karyotypes may prove very difficult. This is fortunately a rare occurrence, about which more must be learned.

D. Mosaicism

Chromosomal mosaicism is generally defined as the occurrence of an identical chromosome abnormality in a portion of cultured amniotic fluid cells from two or more culture vessels.

Pseudomosaicism, on the other hand, is defined as the observation of single or multiple cells found in only one culture vessel, and only cells with a normal karyotype or with different chromosomal variants in other cultures. If cells are grown as primary colonies, the word "entire colony" can be substituted for "cell" in the previous sentence (Boué *et al.*, 1979; L. Hsu, unpublished data; Golbus *et al.*, 1979; Peakman *et al.*, 1979).

The question of mosaicism is perhaps the most frequent and perplexing problem in prenatal cytogenetic diagnosis. The occurrence of more than one fetal karyotype in multiple cells is found in 2–3% of all amniocenteses (Kardon *et al.*, 1972; Bloom *et al.*, 1974; Kohn *et al.*, 1975; Sutherland *et al.*, 1975; Laurence and Gregory, 1976; Hoehn *et al.*, 1978; Hsu *et al.*, 1978). However, the frequency of truly mosaic fetuses, as evidenced by subsequent prenatal studies and/or corroborated postnatally, is perhaps only one-tenth this figure (see previous references). Thus differentiation of true mosaicism from pseudomosaicism is critical.

An initial, consensus criterion for considering a possibility of mosaicism is the observation of the same minority cell type in at least two separate cultures. In practice, at least one of these cultures would contain more than one cell with the second karyotype. The rationale for this addendum is unclear. Throughout, the small number of fetal cells actually sampled ($\leq$ 5–10 colony-forming cells per milliliter of amniotic fluid) reinforces the suspicion that even trace evidence of mosaicism must be given note, that true mosaicism may sometimes be missed, and, if mosaicism is suspected, that the frequency of an unusual karyotype in amniotic cell culture may not reflect its frequency in the fetus.

A natural strategy for dealing with the statistics and differentiation of mosaicism is the use of multiple culture dishes, in each of which multiple primary colonies are examined *in situ*, on coverslips. This approach provides an explicit indication of the number of original fetal cells actually sampled. Perhaps of greater significance, as stressed by Peakman *et al.*, (1979), comparison of cells all presumably belonging to the same colony can usually detect events occurring during culture. In fact, nonuniformity of the karyotype within a colony is the most useful indication of pseudo-, culture-derived mosaicism. Two variants of this situation that still leave uncertainty in interpretation are the observation of just one colony with all cells containing the same abnormality and two colonies, in separate dishes, containing some but not all cells with the same abnormal karyotype. Repeat amniocentesis is sometimes suggested, and the additional data obtained can modify the predictive odds quantitatively. However, a repeat amniocentesis rarely *removes entirely* the mosaicism question.

Additional factors useful in interpreting data on mosaicism are the relative frequencies with which a specific karyotypic abnormality is observed in true or pseudo fetal mosaicism, or in viable, malformed liveborns. That is, chromosomal analysis—like any other laboratory test—especially modifies preexisting odds (Casscells *et al.*, 1978), and the estimate of ultimate interest is the probability that the fetus will give rise to a viable, malformed infant. Detailed tabulations of mosaicism, actually observed in amniotic fluid cultures, have been given by Milunsky (1979). Of particular note is that nearly one-third of all apparent amniotic fluid mosaicism involves trisomy 2 (Fig. 8) (Peakman *et al.*, 1979), which has thus far not been detected in a viable newborn (Borgaonkar and Lillard, 1978). Thus, subject to the disclaimer that one is facing the first, poten-

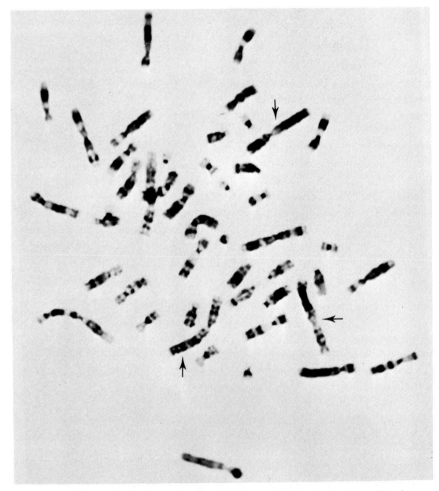

FIG. 8.   A trisomy 2 metaphase cell. This Giemsa–trypsin stained metaphase cell is from an amniotic fluid culture that was predominantly 46,XY, but 3 out of 19 cells were 47,XY,+2, like the one shown. Arrows point to the #2 chromosomes. Thirteen cells from another monolayer culture and 44 cells from six colonies from three other cultures were 46,XY. The overall diagnostic impression was that of pseudomosaicism, the pregnancy was continued, and the child born was phenotypically normal.

tially disastrous, viable mosaicism for trisomy #2, interventive action on trisomy 2 mosaicism is probably not indicated. A similar statement could probably be made for many other autosomal mosaicisms, especially of the larger chromosomes, although current tabulations of observed cytogenetic abnormalities must still be checked (Boué et al., 1976, 1979; Rodriguez et al., 1978; Kardon et al., 1979; Nevin et al., 1979).

Another common mosaicism, trisomy 20 (Fig. 9), poses a converse problem. Mosaicism of trisomy 20 has been observed in both grossly normal and subtly malformed infants (Carbonell et al., 1977; Boué et al., 1979; Mascarello et al.,

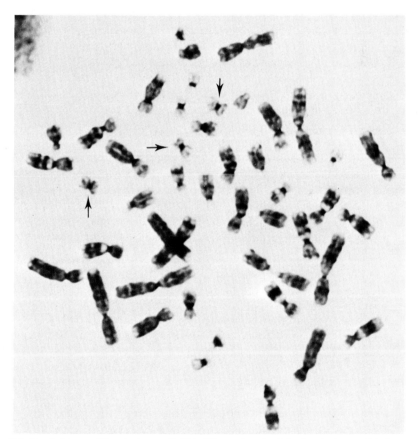

Fig. 9. A trisomy 20 metaphase cell. This Giemsa–trypsin stained metaphase cell is from an amniotic fluid culture that was analyzed as 46,XY/47,XY,+20. Arrows point to the #20 chromosomes. Two colonies were entirely 47,XY,+20, another contained six out of seven cells with an extra #20, and cells from the fourth colony all had two #20s. Twenty-one cells from eight colonies in four other cultures had only two #20s. The mosaicism status of the fetus was considered uncertain; pregnancy termination was elected. Pretermination repeat amniocentesis again revealed some trisomy 20 cells (3 out of 85); attempts to culture abortus tissue were unsuccessful.

1980). Boué *et al.* (1979) have hypothesized that the major source of amniotic fluid trisomy 20 cells is fetal kidney, accounting perhaps for limited physical findings and suggesting the need to attempt culture of fetal kidney if a pregnancy is terminated. A related problem is posed by mosaicism involving X or Y chromosomes (Hsu *et al.*, 1976; Simpson, 1978), for which evaluation of the significance is often a highly subjective, personal matter. The role of a cytogenetics laboratory in such a situation is primarily the provision of data to permit accurate assessment of the various risks. Another question, of some fundamental interest, is whether or not certain chromosomal abnormalities tend to occur primarily on fetal membranes (Cox *et al.*, 1974; Kardon *et al.*, 1979) or arise preferentially during *in vitro* culture of amniotic fluid cells.

Perhaps the major difficulty occurs when the question of mosaicism involves chromosomes #13, #18, or #21, which are those most frequently found in viable, severely malformed newborns (Hook and Hamerton, 1976). In cases involving these chromosomes, the prior odds (that such mosaicism is both viable and significant) are relatively high, and, even with strong negative laboratory data, the final risk to the patient may be uncomfortably high. Possible mosaicism involving these chromosomes probably calls for the development of additional tests (e.g., of DNA content) on multiple amniotic fluid cells, using either flow cytometry or molecular probe studies using sequences specific for individual chromosomes (see chapter by Kurnit *et al.*). Careful tabulation and reporting of laboratory data as well as follow-up information on liveborns, in questions of mosaicism, are needed to provide a better data base for making more accurate risk estimates. One problem related to this goal is the technical difficulty typically observed in confirming the diagnosis of mosaicism following termination of gestation.

E.   Tetraploidy

Tetraploidy is often observed in amniotic fluid cultures (Milunsky, 1979). However, this situation probably reflects artifacts arising during tissue culture and is not typically associated with abnormal live births.

V.   Additional Considerations

A.   Mycoplasma Contamination

Contamination of cell cultures by bacteria, fungal organisms, or mycoplasma is a problem confronted by all tissue culture laboratories. Antibiotics added in small quantity to the initiation of the cultures aids in controlling bacteria, yeast, and other fungal organisms. Contamination by one of these is usually visible by a change in pH or the appearance of cloudiness/opaqueness of the media. Mycoplasma contamination, by contrast, is not always detectable macroscopically. It should be suspected if cell growth abruptly stops or if chromosome breakage is unusually high (Stanbridge, 1971; Kenny, 1973; Schneider et al., 1973). Possible sources of mycoplasma include serum (bovine), trypsin (porcine), clinical samples, or laboratory personnel (human) (Barile et al., 1973). This last contribution can be minimized by avoidance of mouth pipetting (McGarrity, 1976). It is often possible to obtain serum and trypsin that have been prescreened by the supplier, and the serum can be irradiated, in attempts to reduce further the risk of mycoplasma infection. The presence of mycoplasma can be examined by culturing, determination of the ratio (Hayflick, 1965) of ^{3}HUdR to ^{3}HU incorporated into RNA (Schneider et al., 1974a,b), which is decreased in cultures contaminated by mycoplasma. or by immunofluorescence (Kenny, 1973). One in situ method, using A-T specific fluorochromes, is highly sensitive, rapid, and more easily utilized on a routine basis for checking of cell cultures for mycoplasma (Russell et al., 1975; Chen, 1977). Contaminated cultures when fixed and stained with Hoechst 33258 or DAPI reveal small brightly fluorescent bodies surrounding cell nuclei. Cells from uncontaminated control cultures are clear of these bodies. If mycoplasma infection is detected, all likely sources should be removed, incubators emptied and cleaned, and new cultures segregated until absence of the mycoplasma is established.

B. Repeat Samples

Repeat samples may be justified by a number of circumstances. (1) Cell growth is inadequate after 10–14 days of culture; (2) maternal cell contamination is suspected, parental chromosomes are examined, and maternal and putative fetal polymorphic markers are found to be indistinguishable; (3) amniotic fluid AFP is elevated; a repeat amniocentesis for AFP analysis and/or amnioscopy may be indicated; or (4) equipment failure or culture contamination has occurred. This category should obviously be minimized.

Whenever a repeat amniocentesis is considered, attention must be given to the gestational age of the fetus and the associated possibility of obtaining an answer before the legal time limit for a decision to intervene in a pregnancy. Repeat samples are given priority in processing.

C. Follow-Up

Each case is followed through delivery and/or termination. Physicians managing a particular case are requested to provide the laboratory with the date of birth, weight, and sex of the child, as well as any unusual clinical findings noted at birth. If prenatal diagnostic studies indicated or raised the question of pseudomosaicism or true mosaicism, a blood sample after birth is requested to confirm the prenatal data. Similarly, prenatal diagnosis of a chromosomally abnormal fetus necessitates careful, sensitive communication between the laboratory, the referring physicians, and the parents. Help in arranging genetic counseling services is offered the parents. If the pregnancy is to be terminated, both a preabortion amniotic fluid sample and a tissue sample from the abortus are requested, to confirm the diagnosis. It is further advisable to obtain a thorough pathology report. Information thus obtained may be of use both to the referring physician and to the counseling service.

D.   Backup Laboratory

Any laboratory established to provide prenatal diagnosis should have at least one other laboratory willing and able to serve, in an emergency, as a backup facility. Situations falling into the category of "emergency" include technical failure, widespread contamination of cultures, or an extreme overload of cases within a short period of time. Larger institutions might have separate units, distinct from the primary unit, to accommodate this provision. Smaller laboratories will typically depend on outside units. The numbers of samples that can be handled by each unit, the method of sample transport, and the length of the interval during which emergency help can be expected, must be understood clearly by all laboratories involved.

VI.   Future Prospects

A.   Cytology

The major question to be answered in evaluating a cytological preparation of amniotic fluid cells is whether or not a sporadic abnormality is real or artifactual. A related question is whether all contents of a metaphase cell derive from the same cell or whether an "extra" chromosome is actually from another cell. Improved methods of slide preparation should reduce the occurrence of this problem. Sometimes the answer is apparent by comparing the state of chromosome contraction or by examining nearby metaphases. Additional cell-specific "signatures" would be very useful.

Additional information regarding mosaicism might in principle be obtained from the metaphase chromosomes themselves. For example, it might eventually be possible to employ *in situ* hybridization, if appropriate chromosome-specific DNA sequences become available. Additional estimates of the chromosomal content of interphase nuclei, beyond analysis of Barr bodies or Y bodies, would have an analogous use, especially because most cells available are in interphase rather than at metaphase.

B. Flow Cytometry

Flow cytometry offers the opportunity to examine many cells or chromosomes. If biochemical information is necessary, the cells need not be fixed. Resolution of DNA analysis on intact cells is often certainly not sufficient to permit detection of specific aneuploidy (Callis and Hoehn, 1976). However, considerable effort is currently being directed toward obtaining flow karyotypes of isolated metaphase chromosomes (Gray et al., 1975; Carrano et al., 1976, 1979). Though admittedly associated with technical difficulties, this method may prove very useful in quantitating specific mosaicism.

C. DNA Studies

Because the primary goal of chromosome analysis is evaluation of the fetal genotype, the ultimate methodology would seem to be at the DNA level. This could be done in conjunction with specific gene or linkage analyses (see chapter by Kurnit et al.). Both chromosome-specific DNA sequences and a means of quantitating these sequences would be required. Given the rapid progress of gene cloning, restriction-enzyme DNA digestion, and hybridization methods, development of simple, reliable, inexpensive tests of this type might not be an unattainable goal. Recently described methodology for transcervical acquisition of fetal cells from chorionic villi (Rhine and Milunsky, 1978; Williamson et al., 1981) may permit analysis of fetal sex and DNA studies during the first trimester of pregnancy. This approach, the safety of which will require additional evaluation, may prove useful in specific circumstances.

ACKNOWLEDGMENTS

Data presented in this chapter utilized procedures developed with the support of research grants from the National Institutes of Health (GM 21121), the American Cancer Society (CD-36F), and the National Foundation March of Dimes (1-353).

REFERENCES

Arrighi, F. E., and Hsu, T. C. (1971). *Cytogenetics* **10**, 81–86.
Auerbach, A. D., Warburton, D., Bloom, A. D., and Chaganti, R. S. K. (1979). *Am. J. Hum. Genet.* **31**, 77–81.

Aurias, A., Prieur, M., Dutrillaux, B., and Lejeune, J. (1978). *Hum. Genet.* **45**, 259–282.

Barile, M. F., Hopps, H. E., Grabowski, M. W., Riggs, D. B., and Del Guidice. (1973). *Ann. N.Y. Acad. Sci.* **225**, 251–264.

Bernstein, R., Hakim, C., Hardwick, B., and Nurse, G. T. (1978). *J. Med. Genet.* **15**, 136–142.

Bloom, A. D., Schmickel, R., Barr, M., and Burdi, A. R. (1974). *J. Pediatr.* **84**(5), 732–733.

Borgaonkar, D. S., and Lillard, D. R. (1978). "Repository of Chromosomal Variants and Anomalies in Man," Fifth listing, Genetics Center, Dept. of Biol. Sci., North Texas State University, Denton, Texas.

Botstein, D., White, R. L., Skolnick, M., and Davis, R. W. (1980). *Am. J. Hum. Genet.* **32**, 314–331.

Boué, J., Boué, A., and Lazar, P. (1975). *Teratology* **12**, 11–26.

Boué, J., Daketse, M. J., Deluchat, C., Ravise, N., Yvert, F., and Boué, A. (1976). *Ann. Genet. (Paris)* **19**(4), 233–239.

Boué, J., Nicolas, H., Barichard, F., and Boué, A. (1979). *Ann. Genet. (Paris)* **22**(1), 3–9.

Brøndum-Nielsen, K., Dyggve, H., Friedrich, U., Hobolth, N., Lyngbye, T., and Mikkelsen, M. (1978). *Hum. Genet.* **44**, 59–69.

Bruns, G. A. P., Gusella, G. T., Kerp, C., Housman, D., and Gerald, P. S. (1981). *Pediatr. Res.* **15**, 559.

Buckton, K. E., O'Riordan, M. L., Jacobs, P. A., Robinson, J. A., Hill, R., and Evans, H. J. (1976). *Ann. Hum. Genet.* **40**, 99–112.

Callis, J., and Hoehn, H. (1976). *Amer. J. Hum. Genet.* **28**, 557–584.

Carbonell, X., Caballin, M. R., Rubio, A., and Egozcue, J. (1977). *Acta Paediatr. Scand.* **66**, 787–788.

Carr, D. H., and Gedeon, M. (1978). *Can. J. Genet. Cytol.* **20**, 415–425.

Carrano, A. V., Gray, J. W., Moore, D. H., II, Minkler, J. L., Mayall, B. H., Van Dilla, M. H., and Mendelsohn, M. L. (1976). *J. Histochem. Cytochem.* **24**, 348–354.

Carrano, A. V., Gray, J. W., Langlois, R. J., Burkhart-Schultz, K. J., and Van Dilla, M. A. (1979). *Proc. Natl. Acad. Sci. U.S.A.* **76**, 1382–1384.

Caspersson, T., Zach, L., Johansson, C., and Modest, E. J. (1970). *Chromosoma* **20**, 215–227.

Caspersson, T., Lomakka, G., and Zech, L. (1971). *Hereditas* **67**, 89–102.

Caspersson, T., Lindsten, J., Lomakka, G., Moller, A., and Zech, L. (1972). *Int. Rev. Cytol.* **11**, 1–72.

Casscells, W., Schoenberger, A., and Graboys, T. I. B. (1978). *N. Engl. J. Med.* **299**, 999–1001.

Chaganti, R. S. K., Schonberg, S., and German, J. (1974). *Proc. Natl. Acad. Sci. U.S.A.* **71**, 4508–4512.

Chamberlin, J., and Magenis, R. E. (1980). *Hum. Genet.* **53**, 343–347.

Chen, T. R. (1977). *Exp. Cell Res.* **104**, 255–262.

Cox, D. M., Niewczas-Late, V., Riffell, M. I., and Hamerton, J. L. (1974). *Pediatr. Res.* **8**, 679–683.

Czaker, R. (1973). *Humangenetik* **19**, 135–144.

Davies, K. E. (1981). *Human Genet.* **58**, 351–357.

Davies, K. E., Young, B. P., Elles, R. G., Hill, M. E., and Williamson, R. (1981). *Nature* **293**, 374–376.

Dutrillaux, B., and LeJeune, J. (1971). *C. R. Acad. Sci. [D] (Paris)* **272**, 2638–2640.

Dutrillaux, B., and LeJeune, J. (1975). *In* "Advanced Human Genetics" (H. Harris and K. Hirschhorn, eds.), Vol. 5, pp. 119–156. Plenum, New York.

Evans, J. A., Canning, N., Hunter, A. G. W., Martsolf, I. T., Ray, M., Thompson, D. R., and Hamerton, J. L. (1978). *Cytogenet. Cell Genet.* **20**, 96–123.

Felix, J. S., and Doherty, R. A. (1979). *Clin. Genet.* **15**, 215–220.

Fisher, N. L., Starr, E. D., Greene, T., and Hoehn, H. (1980). *Am. J. Med. Genet.* **5**, 285–294.

Francke, U., and Oliver, N. (1978). *Hum. Genet.* **45**, 137–165.

Funderburk, S. J., Spence, M. A., and Sparkes, R. S. (1977). *Am. J. Hum. Genet.* **29**, 136–141.
Gagne, R., and Laberge, C. (1972). *Exp. Cell Res.* **73**, 239–242.
German, J. (1972). *Prog. Med. Genet.* **8**, 61–101.
Gillberg, C., Rasmussen, P., and Wahlstrom, J. (1979). *Lancet* **10**, 1341.
Golbus, M. S., Loughman, W. D., Epstein, C. J., Halbasch, G., Stephens, J. D., and Hall, B. D. (1979). *N. Engl. J. Med.* **300**(4), 157–163.
Goodpasture, C., and Bloom, S. E. (1975). *Chromosoma* **53**, 37–50.
Goodpasture, C., Bloom, S. E., Hsu, T. C., and Arrighi, F. E. (1976). *Am. J. Hum. Genet.* **28**, 559–566.
Gosden, C., Buckton, K., Fotheringham, Z., and Brock, D. J. H. (1981). *Br. Med. J.* **282**, 255–258.
Gosden, C., and Brock, D. J. H. (1978). *J. Med. Genet.* **15**, 262–270.
Gray, J. W., Carrano, A. V., Steinmetz, L. L., Van Dilla, M. A., Moore, D. H., II, Mayall, B. H., and Mendelsohn, M. L. (1975). *Proc. Natl. Acad. Sci. U.S.A.* **72**, 1231–1234.
Gusella, J., Varsany-Breiner, A., Kao, F. T., Jones, C., Puck, T. T., Keys, C., Orkin, S., and Housman, D. (1979). *Proc. Natl. Acad. Sci. U.S.A.* **76**, 5239–5243.
Hayflick, L. (1965). *Tex. Rep. Biol. Med.* **23**, (Suppl. 1), 285–303.
Hecht, F., and Kaiser-McCaw, B. (1979). *Am. J. Hum. Genet.* **31**, 223–225.
Hoehn, H., Bryant, E. M., Karp, L. E., and Martin, G. M. (1974). *Pediatr. Res.* **8**, 746–754.
Hoehn, H., Rodriguez, M. L., Norwood, T. H., and Maxwell, C. L. (1978). *Am. J. Med. Genet.* **2**, 253–266.
Hook, E. B., and Hamerton, J. L. (1976). *In* "Population Cytogenetics" (E. B. Hook and I. H. Porter, eds.), pp. 63–80. Academic Press, New York.
Howard-Peebles, P. N., and Stoddard, G. R. (1979). *Hum. Genet.* **50**, 247–251.
Howard-Peebles, P. N., Stoddard, G. R., and Mims, M. G. (1979). *Am. J. Hum. Genet.* **31**, 214–222.
Hsu, L. Y. F., and Hirschhorn, K. (1977). *In* "New Chromosomal Syndromes" (J. J. Yunis, ed.), pp. 339–368. Academic Press, New York.
Hsu, L. Y. F., Kim, H. J., Hausknecht, R., and Hirschhorn, K. (1976). *Clin. Genet.* **10**, 232–238.
Jenkins, E. C., Brown, W. T., Duncan, C. J., Brooks, J., Ben-Yishai, M., Giordano, F. M., and Nitowsky, H. M. (1981). *Lancet* **2**, 1291.
Jorgenson, K. F., Van de Sande, J. H., and Lin, C. C. (1978). *Chromosoma* **68**, 287–302.
Kardon, N. B., Chernay, P. R., Hsu, L. Y. F., Martin, J. L., and Hirschhorn, K. (1972). *Clin. Genet.* **3**, 83–89.
Kardon, N. B., Lieber, E., Davis, J. G., and Hsu, L. Y. F. (1979). *Clin. Genet.* **15**, 267–272.
Kaufman, R. J., Brown, P. C., and Schimke, R. T. (1979). *Proc. Natl. Acad. Sci. U.S.A.* **76**, 5669–5673.
Keck, M., and Emerit, I. (1979). *Hum. Genet.* **50**, 277–283.
Kenny, G. E. (1973). *In* "Contamination in Tissue Culture" (J. Fogh, ed.), Chap. 5, pp. 107–129. Academic Press, New York.
Knudson, A. G., Meadows, A. T., Nichols, W. W., and Hill, R. (1976). *N. Engl. J. Med.* **295**, 1120–1123.
Kohn, G., Mennuti, M. T., Kaback, M., Schwartz, R. M., Chemke, J., Goldman, B., and Mellman, W. J. (1975). *Israel J. Med. Sci.* **11**(5), 476–481.
Kolata, G. B. (1980a). *Science* **207**, 967–969.
Kolata, G. B. (1980b). *Science* **207**, 970–971.
Kram, D., and Schneider, E. L. (1978). *In* "The Aging Reproductive System" ("Aging," Vol. 4), (E. L. Schneider, ed.), pp. 237–270. Raven Press, New York.
Kram, D., Bynum, G. D., Senula, G. C., and Schneider, E. L. (1979). *Nature* **279**, 531.
Latt, S. A. (1973). *Proc. Natl. Acad. Sci. U.S.A.* **70**, 3395.
Latt, S. A. (1974a). *J. Histochem. Cytochem.* **22**, 478.

Latt, S. A. (1974b). *Proc. Natl. Acad. Sci. U.S.A.* **71**, 3162.

Latt, S. A. (1975). *Somatic Cell Genet.* **1**, 293.

Latt, S. A. (1976). *Proc. Leiden Chromosome Conference* **5**, 367.

Latt, S. A. (1977). *Can. J. Genet. Cytol.* **19**, 603-623.

Latt, S. A. (1978). *Virchow's Arch. Cell Path. (B)* **29**, 19-27.

Latt, S. A. (1981). *In* "Sister Chromatid Exchanges" (S. Wolff, ed.), Wiley, New York (in press).

Latt, S. A., Sahar, E., and Eisenhard, M. E. (1979a). *J. Histochem. Cytochem.* **27**(1), 65-71.

Latt, S. A., Schreck, R. R., Loveday, K. S., and Shuler, C. F. (1979b). *Pharmacol. Rev.* **30**(4), 501-535.

Latt, S. A., Juergens, L. A., Matthews, D. J., Gustashaw, K. M., and Sahar, E. (1980). *Cancer Genet. and Cytogenet.* **1**, 187-196.

Laurence, K. M., and Gregory, P. (1976). *Br. Med. Bull.* **32**, 9-15.

Lebo, R. V., Carrano, A. V., Burkhart-Schultz, K., Dozy, A. M., Yu, L. C., and Kan, Y. W. (1979). *Proc. Natl. Acad. Sci. U.S.A.* **76**, 5804-5808.

Magenis, R. E., Hecht, F., and Lovrien, E. W. (1970). *Science* **170**, 85-87.

Magenis, R. E., Palmer, C. G., Wang, L., Brown, M., Chamberlin, J., Parks, M., Merritt, A. D., Rivas, M., and Yu, P. L. (1977). *In* "Population Cytogenetics" (E. B. Hook and I. H. Porter, eds.), pp. 179-188. Academic Press, New York.

Mascarello, J. T., Chadwick, D. L., and Moyers, T. G. (1980). *Lancet* **1**, 1089.

Matsuura, J., Mayer, M., and Jacobs, P. (1978). *Hum. Genet.* **45**, 33-41.

Mayer, M., Matsuura, J., and Jacobs, P. (1978). *Hum. Genet.* **45**, 43-50.

McDougall, J. K. (1971). *J. Gen. Virol.* **12**, 43-51.

McGarrity, G. J. (1976). *In Vitro* **12**(9), 643-648.

McKenzie, W. H., and Lubs, H. A. (1975). *Cytogenet. Cell Genet.* **14**, 97-115.

Megaw, J. M., Priest, J. H., Priest, R. E., and Johnson, L. D. (1977). *J. Med. Genet.* **14**, 163-167.

Mennuti, M. T., Wu, C. H., Mellman, W. J., and Mikhail, G. (1977). *Am. J. Med. Genet.* **1**, 211-216.

Miller, D. A., Dev, V. G., Tantravahi, R., and Miller, O. J. (1976). *Exper. Cell Res.* **101**, 235-243.

Miller, O. J., Schnedl, W., Allen, J., and Erlanger, B. F. (1974). *Nature* **251**, 636-637.

Miller, O. J., Miller, D. A., Dev, V. G., Tantravahi, R., and Croie, C. M. (1976). *Proc. Natl. Acad. Sci. U.S.A.* **73**, 4531-4535.

Milunsky, A. (1979). *In* "Genetic Disorders and the Fetus" (A. Milunsky, ed.), pp. 93-156. Plenum, New York.

Nevin, N. C., Nevin, J., and Thompson, W. (1979). *Clin. Genet.* **15**, 440-443.

Nevstad, N. P. (1978). *Mutat. Rep.* **57**, 253-258.

Niazi, M., Coleman, D. V., Mowbray, J. F., and Blunt, S. (1979). *J. Med. Genet.* **16**, 21-23.

NICHD National Registry for Amniocentesis Study Group (1976). *J. Am. Med. Assoc.* **236**, 1471-1476.

Nichols, W. W. (1974). *In* "The Cell Nucleus" (H. Busch, ed.), Vol. 2, pp. 437-458. Academic Press, New York.

Papp, Z., and Bell, J. E. (1979). *Clin. Genet.* **16**, 282-290.

Peakman, D. C., Moreton, M. F., and Robinson, A. (1977). *J. Med. Genet.* **14**, 37-39.

Peakman, D. C., Moreton, M. F., Corn, B. J., and Robinson, A. (1979). *Am. J. Hum. Genet.* **31**, 149-155.

Perry, P., and Evans, H. J. (1975). *Nature* **258**, 121.

Perry, P., and Wolff, S. (1974). *Nature* **251**, 156.

Priest, R. E., Priest, J. H., Moinuddin, J. F., and Keyser, A. J. (1977). *J. Med. Genet.* **14**, 157-162.

Priest, R. E., Marimuthu, K. M., and Priest, J. H. (1978). *Lab. Invest.* **39**(2), 106-109.

Ramos, C., Rivera, L., Benitez, J., Tejedor, E., and Sanchez-Cascos, A. (1979). *Hum. Genet.* **49,** 7–10.

Rhine, J. A., and Milunsky, A. (1979). *In* "Genetic Disorders and the Fetus," (A. Milunsky, ed.), pp. 527–538. Plenum, New York.

Riccardi, V. M., Sujansky, E., Smith, A. C., and Francke, U. (1978). *Pediatrics* **61,** 604–610.

Robinson, J. A., Buckton, K. E., Spowart, G., Newton, M., Jacobs, P. A., Evans, H. J., and Hill, R. (1976). *Ann. Hum. Genet.* **40,** 113–121.

Rodriguez, M. L., Luthy, D., Hall, J. G., Norwood, T. H., and Hoehn, H. (1978). *Clin. Genet.* **13,** 164–168.

Rosenberg, L. E., and Kidd, K. K. (1977). *N. Engl. J. Med.* **297,** 1060–1062.

Russell, W. C., Newman, C., and Williamson, D. H. (1975). *Nature* **253,** 461–462.

Sahar, E., and Latt, S. A. (1978). *Proc. Natl. Acad. Sci. U.S.A.* **75,** 5650–5654.

Sahar, E., and Latt, S. A. (1980). *Chromosoma* **79,** 1–28.

Sanchez, D., and Yunis, J. J. (1977). *In* "New Chromosomal Syndromes" (J. J. Yunis, ed.), pp. 1–54. Academic Press, New York.

Schmid, W. (1975). *Humangenetik* **30,** 325–330.

Schnedl, W. (1978). *Hum. Genet.* **41,** 1–9.

Schnedl, W., Dev, V. G., Tantravahi, R., Miller, D. A., Erlanger, B. F., and Miller, O. J. (1975). *Chromosoma* **52,** 59–66.

Schneider, E. L., Epstein, C. J., Epstein, W. L., Betlack, M., and Abbo-Holbasch, G. (1973). *Exp. Cell Res.* **79,** 343–349.

Schneider, E. L., Stanbridge, E. J., Epstein, C. J., Golbus, M., Abbo-Holbasch, G., and Rodger, G. (1974a). *Science* **184,** 477–479.

Schneider, E. L., Stanbridge, E. J., and Epstein, C. J. (1974b). *Exp. Cell Res.* **84,** 311–318.

Schreck, R. R., Dev, V. G., Erlanger, B. F., and Miller, O. J. (1977). *Chromosoma* **62,** 337–350.

Schweizer, D. (1976). *Chromosoma* **58,** 307–324.

Schweizer, D. (1981). *Hum. Genet.* **57,** 1–14.

Schweizer, D., Abros, P., and Andrle, M. (1978). *Exp. Cell Res.* **111,** 327–332.

Scott, A. F., Phillips, J. A., and Migeon, B. R. (1979). *Proc. Natl. Acad. Sci. U.S.A.* **76,** 4563–4565.

Seabright, M. (1971). *Lancet* **2,** 971–927.

Seabright, M. (1973). *Lancet* **1,** 1249.

Sehested, J. (1974). *Humangenetik* **21,** 55–58.

Shapiro, L. R., Wilmot, P. L., Brenholz, P., Leff, A., Martino, M., Harris, G., Mahoney, M. A., and Hobbins, J. (1982). *Lancet* **1,** 99–100.

Siggers, D. C. (1978). *In* "Prenatal Diagnosis of Genetic Disease," pp. 1–11. Blackwell, Oxford.

Simoni, G., Larizza, L., Sacchi, N., Della Valle, G., Dambrosio, F., and De Carli, L. (1979). *Hum. Genet.* **49,** 327–332.

Simpson, J. L. (1978). *Hum. Genet.* **44,** 1–49.

Simpson, N. E., Dallaire, L., Miller, J. R., Siminovich, L., Hamerton, J. L., Miller, J., and McKeen, C. (1976). *Can. Med. Assoc. J.* **115,** 739–746.

Stanbridge, E. (1971). *Bacteriol. Rev.* **35**(2), 206–227.

Stetka, D. G., and Wolff, S. (1976). *Mutat. Res.* **41,** 343–350.

Stetten, G., Sroka-Zaczek, B., and Corson, V. L. (1981). *Hum. Genet.* **57,** 357–359.

Sumner, A. T. (1972). *Exp. Cell Res.* **75,** 304–306.

Sutherland, G. R. (1977). *Science* **197,** 265–266.

Sutherland, G. R. (1979a). *Am. J. Hum. Genet.* **31,** 125–135.

Sutherland, G. R. (1979b). *Am. J. Hum. Genet.* **31,** 136–148.

Sutherland, G. R., Bowser-Riley, S. M., and Bain, A. D. (1975). *Clin. Genet.* **7,** 400–404.

Tompkins, D., Hunter, A., and Roberts, M. (1979). *Am. J. Med. Genet.* **4,** 17–26.

Tommerup, H., Puolsen, H., and Brondum-Mielson, K. (1981). *J. Med. Genet.* **18,** 374–376.

Van de Sande, J. H., Lin, C. C., and Jorgenson, K. F. (1977). *Science* **195,** 400–402.

Verma, R. S., and Lubs, H. A. (1975). *Am. J. Hum. Genet.* **27,** 110–117.

Vogel, W., Schempp, W., and Sigwarth, I. (1978). *Hum. Genet.* **45,** 193–198.

Williamson, R., Eksdale, J., Coleman, D. V., Niazi, M., and Modell, B. M. (1981). *Lancet* **2,** 1125–1129.

Wolf, S. F., Mareni, C. E., and Migeon, B. R. (1980). *Cell* **21,** 95–102.

Wolff, S. (1977). *Ann. Rev. Genet.* **11,** 183.

Yunis, J. J. (1976). *Science* **191,** 1268–1270.

Yunis, J. J., Sawyer, J. R., and Ball, D. W. (1978). *Chromosoma* **67,** 293–307.

Yunis, J. J., Ball, D. W., and Sawyer, J. R. (1979). *Hum. Genet.* **49,** 291–306.

Chapter 4

Prenatal Diagnosis of Open Neural Tube Defects

JAMES E. HADDOW

Foundation for Blood Research
Scarborough, Maine

AND

WAYNE A. MILLER

Prenatal Diagnostic Laboratory
Massachusetts General Hospital
Boston, Massachusetts

METHODS IN CELL BIOLOGY, VOL. 26

I. General Information about Neural Tube Defects

A. Prevalence

Spina bifida and anencephaly, which collectively account for nearly all neural tube defects (NTD), are serious fetal malformations resulting from incomplete closure of the neural tube during embryogenesis. The two occur in approximately a 1:1 ratio, and roughly 20% of spina bifida lesions are skin-covered. Their combined rate of occurrence in the United States, approximately 2 per 1000 live births, places them among the most common of major fetal defects (Centers for Disease Control, Congenital Malformations Surveillance Report, 1980). Prevalence has been shown to vary depending on ethnic origins and socioeconomic status. The highest reported prevalence of these conditions is found in people of Celtic origin in the United Kingdom, whereas black populations have a low prevalence.

B. Genetics

NTD have been classified as multifactorial disorders. Multifactorial disorders do not follow Mendelian laws of inheritance and are believed to be caused by a combination of genetic and environmental factors. The resulting patterns of occurrence and recurrence are complex (Wald and Cuckle, 1980). For instance, in multifactorial inheritance, the recurrence risk is linked to the occurrence risk, so that a white woman in the United States (NTD occurrence risk 2 per 1000) has a recurrence risk of 20 per thousand, whereas a woman in Glasgow (NTD occurrence risk 5 per thousand) has a recurrence risk of roughly 50 per thousand. A second non-Mendelian characteristic of multifactorial inheritance is that recurrence risk becomes steadily greater in an individual after each succeeding affected pregnancy. As an example, a white woman in the United States now with two NTD-affected pregnancies would have a recurrence risk of 40 per thousand. The risk in Glasgow under those conditions becomes 100 per thousand.

C.   Severity

Anencephaly is not compatible with life, and affected infants rarely live for more than a few hours after delivery. Survival and morbidity figures for spina bifida are more variable, depending, to some extent, on medical management. A recent survey at Oxford (Althouse and Wald, 1980) demonstrates that approximately one-third of infants with open lesions survive for 5 years at a center where selective treatment is carried out. Of those surviving beyond 5 years, 85% are severely handicapped, 10% are moderately handicapped, and the remainder have no handicap. This group of survivors spends an average of 6 months in the hospital during the first 5 years and has an average of six surgical procedures.

II.   Prenatal Diagnosis of Neural Tube Defects in High-Risk Women

A.   Alpha-Fetoprotein (AFP)

The discovery that amniotic fluid AFP levels were elevated in the presence of open NTD (Brock and Sutcliffe, 1972) ushered in a new era of prenatal diagnosis. AFP, normally present in high concentrations in fetal circulation, crosses into amniotic fluid from exposed membrane surfaces on the fetus such as are found with open NTD. Recognition of this occurrence allowed, for the first time, a substance to be measured routinely in second-trimester amniotic fluid samples by an immunochemical test for the purpose of detecting major physical defects in the fetus.

Two other major fetal lesions, omphalocele (Kunz and Schmid, 1976) and congenital nephrosis (Kjessler et al., 1975), have also been reliably diagnosed via AFP measurements in amniotic fluid. The former occurs at a rate of between 3 and 4 per 10,000 (Report of the Working Group on Maternal Serum Alpha-Fetoprotein Screening, 1981) whereas the latter is very uncommon except in the Finnish population. Both of these conditions usually produce elevations in amniotic fluid AFP levels and are important to consider in differential diagnosis. AFP crosses from exposed omphalocele membrane surfaces in a manner analogous to NTD, whereas in congenital nephrosis AFP enters amniotic fluid from damaged kidneys. Another serious problem, unrecognized or impending fetal demise, may also lead to significant amniotic fluid AFP elevations.

B.   The Importance of Gestational Dating

Mean AFP concentrations in amniotic fluid fall steadily throughout the second trimester, emphasizing the need to document gestational age before interpreting test results. Pregnancies are dated, by convention, from the first day of the last menstrual period, and the three ways of obtaining dates include (1) history, (2) physical examination, and (3) ultrasound measurements. In most instances, acceptable dating can be obtained historically, but sometimes the physician must make an estimate using only uterine size. Ultrasound dating is now available for nearly all women having amniocentesis, as an added parameter. However, recent observations on biparietal diameters in fetuses with open spina bifida have given rise to recommendations that dating by history ought to take precedence over ultrasound measurements when interpreting amniotic fluid AFP results (Wald *et al.*, 1980). Whatever the means of dating, it is important to obtain as accurate information as possible, both when establishing normal AFP ranges in amniotic fluid and when interpreting clinical results.

C.   Sources of AFP in Amniotic Fluid

AFP is the major fetal serum protein during the early weeks of pregnancy, occurring in concentrations as high as 300 mg/100 ml at the twelfth week of gestation. Thereafter it falls steadily as albumin levels begin to rise. The molecular structures of AFP and albumin are similar, even though the two are immunologically distinct (Ruoslahti, 1978). The major normal source of AFP in amniotic fluid is fetal urine; the fetal kidney allows significant amounts to filter from fetal blood (Macri and Weiss, 1976). The increased amounts of AFP found in amniotic fluid in the presence of NTD are thought to result from transudation across fetal blood vessels on the NTD exposed membrane surfaces. AFP is manufactured in the fetal liver and the yolk sac and appears immunologically identical from these two sources, but liver-derived AFP is glycosylated, whereas yolk sac-derived AFP is not (Smith, C. J. *et al.*, 1979). For practical purposes, AFP can be considered fetospecific; the normal nonpregnant adult has circulating AFP levels no higher than 10 ng/ml.

D.   False-Positive AFP Results

Within a very short time after the introduction of AFP testing in amniotic fluid, women with a history of neural tube defect-affected pregnancies began to be offered amniocentesis with subsequent pregnancies. In addition, AFP measurement was introduced as an additional test in amniotic fluid samples from women having chromosome studies, and false-positive AFP results began to be reported. The major source for these spurious elevations was identified as fetal blood contamination, and as a result, AFP laboratories began routinely inspecting samples for blood and recording total RBCs, hematocrit, and fetal versus maternal cells. Furthermore, in clear amniotic fluid samples with AFP elevations, Hemoglobin F was measured as an indirect indicator of fetal cells that might have been removed before analysis. Appreciation for the role of fetal blood contamination in producing false-positive AFP results helped greatly to reduce misdiagnoses.

Pitfalls also were appreciated, however, on the side of overinterpretation of the significance of fetal blood. For instance, an opaque amniotic fluid sample that, when centrifuged, produces a small button of fetal RBCs, is not sufficiently contaminated to contribute significantly to the measured value of AFP. Furthermore, the presence of hemoglobin F in a sample known to be clear but with a grossly elevated AFP level, should not rule out the possibility of a fetal neural tube defect. About 40% of anencephalic and 20% of open spina bifida pregnancies are associated with bloodstaining (Wald and Cuckle, 1980). Brown samples also appear on occasion. These latter rarely have intact red cells but may have detectable hemoglobin F. Rather than being procedure-related, these brown samples are felt to indicate an earlier spontaneous hemorrhage.

E.   Stability of AFP

Alpha-fetoprotein is very stable in amniotic fluid, and samples can be shipped unrefrigerated for AFP analysis. For reasons already stated, it is generally recommended that uncentrifuged fluid be sent for analysis, and, if bloodstaining is present, that the sample be protected from freezing.

F.   Amniotic Fluid versus Maternal Urine

Rarely, a second-trimester amniotic fluid sample has unmeasurably low AFP levels. When that happens, there should be an immediate suspicion that the sample is maternal urine rather than amniotic fluid. Because, in contrast to urine, amniotic fluid ordinarily contains glucose and protein, differentiation from urine ought not to be difficult.

III.   The Second U.K. Collaborative Study

A.   Sensitivity of Amniotic Fluid AFP Testing

A major advance in understanding the sensitivity of amniotic fluid AFP measurement came with the publication of the Second Report of the U.K. Collaborative Study (1979). This study was a cooperative effort involving 17 U.K. laboratory centers and sought to define the overlap in AFP levels between NTD and non-NTD pregnancies. Given the different mass unit standards in use at the various participating laboratories, it became necessary to convert all values into multiples of the median (MOM), in order to integrate results. Retrospective analysis of the results for each gestational week between 13 and 24 established that a sliding cutoff point would be necessary to maximize diagnostic efficiency and minimize false positives.

B.   Specificity and False Positives

Ninety-eight percent of all open neural tube defects could be identified by using cutoffs of 2.5 MOM at 13–15 weeks, 3.0 MOM at 16–18 weeks, 3.5 MOM at 19–21 weeks, and 4.0 MOM at 22–24 weeks. Using these cutoffs, a theoretical *practical false-positive rate* was developed, based on how frequently a viable pregnancy might be terminated due to a single false-positive amniotic fluid AFP result in the absence of other clinical considerations or diagnostic studies. This estimated rate was 0.48% if bloodstained fluids were included and 0.27% if they were not. The pregnancies actually terminated in the U.K. study as a result of false-positive AFP results totaled 0.06%, indicating either that higher cutoff lines had been used in practice or that additional clinical and diagnostic parameters were being utilized. The collaborative study's definition of blood-staining included samples that were brown or green (i.e., had evidence of an earlier hemorrhage) as well as red. This is important because bloodstaining associated with elevated amniotic fluid AFP levels, whether procedure-related or not, appears to carry a significant risk for subsequent spontaneous fetal loss, as can be seen in Table I. Risk of miscarriage is great with all falsely elevated amniotic fluid AFP levels, and especially those in which AFP levels are very high. For instance, although not displayed in Table I, 28% of the pregnancies with bloodstained samples and AFP levels between 2.5 and 5.9 × median miscarried, whereas 88% of those with values at or above 6 × median terminated spontaneously.

TABLE I

RELATIONSHIP BETWEEN AMNIOTIC FLUID AFP LEVELS, BLOODSTAINED FLUID, AND SUBSEQUENT MISCARRIAGE IN PREGNANCIES WITHOUT FETAL DEFECTS[a]

AFP level	Character of sample	Miscarriages (%)
<2.5 × Median	Clear	230/11,820 (1.9)
	Bloodstained	36/1182 (3.0)
≥2.5 × Median	Clear	6/34 (17.6)
	Bloodstained	24/49 (49.0)

[a] Data abstracted from the Second U.K. Collaborative Study (1979) and from appendix material provided by Drs. Nicholas J. Wald and Howard S. Cuckle.

C. False-Positive Reduction via Repeat Amniocentesis

The value of repeat amniocentesis to reduce false positives was supported by the collaborative study. Ten out of thirteen women with elevated AFP values and bloodstained samples were found to be normal after resampling, and the three whose AFP values remained elevated were retested within 1 week, an interval believed to be too short for meaningful comparison. All 16 women with NTD-affected pregnancies who had repeat amniocentesis continued to show AFP elevations. The practice of repeating amniocentesis continues to be an important clinical option, but the advent of a new diagnostic study, acetylcholinesterase analysis, may reduce the need for the second procedure. This test appears capable of distinguishing between false positives and true positives in nearly all cases and will be discussed later in this chapter. If studies such as this are established as helpful in discriminating between true- and false-positive AFP elevations, the additional risks from a second amniocentesis might be avoided.

IV. Prospective Experiences in One Laboratory

A. Analysis of Positive AFP Results

Thirteen neural tube defects have been identified at the Foundation for Blood Research among the first 2500 women studied, and all of these AFP results have been significantly above the U.K. cutoff line. Our experience with false-positive AFP results is summarized in Fig. 1. This represents only amniotic fluid samples processed prospectively for clinical diagnosis and includes a total of 2500 patients having amniocentesis during the second trimester. Roughly 95% of these women have had the procedure done for advanced maternal age with the remainder being at risk for having NTD-affected fetuses, either by history or by serum screening. In this small series the pattern is similar to the U.K. Collaborative Study experience in that 0.32% of false-positive results from first samples are above the U.K. cutoff; but contrasts with U.K. results in that all of those samples are bloodstained. The miscarriage rate is high (25%) in these false positives, and in two instances where repeat sampling has been done, there have been normal AFP results.

Also included in Fig. 1 are all of the AFP values between 3 standard deviations above the mean and the U.K. cutoff line, totaling 0.68% for first samples. Approximately half of the samples in this zone are bloodstained, and 23% of the pregnancies are lost spontaneously. The single termination of a pregnancy unaffected by NTD (a star in the figure) showed a malnourished fetus and a grossly infarcted placenta, yielding a true false-positive rate of 0.04%. Of the eight women having repeat amniocentesis in this group, seven yielded lower AFP

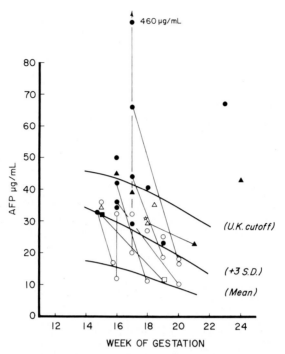

Fig. 1.   Experience with false-positive amniotic fluid AFP values at the Foundation for Blood Research. The risk of stillbirth or miscarriage is high in pregnancies associated with amniotic fluid AFP levels greater than 3 standard deviations above the mean. Where two AFP observations have been made on the same pregnancy, a line connects them. The single vertical line connects two aliquots analyzed from the same amniocentesis, with the higher value associated with gross fetal blood contamination. ○, Normal delivery at term; △, stillbirth or miscarriage; ● ■ ▲, fetal blood in sample; □, premature delivery; ☆, induced abortion.

results, whereas the eighth subsequently miscarried. If trends identified here are confirmed with larger series, miscarriage risk can be assigned in the zone between 3 standard deviations above the mean and the U.K. cutoff line, even if the higher U.K. cutoff line is chosen for diagnosing NTD.

B.   Acetylcholinesterase—A Newer Diagnostic Test for NTD in Amniotic Fluid

A recent report indicates that identification of a specific molecular form of acetylcholinesterase (AChE) in amniotic fluid can be useful both in diagnosing neural tube defects and in identifying false-positive AFP results (Smith, A. D. et al., 1979). A positive test indicates that a fetal lesion is present, and on some occasions, this assay will detect an open NTD even when alpha-fetoprotein levels are normal. Conversely, the specific AChE band is absent as a rule in bloodstained samples from unaffected pregnancies, even when AFP is elevated. Table II summarizes our laboratory's preliminary experience with this new test and provides documentation of its reliability.

A summary of the experience of other investigators (Report of the Working Group on Amniotic Fluid Diagnostic Studies, 1981), utilizing this technique shows similar results, documenting that the qualitative AChE assay is the best ancillary method currently available to identify open neural tube defects *in utero*. Although the specific AChE band is nearly always present in cases of open NTD and absent in fluids where fetal blood contamination is the cause of the AFP elevation, the assay is less useful in differentiating between other fetal causes of elevated amniotic fluid AFP. The band is often, but not always, present in omphalocele (our own small series in Table II is too small to define this), sometimes present in fetal demise, and absent in congenital nephrosis. In order to define the discriminatory power of this assay more completely, a further collaborative study is currently under way.

C.   Integration of Amniotic Fluid Diagnostic Processes for Open NTD Detection

Figure 2 summarizes the current management of second-trimester amniotic fluid samples received at the Foundation for Blood Research for diagnostic AFP testing. Efforts are now under way to diagnose AFP-related fetal disorders more precisely, to the point where the size of a given lesion may be defined. Biochemical studies in amniotic fluid can carry such characterization only so far, after which visualizing techniques, including most especially ultrasonography, must

TABLE II

COMPARISON OF AChE AND AFP TEST RESULTS IN SELECTED BANKED AMNIOTIC FLUID SAMPLES FROM PREGNANCIES OF KNOWN OUTCOME

	No.	AChE Positive	AFP Positive[a]
No fetal malformation			
Blood-free	128	0	3
Maternal blood present	14	0	0
Fetal blood present	11	1	10
Fetal malformation			
Anencephaly	36	36	36
Open spina bifida	14	13	13
Omphalocele	5	5	5

[a] $\geq +4$ SD

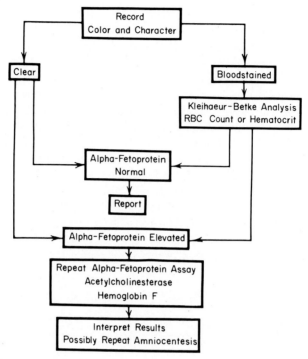

Fɪɢ. 2. The present protocol at the Foundation for Blood Research for managing biochemical testing on amniotic fluid samples sent for AFP analysis.

take over. Refinements in ultrasound technology have allowed highly skilled operators to visualize individual fetal vertebrae during the second trimester and to identify bowel obstruction and omphalocele. A comprehensive discussion of this subject appears elsewhere in this volume. Given these rapidly emerging diagnostic refinements, it may soon be possible not only to confirm a diagnosis made biochemically but also to state its extent and prognosis.

V.   Biochemical Testing Methodology

A.   Measurement of Amniotic Fluid AFP

Electroimmunodiffusion (''rocket'' or EID) was the first technique used to measure AFP in amniotic fluid (Laurell, 1966), and this continues to be the method of choice in most prenatal diagnosis laboratories. In this assay, specific antibody (in this case anti-AFP) is mixed with agarose gel in appropriate concentration, and the gel is then cast as a slab. Holes are punched along one side, followed by addition of measured amounts of standard curve and of amniotic fluid samples. An electrical current is then applied to drive proteins into the gel, where AFP and anti-AFP react to form a precipitate. This reaction continues until AFP is exhausted, and the resulting precipitate is shaped like a rocket. The gel is washed to remove extraneous protein, stained, and the rockets are then measured (Fig. 3). A linear relationship exists between the height of the rocket peak and the amount of AFP present in the sample. Careful adjustment of antibody concentration is critical if rockets are to be optimal, because too little will produce large, indistinct rockets, whereas too much will produce dense, stubby rockets. At both extremes, assay reliability is lessened. When the assay is functioning properly, coefficients of variation less than ±8% can be readily achieved, and this is more than adequate for reliable clinical diagnosis.

1. ELECTROIMMUNODIFFUSION PROTOCOL FOR MEASURING AFP IN SECOND-TRIMESTER PREGNANCY AMNIOTIC FLUID

Reagents

Acetic acid, glacial	Ethanol, absolute
Coomassie brilliant blue R	Goat antiserum to AFP
Diethylbarbituric acid	SeaKem agarose ME
Distilled water	Sodium barbital
	Sodium chloride

Working Solutions

AFP reference standard—Prepare working AFP standards of 20, 15, 10, 5, 2.5, and 1.25 mg/liter by diluting cord serum standard in B2 buffer.

Agarose—12 g/liter SeaKem agarose ME and 7.5 ml of goat antiserum with full-strength B2 buffer to final volume of 1 liter

B2 buffer—2.79 g/liter diethylbarbituric acid and 15.4 g/liter sodium barbital with pH adjusted to 8.6

Coomassie stain—2 g Coomassie brilliant blue R, 400 ml ethanol, 100 ml acetic acid, 500 ml distilled water

Destain—400 ml ethanol, 100 ml acetic acid, 500 ml distilled water

Saline—9 g NaCl per liter

Sample diluting buffer—Full-strength B2 buffer

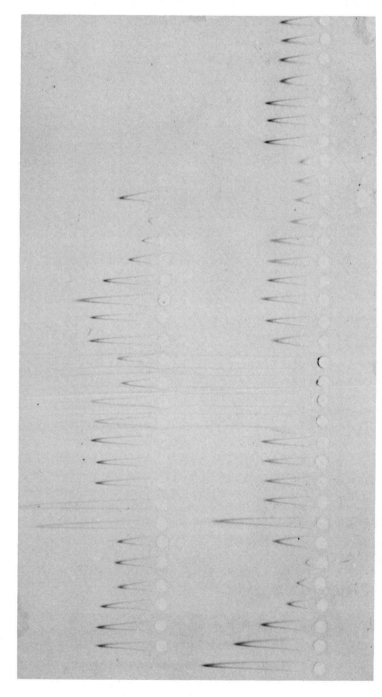

Fig. 3. A typical electroimmunodiffusion study for assaying amniotic fluid AFP. The first six wells on the left-hand side of the lower row contain the standard curve, and the remaining wells contain clinical samples. Wells 13–16 in the lower row contain fluid from a case of anencephaly, showing markedly increased amounts of AFP.

Equipment

Absorbant paper, Gelman
Beaker—0.25 liter
Clips, bulldog
Electrophoresis (MRA, water-cooled) apparatus
Filter paper
Flask, Erlenmeyer, 2-liter
Frames, spacer
Gelbond
Mixer, magnetic
Mixer, vortex
pH meter
Pipets, glass serological (one), and 1-ml and 10-ml MLA
Glass plates
Power source, Gelman
Vacuum pump
Punch, 3 mm
Scale
Test tubes, disposable
Test tube holder
Tray, 0.05 liter (two), and 2-liter

Sample Preparation:
Less than 19 weeks gestation: sample diluted 1:2 (B2 buffer)
19 weeks gestation or greater: sample not diluted

Procedure

Make a sandwich mold with glass plates, spacer frames, and gelbond. Dissolve agarose in buffer (100 ml) by boiling twice; then cool to 40°C. Heat water in 250-ml beaker to 50°C for warming 0.15 ml goat AFP antiserum to which 20 ml of the warm agarose solution is added. Mix gently and pipet into mold. Cool 1 hour at 20°C. Remove gel from mold and punch wells along the cathode border, 10 mm from edge and at least 5 mm apart. Remove plugs with suction and mount gel with water seal on MRA apparatus whose tanks have been filled with full-strength B2 buffer. Connect gel to buffer tanks with 3-in. wide wicks made from Gelman absorbant paper.

Attach electrodes and apply standards, samples in duplicate and controls within 5 minutes (using 5-μl MLA pipet). Apply 100 V for 16 hours. Remove plate, cover agarose with damp filter paper, layer several paper towels on top, and press with a 10-lb weight for 10 minutes. Remove filter paper and submerge in tray filled with normal saline for 30 minutes. Repeat press and wash cycle three times. At the end of the third press, rinse plate with tap water, air-dry, and stain for 30 minutes. Wash with tap water and destain until background is clear (15 minutes). Air-dry and measure peak heights of rockets from top of well. Plot standard curve as concentration versus peak height and read unknowns.

Amniotic fluid AFP testing can also be carried out successfully by radioimmunoassay, a method discussed later, in the section on serum AFP measurement. The only major objection to this approach can be avoided by accounting for potential inaccuracies resulting from two sources: imprecise dilution and improper diluents. Occasionally, radial immunodiffusion (RID) is utilized for AFP analysis. This technique produces larger coefficients of variation than EID and is not recommended for general use. Once the assay is working satisfactorily, the laboratory should establish its normal ranges for each gestational week, based on a minimum of 50 amniotic fluid samples per week; this number allows a stable median to be derived.

B.   Detection of Blood Contamination

1.   FETAL VERSUS MATERNAL RED CELLS

This differentiation is made possible by the Kleihauer–Betke method (Kleihauer *et al.*, 1957). This technique utilizes the principle that fetal hemoglobin is highly resistant to an acid environment in contrast to adult hemoglobin. Fixed smears of red blood cells are exposed to an acid citrate buffer (pH 3.3). At this pH adult hemoglobin is eluted from the cells, leaving a ghostlike stroma. Fetal cells can then be stained with eosin, making quantitation possible.

2.   MEASUREMENT OF HEMOGLOBIN F

Counterimmunoelectrophoresis is the procedure of choice. This is a qualitative technique that utilizes the principle that IgG migrates oppositely in an electrical field from most other major proteins. An aliquot of amniotic fluid is placed in a well (in agarose gel) next to a second well containing hemoglobin F (Fig. 4). Hemoglobin F antiserum is then added to a third well, placed to form the peak of a triangle with the two other wells as the base. An electrical current then forces proteins from the antibody and samples together. If hemoglobin F is present, a precipitate will be formed as a U-shaped continuous line between the sample and the hemoglobin F standard, proving immunologic identity. It is possible, but unnecessary, to carry out quantitative hemoglobin F measurement by rocket.

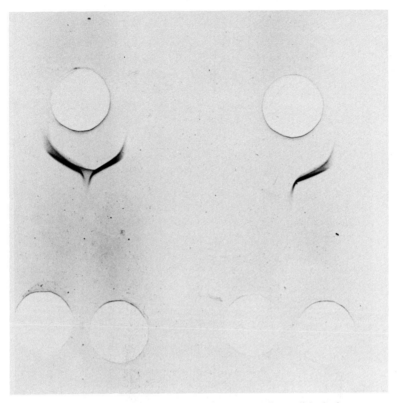

Fig. 4. Counterimmunoelectrophoresis for hemoglobin F. The first well in the lower row contains an aliquot of amniotic fluid contaminated with fetal blood; the second, a preparation of hemoglobin F (the positive control). The well above them contains hemoglobin F. The anode is at the top, and electrophoresis has forced the antigen and antibody together. The continuous U-shaped precipitate establishes immunologic identity between the unknown and the standard. In the study on the right, samples are arranged as in the first study except that the amniotic fluid sample has no hemoglobin F.

C. Acetylcholinesterase—Qualitative Method

The technique currently employed is polyacrylamide gel electrophoresis of an aliquot of amniotic fluid, followed by development with substrate to make the bands visible. A detailed protocol is available in the literature (Haddow *et al.*, 1981a). A specific inhibitor can be added to the reaction mixture to differentiate acetylcholinesterase from pseudocholinesterase, and the test is positive if the characteristic AChE band is present (Fig. 5).

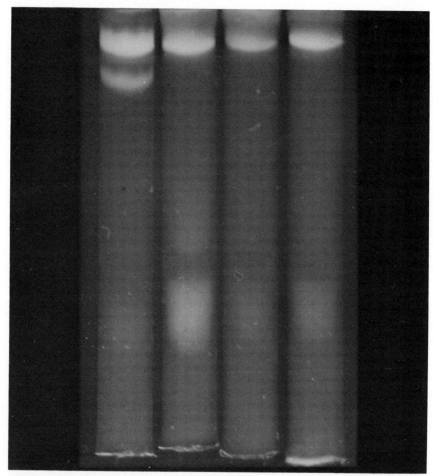

Fig. 5.   Qualitative acetylcholinesterase analysis by gel electrophoresis. The anode is at the bottom. All gels have been developed with acetylthiocholine, producing white precipitates. The first gel on the left contains an amniotic fluid aliquot from a case of open spina bifida. The top band is pseudocholinesterase; the band immediately below it is the molecular form of acetylcholinesterase found with open NTD. The second gel is from the same case, but an inhibitor specific for acetylcholinesterase has been added prior to development with acetylthiocholine. Pseudocholinesterase continues to react with substrate under these conditions, and the band remains. The third and fourth gels contain aliquots from a sample sufficiently contaminated with fetal blood to have a falsely elevated AFP level (the far right-hand gel has inhibitor added), showing that no acetylcholinesterase band is present.

D. Diagnostic Techniques under Investigation

Three analytic processes are presently being evaluated for possible use as adjuncts to, or substitutes for, amniotic fluid AFP measurement. The first two, Con-A fractionation of AFP and rapidly adhering cell analysis, offered the best promise as ancillary tests until the advent of the AChE assay. They are presented here because certain centers will continue to use them at least for research purposes. Most investigators are now convinced that the qualitative AChE assay is a better alternative. The third approach involves testing for neuronal-specific proteins, a promising new area of investigation, but still at an early stage of development.

1. RAPIDLY ADHERING (RA) CELL ANALYSIS

RA cell analysis utilizes morphologic analysis of the amniotic fluid cells that attach to the culture vessel within 24 hours of plating. Sutherland *et al.* (1973) originally observed large numbers of such RA cells in association with NTD fetuses. Gosden and Brock (1977a,b, 1978a) then defined the quantitative aspect of this method and went on to identify several distinct RA cell types, including some that appeared to be associated with NTD. These RA cell types were more diverse than the three basic cell morphologies—fibroblasts, epithelioid, amniotic fluid type (spindle cell)—found in established amniotic fluid cell cultures. Applying this technique to amniotic fluid samples obtained from a high-risk population, they were able to identify NTD and other fetal defects. In another study, Gosden and Brock reported that certain RA cell types may identify unfavorable intrauterine environments that lead to fetal loss, premature delivery, and intrauterine growth retardation (1978b).

At the Massachusetts General Hospital a similar prospective study has been carried out in a low-risk population, using a modified and shortened technique, and it has been found helpful in discriminating between true- and false-positive AFP elevations (Miller, 1979; Miller and Carroll, 1979). The major drawback to this technique is the subjective nature of morphologic analysis, coupled with the wide variety of RA cell types. With experience, however, the differences between normal and NTD-associated RA cell types are clear in most cases.

a. RA Cell Analytic Method. First, 1 ml of amniotic fluid is centrifuged, the supernatant removed, and the cells resuspended in 0.5 ml of MEM media supplemented with 20% fetal calf serum. The cell suspension is then plated on a 22-mm^2 coverslip in a 35-mm Falcon plastic petri dish. Care is taken that the cell suspension remains intact on the coverslip. The coverslips are then incubated for 20–24 hours at 37°C in a 5% CO_2 atmosphere. The coverslips are rinsed in phosphate-buffered saline, fixed in absolute methanol, and stained with Giemsa. Each coverslip is mounted on a slide, and the total number and morphology of RA cells are recorded. A case is considered abnormal if there are greater than 1500 RA cells and if the ratio of abnormal to normal cells is greater than 10:1.

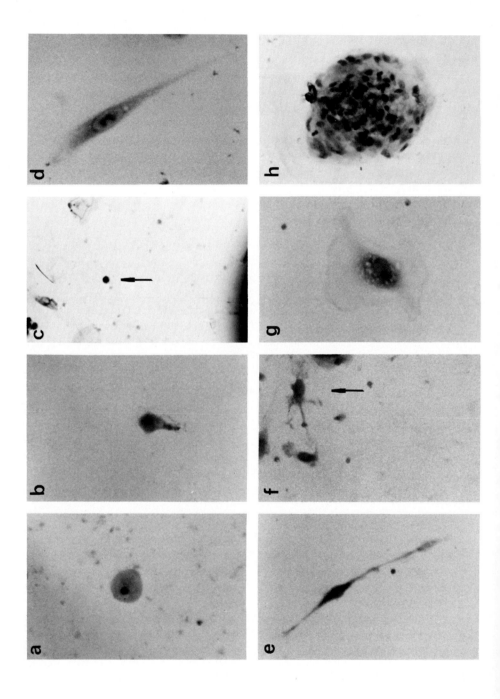

b. Morphologic Analysis of RA Cells. This relies heavily on proper classification of the eight major cell types shown in Fig. 6. Among the normal cell types, uninucleate cells are found most often after placental trauma, and blood cells as a procedure-related complication. Blood cells can confound this analysis when present in large numbers. We note them, but do not include them in the count. Fibroblasts are occasionally vacuolated but are clearly distinguishable from either bipolar or multiple pseudopodia cells found with NTD. This class exhibits the greatest variation and could probably be further subdivided. Lack of experience in examining amniotic fluid RA cells and failure to adhere to protocol can lead to difficulties in interpretation. For example, our studies have shown significant increases in the number of cells and changes in morphology on replicate coverslips harvested at 48 and 72 hours when compared to 24-hour coverslips from the same case.

c. Possible Applications. Applied prospectively, RA cell analysis is tedious and expensive. It does not seem to offer any advantage over the newly developed AChE isoenzyme assay as a confirmatory test for NTD. However, recognition of the many cell types in amniotic fluid cultures identifies a new area for research. Current culture techniques apparently select for or enhance the growth of certain relatively undifferentiated cell types. The range of genetic expression of these cell types is limited. Development of techniques for the selection and culture of the more specialized cell types known to be present in amniotic fluid samples could greatly expand the applicability of amniocentesis for prenatal genetic diagnosis.

2. CONCANAVALIN-A FRACTIONATION OF AFP

This procedure involves separation of the glycosylated (liver-derived) and non-glycosylated (yolk sac-derived) fractions of AFP by column or two-dimensional crossed-affinity electrophoresis. Elevated AFP values associated with open NTD have a low percentage of nonglycosylated AFP, whereas clear amniotic fluid samples with false-positive AFP values have high percentages of nonglycosylated AFP (Hindersson *et al.*, 1979; Ruoslahti *et al.*, 1979; Smith, C. J. *et al.*, 1979; Nørgaard-Pedersen *et al.*, 1980). The major problem with this technique is that AFP elevation caused by fetal blood contamination often has a relatively low percentage of nonglycosylated AFP similar to that found when

---

FIG. 6. Morphologic cell types of rapidly adhering (RA) cells. The four major categories of normal RA cells are shown in a–d. (a) Epithelioid: small nucleus, hexagonal to round, with uniformly stained cytoplasm. (b) Uninucleate: a darkly stained, eccentric nucleus and small amount of uniformly stained cytoplasm. (c) Blood: small round cells with darkly stained cytoplasm. (d) Fibroblasts: triangular cells, occasionally vacuolated. Pictures e–h depict the four major categories of NTD cells. (e) Bipolar: darkly stained nuclei and small amount of cytoplasm. (f) Multiple pseudopodia: filamentous pseudopodia and vacuoles. (g) Large vacuolated: irregularly shaped with foamy, vacuolated cytoplasm. (h) Giant multinucleate: either true multinucleate or tight aggregates.

fetal NTD are present. Since fetal blood contamination is a major cause of non-NTD-related AFP elevations, Con-A fractionation therefore offers little advantage in the majority of cases where a discriminatory test is necessary. Some laboratories apply a correction factor for blood contamination of the amniotic fluid sample, making assumptions about the concentration of total AFP and the Con-A fractions in fetal serum. These assumptions can lead to serious interpretive errors.

3.   NEURONAL-SPECIFIC PROTEINS

Two of the neuronal-specific proteins are currently being studied for their potential usefulness in diagnosing open NTD (Report of the Working Group on Amniotic Fluid Diagnostic Studies, 1981). Nørgaard-Pedersen has identified a synaptic membrane D_2 protein that can be assayed by counterflow immunoelectrophoresis. Preliminary data show the presence of this protein in affected pregnancies and its absence in unaffected pregnancies. Marangus has developed a radioimmunoassay for brain-specific enolase, also known as 14-3-2 protein. It is not yet known whether this substance is present in amniotic fluid from affected pregnancies. The rationale for pursuing this line of investigation is that these neuronal-specific proteins may provide greater diagnostic specificity.

VI.   Maternal Serum AFP Levels as a Means of Screening for Neural Tube Defects

A.   Rationale

Until now this chapter had been restricted to NTD diagnosis via amniotic fluid AFP measurement. Though very reliable, this approach is capable of identifying less than 5% of open neural tube defects born in a given year, even if all pregnant women with defined risks were to take advantage of amniocentesis and have AFP measured in amniotic fluid samples. This is because more than 95% of all neural tube defects born each year occur in families with no preceding indication of risk. The potential significance of a maternal serum screening test would be to reach out to the remaining pregnant women and provide a means for selecting from among them a small group whose risk would be sufficiently great to warrant further diagnostic procedures, including amniocentesis. Between 1972 and 1974, elevated Maternal Serum AFP (MSAFP) levels in association with open neural tube defects were reported by several groups (Hino et al., 1972; Leek et al., 1973; Brock et al., 1973, 1974; Harris et al., 1974; Seller et al., 1974; Wald et al., 1974). This was followed by a multicenter collaborative study aimed at defining the sensitivity and specificity of MSAFP measurements and identifying the optimal time for testing.

B.   The U.K. Collaborative Study on MSAFP Screening

1.   ESTABLISHING A COMMON INTERLABORATORY CURRENCY

At the time of the Report of the First U.K. Collaborative Study (1977), which involved 19 centers, no single AFP laboratory reference preparation was in general use. Furthermore, there was some question as to whether mass unit comparisons could be reliably made even in the presence of such a standard. As a result, it was decided that all data be expressed as multiples of the median (MOM). Using this approach, it became possible to characterize the maternal serum AFP distributions of non-NTD singleton populations, non-NTD twin populations, and populations of open spina bifida and anencephaly. From these data, conclusions could be drawn about diagnostic efficiencies and false-positive rates at different multiples of the median, providing a rational basis for subsequent screening policies. The use of MOM is now widely accepted as a means of expression in individual laboratories for clinical purposes.

2.   OPTIMAL TIME FOR TESTING

The first day of the last menstrual period is, by convention, the starting point for calculating gestational weeks. The Collaborative Study used completed weeks to express its results (e.g., 13 weeks and 0 days through 13 weeks and 6 days = 13 weeks). Data from 18,684 singleton and 163 twin non-NTD pregnancies were combined with 301 pregnancies with fetal NTD (146 with anencephaly, 142 with spina bifida, and 13 with encephalocele). All of the sera were collected at between 10 and 24 weeks gestation, and only results from the first sample obtained for a given pregnancy were used for analysis. The greatest percentage of open NTD could be detected at between 16 and 18 weeks gestation. Prior to that time, diagnostic efficiency was very poor, whereas after that time there appeared to be some diminution in sensitivity.

3.   MSAFP SENSITIVITY FOR OPEN NTD AT 16–18 WEEKS

Under conditions of the Collaborative Study, 88% of cases of anencephaly and 79% of cases of open spina bifida were associated with maternal serum AFP levels equal to or greater than 2.5 MOM at between 16 and 18 completed gestational weeks. Sensitivity could be increased to 90% and 91%, respectively, at a cutoff equal to or greater than 2.0 MOM, but only at the expense of increasing the false-positive rate.

4.   TWIN DETECTION AT 16–18 WEEKS

At or above 2.5 MOM, 26% of twin pregnancies could be detected, and this figure increased to 47% if 2.0 MOM were used.

5.   AFP ELEVATIONS IN SINGLETON, NON-NTD PREGNANCIES AT 16–18 WEEKS

These are considered false positives, even though a variety of high-risk pregnancy conditions have been found in this group, other than those addressed by the Collaborative Study. A total of 3.3% of singleton, non-NTD pregnancies were found to have MSAFP values at or above 2.5 MOM, and this rose to 7.2% if the cutoff was lowered to 2.0 MOM. From this it is possible to see that a variety of consequences are possible in a given screening program, largely dependent on its choice of a cutoff line. Data are also available for percentages of NTD, twins, and false positives at higher cutoffs in the Collaborative Study report.

6.   RELIABILITY OF COLLABORATIVE STUDY DATA

A number of centers in the United Kingdom and the United States now have gained experience from prospective MSAFP screening. To date, no significant discrepancies have been found with predicted consequences of screening (Report of the Working Group on Maternal Serum Alpha-Fetoprotein Screening, 1981).

C.   Passage of Fetal AFP into the Maternal Circulation

Under normal conditions, most fetally derived AFP reaches the maternal circulation indirectly, being first filtered through the fetal kidneys into amniotic fluid and then diffusing transamniotically. Amnions appear to vary in porosity from pregnancy to pregnancy, some restricting AFP diffusion markedly and others allowing relatively large amounts to pass (Haddow *et al.*, 1979). MSAFP levels increase steadily during the second trimester, a seeming paradox when coupled with the fact that amniotic fluid AFP levels decrease steadily during the same time period. One theoretic explanation for this phenomenon would be that the rapidly expanding surface area of the amnion allows more AFP to diffuse. Elevated MSAFP levels arising from fetal NTD are most probably produced by transamniotic diffusion.

Transplacental passage of fetal AFP into the mother also occurs in conjunction with feto–maternal hemorrhage, either spontaneously or as a result of amniocentesis (Hay *et al.*, 1979; Los *et al.*, 1979); it is not known whether AFP traverses the placental barrier directly under other conditions. AFP from this latter source may partially explain elevated MSAFP levels in the absence of fetal malformations, and it is also possible that such elevations will occur as a result of a very porous amnion.

Recently, two groups have demonstrated that maternal weight influences MSAFP concentration (Report of the Working Group on Maternal Serum Alpha-Fetoprotein Screening, 1981; Haddow *et al.*, 1981b), presumably as a reflection of differences in maternal blood volume. As might be expected, mean MSAFP values become steadily lower as maternal weight increases. It may be possible to apply this biological characteristic when interpreting MSAFP results, but further work must be carried out before such refinements can be introduced routinely.

D.   MSAFP Assay Technique and Interpretation

1.   RADIOIMMUNOASSAY (RIA)

This is the only technique presently in general use that is capable of measuring AFP reliably in maternal serum. AFP concentrations normally range between the low and middle nanograms-per-milliliter range during the mid-second trimester. A variety of RIAs, including competitive double-antibody assays and solid-phase assays, all have proved successful. It is generally agreed that radioimmunoassays for AFP can be made to perform uniformly well and that AFP represents one of the more reliably measured substances in RIA systems (Knight, 1980).

a.   RIA Protocol for Measuring AFP in Second-Trimester Pregnancy Sera

Reagents

Goat antiserum to AFP	Purified AFP
Human male serum	Anti-goat antiserum
Normal goat serum (NGS)	Sodium barbital
Polyethylene glycol MW 6000	sodium chloride

Working Solutions

AFP antibody—Dilute goat anti-AFP in NGS buffer to give binding of 30–50% count of label input.

AFP standards—Use cord serum secondary standards that have been calibrated against World Health AFP standard (72/225), diluted in normal male serum (<2 KIU/liter) to 15, 30, 60, 90, 120, and 240 KIU/liter.

Assay buffer—0.005 mol/liter sodium barbital buffer pH 7.5, containing 50 ml/liter normal male serum (<2 IU/ml AFP) and 0.15 mol/liter sodium chloride

Normal goat serum buffer (NGS buffer), 0.25% normal goat serum—Dilute normal goat serum in assay buffer to final concentration of 0.25% (v/v).

Polyethylene Glycol—69 g/liter of PEG MW 6000 dissolved in distilled water

Rabbit anti-goat gamma globulin—Dilute in assay buffer to a concentration that precipitates maximum count in zero AFP assay tubes.

Tracer—Dilute ^{125}I-labeled AFP with assay buffer to an activity of approximately 20,000 cpm in 100 μl.

Procedure

Pipet 0.1 ml of samples, control pools, and standards into 10 × 75-mm disposable plastic tubes.

Pipet 0.1 ml of 0.25% NGS buffer into nonspecific binding tubes (NSB), followed by 0.1 ml of human male serum (<2 IU/ml) and 0.5 ml of assay buffer.

Add 0.1 ml ^{125}I-labeled AFP (20,000 cpm/0.1 ml) to all tubes.

Add 0.5 ml of assay buffer to all tubes except NSB tubes.

Add 0.1 ml of goat anti-AFP antibody previously diluted in NGS buffer to all tubes except NSB tubes.

Shake all tubes and incubate overnight at room temperature (16–24 hours).

Add 0.1 ml of diluted anti-goat antiserum to all tubes (optimum titer determined previously).

Shake all tubes and incubate for 45 minutes at 37°C.

Add 1.0 ml of 6.9% polyethylene glycol 6000 to each tube and shake well.

Centrifuge all tubes at 4°–8°C at 3000 rpm for 20 minutes.

Aspirate or decant supernatant and count the radioactivity of the bound ^{125}I-labeled AFP.

Calculations

Percent bound is calculated as follows:

$$\frac{\text{Standard or sample cpm} - \text{NSB cpm}}{\text{Zero standard cpm} - \text{NSB cpm}} \times 100 = \% \text{ bound (B/B)}$$

Plot % bound of standards versus concentration of AFP on logit-log paper to obtain dose–response curve. Read sample and control values from dose–response curve.

2. THE NINETIETH PERCENTILE OVER THE MEDIAN

The U.K. Collaborative Study (1977) has developed a ratio of the ninetieth percentile to the median, which demonstrates that NTD detection is influenced only to a minor degree when the AFP assay is performed with more or less precision. The major impact of imprecision is on the classification of singleton, non-NTD pregnancies, where a significantly greater number will be said to have elevated AFP levels with a less precise assay, at any given cutoff line.

3.   Quality Control

A quality-control scheme exists in the United Kingdom to monitor performance of the AFP assay and to provide advice, when needed and asked for (Cameron, 1978). Overall improvement in AFP assay performance over time has been documented by the scheme, and it is felt that the quality-control program has contributed to this. Besides encouraging good laboratory technique, the scheme can help an individual laboratory to identify rapidly when its assay is deteriorating. The external monitoring service emphasizes that its purpose is to encourage careful internal laboratory quality-control procedures, not to replace them. Further recommendations for quality control, including epidemiologic considerations, are contained in a report of a workshop sponsored by the National Institute of Child Health and Human Development (1980).

4.   Reference Materials

The World Health Organization (WHO) has prepared a lyophilized AFP standard 72/225 from cord serum with a value assigned in International Units. A British reference preparation has been similarly manufactured. The WHO preparation has been made available to manufacturers and scientists so that most laboratories are now able to compare results by conversion of mass units to International Units. The United States is currently in the process of making its own reference material, based on the WHO standard (Reimer, 1980).

5.   The Distribution of MSAFP Concentrations in the Second Trimester

Median MSAFP values rise throughout the second trimester. This is directly in contrast to median amniotic fluid AFP values during the same time period. It has been recommended that 100 maternal serum samples be assayed for each gestational week between 16 and 20 by a laboratory planning to establish AFP testing capabilities (Report of a Workshop Sponsored by the National Institute of Child Health and Human Development, 1980). This is a sufficient number to allow medians to be calculated confidently, after which cutoff points can be established. The need for accurate gestational dating is clearly apparent, both for constructing a normal curve and for interpreting clinical results.

6.   Menstrual Dates versus Ultrasound Dates for Maternal Serum AFP Interpretation

Biparietal diameters of spina bifida fetuses are smaller, on average, than established norms at a given gestational week in the second trimester (Wald *et al.*, 1980). This characteristic would cause spina bifida pregnancy dates to be underestimated by ultrasound. As a result, the maternal serum AFP level would appear higher, leading to an increased percentage of open spina bifida cases being identified. This advantage would be lost if ultrasound dating were also used for amniotic fluid interpretation, but would be maintained if menstrual dates were used for the latter interpretation.

7.　PROBLEMS OTHER THAN OPEN NTD ASSOCIATED WITH ELEVATED MSAFP LEVELS

Open ventral fetal lesions (omphalocele and gastroschisis) are among the other major defects identified through MSAFP elevations. Approximately 80% of these are associated with MSAFP levels at or above 2.5 MOM. Congenital nephrosis, a rare condition except in Finland, has also been documented as being associated with elevated maternal serum AFP levels. Pregnancies with MSAFP values greater than 3 MOM have roughly one chance in seven of a low-birth-weight outcome (Brock *et al.*, 1977; Wald *et al.*, 1977a,b). Although only a small portion of the total low-birth-weight outcomes are thus accounted for, this nevertheless defines a significant risk in a small group of pregnancies, possibly explained by feto–maternal hemorrhage. Women with elevated serum AFP levels also have approximately a 6-fold increased risk for miscarriage (Wald *et al.*, 1977b), and feto–maternal hemorrhage might also explain that phenomenon. In the U.K. Collaborative Study (1977), nearly half of all twin pregnancies were associated with MSAFP values greater than 2.5 MOM. At times, amniocentesis itself can produce rises in MSAFP levels, thus complicating interpretation of analyses from samples obtained after the procedure (Chard *et al.*, 1976).

8.　LOW MSAFP VALUES

Several pregnancy conditions, including hydatidiform moles, fetal demise, pseudopregnancy, and gross overestimation of dates, have been identified in association with low MSAFP levels (Report of the Working Group on Maternal Serum Alpha-Fetoprotein Screening, 1981). Many times the condition has been unsuspected until the AFP report. Therefore, it appears worthwhile to call attention to low MSAFP values for clinical purposes. One center (Oxford) has documented that a higher rate of induced labor occurs in women with low serum AFP values, leading to low-birth-weight outcomes. In this situation the low MSAFP value is a reflection of the clinician's having overestimated gestational age.

E.   Integration of MSAFP Screening with Ultrasonography and Amniocentesis

Sufficient MSAFP screening experience has accumulated both in the United Kingdom and in the United States to document that an organized protocol for patient management is important if services are to be delivered effectively (Haddow and Macri, 1979). This aspect of screening has been discussed at several conferences, and the necessary elements have been well defined.

Besides the necessity to assure that laboratory services are reliable and prompt, there should be a system to report elevated MSAFP values rapidly and to direct the physician and patient stepwise through the diagnostic process within a relatively brief time, allowing for the option to terminate the pregnancy, if necessary. Even though logistical problems occur due to the need to work with many individual physician offices, it is possible to solve most of them satisfactorily. The ability to respond to individual patient needs must be a primary consideration, and this can best be accomplished through an organized regional system that takes cost efficiency and quality control into account. Some programs may recommend a second blood sample for AFP analysis; all will recommend sonography for dating, twin identification, and assessment of viability. In the event that amniocentesis is indicated, processing and reporting of the amniotic fluid sample will have to be carried out rapidly. Throughout the process, information and counseling will have to be made available to the patient and physician.

REFERENCES

Althouse, R., and Wald, N. J. (1980). *Arch. Dis. Child.* **55,** 845–850.

Brock, D. J. H., and Sutcliffe, R. G. (1972). *Lancet* **2,** 197–199.

Brock, D. J. H., Bolton, A. E., and Monaghan, J. M. (1973). *Lancet* **2,** 923–924.

Brock, D. J. H., Bolton, A. E., and Scrimgeour, J. B. (1974). *Lancet* **1,** 767–769.

Brock, D. J. H., Barron, L., Jelen, P., Watt, M., and Scrimgeour, J. B. (1977). *Lancet* **2,** 267–268.

Cameron, E. H. D. (1978). *In* "Alpha-Fetoprotein Serum Screening in Pregnancy. Proceedings of the Second Scarborough Conference" (J. E. Haddow and J. N. Macri, eds.), pp. 157–165. Foundation for Blood Research, Scarborough, Maine.

Centers for Disease Control (1980). "Congenital Malformations Surveillance Report," April 1978–March 1979, p. 4.

Chard, T., Kitau, M. J., Ledward, R., Coltart, S., Embury, S., and Seller, M. J. (1976). *Br. J. Obstet. Gynaecol.* **83,** 33–34.

Gosden, C. M., and Brock, D. J. H. (1977a). *Lancet* **1,** 919–922.

Gosden, C. M., and Brock, D. J. H. (1977b). *Clin. Genet.* **12,** 193–201.

Gosden, C. M., and Brock, D. J. H. (1978a). *J. Med. Genet.* **15,** 262–270.

Gosden, C. M., and Brock, D. J. H. (1978b). *Br. Med. J.* **2,** 1186–1189.

Haddow, J. E., and Macri, J. N. (1979). *J.A.M.A.* **242,** 515–516.

Haddow, J. E., Macri, J. N., and Munson, M. E. (1979). *J. Lab. Clin. Med.* **94,** 344–347.

Haddow, J. E., Morin, M. E., Holman, M. S., and Miller, W. A. (1981a). *Clin. Chem.* **27,** 61–63.

Haddow, J. E., Kloza, E. M., Knight, G. J., and Smith, D. E. (1981b). *Clin. Chem.* **27,** 133–134.

Harris, R., Jennison, R. F., Barson, A. J., Laurence, K. M., Ruoslahti, E., and Seppala, M. (1974). *Lancet* **1,** 429–433.

Hay, D. L., Barrier, J. U., Davison, G. B., Buttery, B. W., Horacek, I., Pepperell, R. J., and Fliegner, J. R. H. (1979). *Br. J. Obstet. Gynaecol.* **86,** 516–520.

Hindersson, P., Toftager-Larsen, K., Nørgaard-Pedersen, B. (1979). *Lancet* **2,** 906.

Hino, M., Koki, Y., and Nishi, S. (1972). *Igaku No Ayumi* **82,** 512–515.

Kjessler, B., Johansson, S. G. O., Sherman, M., Gustavson, K.-H., and Hultquist, G. (1975). *Lancet* **1,** 432–433.

Kleihauer, E., Braun, H., and Betke, K. (1957). *Klin. Wochenschr.* **35,** 637–638.

Knight, G. J. (1980). Foundation for Blood Research, Scarborough, Maine. Personal communication.

Kunz, J., and Schmid, J. (1976). *Lancet* **1,** 47.

Laurell, C.-B. (1966). *Anal. Biochem.* **1,** 45–49.

Leek, A. E., Ruoss, C. F., Kitau, M. S., and Chard, T. (1973). *Lancet* **2,** 385.

Los, F. J., deWolf, B. T. H. M., and Huisses, H. J. (1979). *Lancet* **2,** 1210–1212.

Macri, J. N., and Weiss, R. R. (1976). *In* "XXIV Colloquium. Protides of the Biological Fluids," p. 88, Brugge, Belgium.

Miller, W. A. (1979). *In* "Alpha-Fetoprotein Serum Screening in Pregnancy: Proceedings of the Second Scarborough Conference" (J. E. Haddow and J. N. Macri, eds.), pp. 157–165. Foundation for Blood Research, Scarborough, Maine.

Miller, W. A., and Carroll, R. (1979). *In* "Proceedings of the American Society of Human Genetics," p. 78a, Minneapolis, Minnesota.

Nørgaard-Pedersen, B., Toftager-Larsen, K., Philip, J., and Hindersson, P. (1980). *Clin. Genet.* **17,** 355–362.

Reimer, C. (1980). Centers for Disease Control, Atlanta, Georgia. Personal communication.

Report of the U.K. Collaborative Study on Alpha-Fetoprotein in Relation to Neural-Tube Defects (1977). *Lancet* **1,** 1323.

Report of the Working Group on Amniotic Fluid Diagnostic Studies (1981). *In* "Alpha-Fetoprotein Screening. The Current Issues. Report of the Third Scarborough Conference" (J. E. Haddow and N. Wald, eds.) Foundation for Blood Research, Scarborough, Maine.

Report of the Working Group on Maternal Serum Alpha-Fetoprotein Screening (1981). *In* "Alpha-Fetoprotein Screening. The Current Issues. Report of the Third Scarborough Conference" (J. E. Haddow and N. Wald, eds.) Foundation for Blood Research, Scarborough, Maine.

Report of a Workshop Sponsored by the National Institute of Child Health and Human Development (NICHD) (1980). *Clin. Chim. Acta.* **105,** 9–24.

Ruoslahti, E. (1978). *In* "Prevention of Neural Tube Defects" (B. F. Crandall and M. A. B. Brazier, eds.), pp. 9–12. Academic Press, New York.

Second Report of the U.K. Collaborative Study on Alpha-Fetoprotein in Relation to Neural Tube Defects (1979). *Lancet* **2,** 651–661.

Seller, M. J., Singer, J. D., Coltart, T. M., and Campbell, S. (1974). *Lancet* **1,** 428–429.

Smith, A. D., Wald, N. J., and Cuckle, H. S. (1979). *Lancet* **1,** 685–688.

Smith, C. J., Kelleher, P. L., Belanger, L., and Dallaire, L. (1979). *Br. J. Med.* **1,** 920–921.

Sutherland, G. R., Brock, D. J. H., and Scrimgeour, J. B. (1973). *Lancet* **2,** 1098–1099.

Wald, N. J., Brock, D. J. H., and Bonnar, J. (1974). *Lancet* **1,** 765–767.

Wald, N. J., Barker, S., Cuckle, H. S., Brock, D. J. H., and Stirrat, G. M. (1977a). *Br. J. Obstet. Gynaecol.* **84,** 357–362.

Wald, N. J., Cuckle, H. S., Stirrat, G. M., Bennett, M. J., and Turnbull, A. C. (1977b). *Lancet* **2,** 268–270.

Wald, N. J., Cuckle, H. S., and Haddow, J. E. (1980). *Lancet* **2,** 690.

Wald, N. J., and Cuckle, H. S. (1980). *Br. J. Hosp. Med.* **23,** 473–489.

Chapter 5

Prenatal Diagnosis of Inherited Metabolic Diseases: Principles, Pitfalls, and Prospects[1]

GREGORY A. GRABOWSKI AND ROBERT J. DESNICK

Division of Medical Genetics
Mount Sinai School of Medicine
New York, New York

[1]Supported in part by grants (1-578 and 5-281) from the March of Dimes Birth Defects Foundation, a grant from the Muscular Dystrophy Association, and grants (GM 25279 and AM 26824) from the National Institutes of Health. G.A.G. is the recipient of an NIH Clinical Investigator Award (1 K08 HD00386) and a grant (RR-71) from the Division of Research Resources, General Clinical Research Centers Branch, National Institutes of Health, Bethesda, Maryland.

95

I. Introduction

During the past 20 years, major advances have been made in the identification, delineation, and understanding of inherited metabolic diseases (Stanbury *et al.*, 1978; Bondy and Rosenberg, 1980). The specific enzymatic defects have been identified in over 150 of the more than 400 catalogued inborn errors of metabolism (McKusick, 1978). Application of sophisticated biochemical, immunologic, and tissue-culture methods have provided precise metabolic diagnosis of affected individuals and accurate identification of carriers for the disease-causing genes. Increased understanding of the molecular and cellular pathology in specific disorders has provided the rationale for experimental strategies designed to treat these diseases (Desnick, 1981; Desnick and Grabowski, 1981), many of which are compatible with life, albeit severely debilitating. However, our therapeutic armamentarium is painfully limited, and the affected patients and their families have become increasingly disappointed by the absence of specific therapy.

Lacking the means to successfully treat or cure these devastating disorders, many parents who have had an affected child choose not to risk another pregnancy (Kaback *et al.*, 1977a,b). For these parents and for other at-risk couples identified by carrier-screening programs (Kaback, 1981), the development of methods to determine the health of the fetus prenatally has become a major consideration in their reproductive planning. Indeed, the advent of prenatal diagnosis for inherited metabolic disorders, in which the chance for an affected child is usually 25%, has enabled at-risk parents to selectively have only unaffected offspring. For such families, particularly those in which the firstborn was afflicted, the ability to monitor subsequent pregnancies and the option to prevent the birth of affected offspring has been an important component in maintaining the integrity and psychologic well-being of the family unit.

Thus the purpose of this article is to identify the inherited metabolic disorders in which the prenatal diagnosis has been reliably *made,* to indicate the disorders in which prenatal diagnosis is *feasible* using currently available procedures, and finally, to specify those disorders in which the prenatal diagnosis may be *plausible* using experimental methods for obtaining certain fetal tissues and/or by the future application of newer immunologic or molecular technologies to demonstrate the metabolic or genetic defect.

II.   Principles of Prenatal Metabolic Diagnosis

The prenatal diagnosis of an inherited metabolic disease is based on the demonstration of the metabolic or cellular defect in fetal tissues or fluids. Amniotic fluid cells, safely obtained by transabdominal amniocentesis (NICHD National Registry for Amniocentesis Study Group, 1976; Simpson *et al.,* 1976; MRC Working Party on Amniocentesis, 1978; Aula *et al.,* 1979b) and grown by standard tissue-culture techniques, have proved the most reliable fetal diagnostic source for most diseases. In certain disorders the metabolic or cellular defect is not expressed in the cultured amniotic cells or in the amniotic fluid, and more invasive techniques may be required to obtain other fetal tissues for diagnostic studies. In most disorders the laboratory diagnosis has been based on the demonstration of the specific enzymatic deficiency. Certain disorders have been diagnosed by the chemical analysis of the amniotic fluid or by newer techniques including characterization of fibroblast HLA haplotypes (Pollack *et al.,* 1979; Rosenmann *et al.,* 1980), the use of recombinant DNA techniques (Kan and Dozy, 1978; Kan *et al.,* 1980; Orkin *et al.,* 1978), or the characterization of enzymes or proteins in fetal blood components (see Chap. 7). The requisites and laboratory diagnostic techniques for the prenatal diagnosis of inherited metabolic diseases are discussed in the following section.

A.   Requisites for Prenatal Metabolic Diagnosis

1.   GENETIC COUNSELING

Although it is not the purpose of this article to discuss genetic counseling, it should be clearly recognized that fundamental to the prenatal diagnosis of any disorder is the provision of nondirective genetic counseling. It is essential that the at-risk couple be informed of all their reproductive options. If they choose to undergo prenatal diagnostic studies, they must understand the risks of the procedures required to obtain the appropriate specimens for analysis. Discussions of the ethical, moral, and legal aspects of prenatal diagnosis are available (Friedman, 1974; Fletcher, 1979; Milunsky, 1976, 1979; Powledge and Fletcher, 1979; Thompson, 1979).

2.   PRECISE DIAGNOSIS

Prior to undertaking the prenatal diagnosis of any inherited metabolic disease, it is essential to establish or confirm the specific diagnosis. Efforts must be directed to eliminating the possibility of misdiagnosis due to phenotypic, metabolic, or genetic heterogeneity. The precise enzymatic defect must be demonstrated in the proband or other affected relatives (preferably in cultured skin fibroblasts, if expressed). If the proband is deceased, the heterozygosity of both parents for the disease-causing gene must be determined. In all assays for homozygosity or heterozygosity, care must be taken to demonstrate simultaneously the metabolic defect using the appropriate substrate or reference standards in sources from confirmed cases and normal controls under the same conditions, cell density, and so on. Laboratories not previously experienced in a specified assay should consult with and split samples with expert laboratories in order to ensure proper diagnosis.

3. CONFIRMATION OF PARENTAL HETEROZYGOSITY

Even when the precise diagnosis of the proband has been established, the heterozygosity of both parents should be confirmed for autosomal recessive disorders. Heterozygote status for X-linked traits and for dominantly inherited metabolic disorders (e.g., various porphyrias) also must be enzymatically or biochemically documented. These assays are useful because they establish the levels of the critical enzyme or metabolite in the obligate heterozygotes and facilitate interpretation of the fetal diagnosis.

4. DEMONSTRATION OF GENE EXPRESSION IN FETAL SOURCES

It is essential that the specific enzyme or metabolite to be determined is expressed in the fetal source. This is particularly true for amniotic fluid cells, because a culture may be primarily epithelial rather than fibroblastic. The range of normal values as well as the assay sensitivity and reproducibility must be established; this requirement is also essential for cell or tissue sources other than amniocytes.

For certain disorders, the prenatal diagnosis can be made or supported by more than one determination. For example, (1) two different substrates may be used to measure the enzymatic activity; (2) the enzymatic activity may be visualized by electrophoretic or isoelectric-focusing techniques; or (3) the concentrations of the substrate and/or product may be determined in cultured amniotic cells or amniotic fluid. Every effort should be made to carry out these studies to support the diagnosis.

5. CONFIRMATION OF THE PRENATAL DIAGNOSIS

Following the termination of a fetus diagnosed as affected, studies should be performed to confirm the diagnosis. The increasing use of the dilatation and extraction procedure not only affords the woman a safe and rapid termination without the induction of labor (Grimes *et al.*, 1977), but it also permits confirmation of the prenatal diagnosis with suitable specimens for metabolic and ultrastructural studies. When the parents have decided to carry an affected pregnancy to term, preparations should be made to confirm the diagnosis and institute appropriate therapeutic intervention immediately after delivery. Monitored fetuses that were diagnosed as unaffected also should be confirmed by obtaining placental tissue, amnion, and/or cord blood at delivery. Studies that require fibroblasts can be easily obtained from males that are circumcised. The results of the confirmatory studies on both affected fetuses and unaffected newborns should be transmitted to the referring physician and parents as soon as possible.

B. Methods for Prenatal Metabolic Diagnosis

1. Enzyme and Metabolite Analyses

For disorders in which the specific enzymatic defect can be demonstrated in cultured skin fibroblasts, the prenatal diagnosis usually can be accomplished using cultured amniotic cells. Care must be taken to determine the normal levels of the specified enzyme in both fibroblast-like and epithelial-like amniotic cells grown under identical culture conditions (i.e., cell density, number of passages, etc.). For unstable enzymes, such as β-hexosaminidase A and α-galactosidase A, adequate amounts of cell protein or additional albumin must be used to ensure adequate enzyme stability during assay.

The use of uncultured amniotic cells or cell-free amniotic fluid has been reported for the diagnosis of several inborn errors by determination of the specific enzyme or metabolites (Matalon *et al.*, 1970; O'Brien *et al.*, 1971; Christamanou *et al.*, 1978). However, particular care is required in the interpretation of data from these sources. For example, enzyme levels determined directly on uncultured amniocytes may give low specific activities because only a few cells are viable. If an enzyme or metabolite is unstable, direct assay of amniocytes or amniotic fluid may give uninterpretable values, perhaps leading to a false-positive diagnosis (e.g., Davidson and Rattazzi, 1972). Also, erroneous false-negative results may result from an undetected admixture of fetal and maternal cells. In addition, the levels of soluble enzymes or metabolites in amniotic fluid must be compared to values from adequate numbers of normal control fluids matched for gestational age by ultrasound, because these levels may increase or decrease with advancing gestation as well as in twin pregnancies.

Newer methods have been designed to increase the sensitivity and accuracy of diagnostic assays as well as to decrease the psychologically burdensome period from amniocentesis to diagnosis. These include the use of enzyme microassays using single or small numbers of cultured cells (see Chap. 8) or assays in cultured cells *in situ* following endocytosis of fluorescent or fluorogenic natural substrates (Gatt, 1981, personal communication).

The characterization and visualization of the specified enzyme or isozyme by isoelectric-focusing and electrophoretic techniques provide diagnostic information that is clearly superior to enzymatic activity levels alone. Application of immunologic techniques, including quantitative radioimmunoassay or rocket-immunoelectrophoretic procedures, provide specific assays that are not complicated by the presence of other isozymes that may metabolize the artificial or natural substrates used for direct enzyme determinations. When immunologic techniques are used to specifically quantitate enzyme protein, prior studies of the defective enzyme in the same or similar source from the proband must be accomplished in order to determine the presence of cross-reactive immunologic material (CRIM-positive) or absence of the enzyme protein (CRIM-negative) (Anderson and Desnick, 1981). In the future, it is likely that monoclonal antibodies will be available for many of the enzymes involved in these disorders. The CRIM status for a given enzymatic defect can be characterized in each family using a battery of monoclonal antibodies with different specificities toward the normal protein. In this way, an antigenic profile of the defective enzyme protein can be established, and qualitative as well as quantitative differences from the normal protein (if any) may be useful diagnostically. It is conceivable that monoclonal antibody batteries for a large variety of enzyme proteins will become available in the near future (either commercially or from individual investigators) and that prenatal diagnostic studies for certain metabolic disorders will be made using the same standardized, sensitive reagents in all laboratories. Such studies will not only facilitate rapid prenatal diagnoses, but also provide increased characterization of the antigenic architecture of various defective proteins.

2. FETOSCOPY FOR FETAL BLOOD ASPIRATION AND SKIN BIOPSY

Use of the fiberoptic fetoscope has permitted the direct visualization of the fetus and placenta (Valenti, 1972; Hobbins *et al.*, 1974; Benzie and Doran, 1975; Hobbins, 1979). Midtrimester fetoscopy has been successfully performed to facilitate the collection of fetal blood (Kan *et al.*, 1974; Hobbins and Mahoney, 1974; Golbus *et al.*, 1976; Rodeck and Campbell, 1978, 1979) and fetal skin (Valenti; 1972; Golbus *et al.*, 1980; Rodeck *et al.*, 1980). Several different techniques for obtaining fetal blood have been used, including blind placental aspiration, puncture of a vessel on the chorionic plate, and, more recently, direct aspiration from the cord. The latter procedure allows the collection of fetal blood without contamination by maternal cells or amniotic fluid (Rodeck, 1980).

Fetal blood aspiration has been used successfully for the prenatal diagnosis of hemophilia due to Factor VIII (Firshein *et al.*, 1979) and Factor IX deficiency

(Holmberg, 1980), von Willebrand's disease (Rodeck *et al.*, 1979), and various hemoglobinopathies (see Chap. 7) including β-thalassemia and sickle cell disease (Hobbins and Mahoney, 1974; Kan *et al.*, 1977; Fairweather *et al.*, 1978, 1980). Further applications of this technique are obvious, especially for the prenatal diagnosis of metabolic defects expressed in erythrocytes, leukocytes, platelets, and/or plasma (see Chap. 7). These sources should be used for direct assay of the primary defect because the measurement of a secondary alteration (e.g., serum creatinine phosphokinase in Duchenne muscular dystrophy) may prove unreliable (Golbus *et al.*, 1979). However, fetal blood aspiration has proved valuable for the prenatal diagnosis of chronic granulomatous disease by the demonstration of defective nitroblue tetrazolium reduction and superoxide dismutase generation in fetal granulocytes (Newburger *et al.*, 1979). In addition, fetal blood aspiration has proved useful for the diagnosis of inborn errors that can be detected in cultured amniocytes (i.e., galactosemia), when the patient scheduled so late that the amniotic cell culture result could not be available before 24 weeks gestation (Fenson *et al.*, 1979). Finally, in two cases of severe Rhesus isoimmunization, fetoscopy has been used to infuse blood directly into umbilical vessels at either the umbilicus or the placental cord insertion, indicating the ability to administer blood or other therapeutic agents into the fetal circulation (Rodeck *et al.*, 1981).

The recent demonstration that fetal skin can be biopsied under fetoscopic guidance (Golbus *et al.*, 1980; Rodeck *et al.*, 1980) has opened the possibilities for the prenatal diagnosis of metabolic abnormalities with dermatologic manifestations. The diagnosis of epidermolysis bullosa lethalis was accomplished by electron microscopy of a fetal skin biopsy at 18 weeks gestation (Rodeck *et al.*, 1980). Similarly, the diagnosis of congenital bullous ichthyosiform erythroderma, a dominantly inherited trait, was made by light- and electron-microscopic examination of a fetal skin biopsy (Golbus *et al.*, 1980). These prototype diagnoses have shown the feasibility and relative safety of fetal skin biopsies and indicate that this technique may be useful for other dermatogenoses. A further recent extension of fetoscopy has been the successful percutaneous needle biopsy of fetal liver and the diagnosis of ornithine carbamyltransferase deficiency (Rodeck, 1981, personal communication). A more comprehensive review of the application of fetoscopy and the fetoscopic-guided collection of fetal blood and tissues is presented in Chapter 7.

3. LINKAGE STUDIES

Another approach for the prenatal diagnosis of metabolic defects that are not expressed in cultured amniotic cells is the use of linkage analysis. For example, the gene for 21-hydroxylase deficiency (the metabolic defect in one form of congenital adrenal hyperplasia) is closely linked to the HLA-B locus on chromosome 6 (Levine *et al.*, 1978). HLA genotyping of family members has permitted the identification of heterozygous and previously undiagnosed homozygous affected siblings. Because the HLA genotype of cultured amniotic cells can be determined, this marker already has proved useful for the prenatal diagnosis of 21-hydroxylase deficiency in several at-risk families (Pollack *et al.*, 1979; Rosenmann *et al.*, 1980). It should be noted that the genes for other recessively inherited forms of congenital adrenal hyperplasia are not closely linked to this marker (New *et al.*, 1979; Mantero *et al.*, 1980). To date, linkage to the HLA complex has been established for only three other monogenic disorders, dominantly inherited spinocerebellar ataxia (Jackson *et al.*, 1977), recessively inherited idiopathic hemochromatosis (Simon *et al.*, 1977a), and inherited hypertrophic cardiomyopathy (Darsee *et al.*, 1979). For these disorders, HLA genotyping might provide useful prenatal diagnostic information. However, for other disorders that have HLA-disease associations—including those of nongenetic, multifactorial, or monogenic etiologies—this approach will not be useful because close genetic linkage is required. As point in fact, an association between certain HLA antigens and recessively inherited nephropathic cystinosis has been established, but close linkage between these loci could not be demonstrated (Steinherz *et al.*, 1981), thereby precluding the use of fibroblast HLA genotyping for prenatal diagnosis.

Experience with linkage studies for the prenatal diagnosis of myotonic dystrophy is instructive. The gene for this dominantly inherited disease is closely linked to the ABH secretor locus (Renwick and Bolling, 1971). By determining the fetal secretor type from amniotic fluid, it has been estimated that the diagnosis of myotonic dystrophy can be made with at least 75% certainty in about 10–35% of at-risk pregnancies (Omenn and Schrott, 1973; Insley *et al.*, 1976). To date, two prenatal diagnoses for myotonic dystrophy by fetal ABH-secretor linkage studies have been reported (Omenn and Schrott, 1973; Insley *et al.*, 1976). Of these, one was diagnosed as affected and subsequently terminated; the other was diagnosed as normal (Insley *et al.*, 1976). Unfortunately, it is not possible to confirm an affected diagnosis in the fetus, and because onset of the disease is delayed, a normal diagnosis cannot be verified for years. Although the linkage is close, the inability to confirm the diagnoses and the fact that so few at-risk families can benefit from linkage studies, illustrate the limitations of this approach. However, it should be noted that the number of human genes being assigned to specific subchromosomal regions is increasing at an accelerating rate (Evans *et al.*, 1979). Therefore, it is likely that the identification of closely linked markers that are expressed in cultured amniotic cells, amniotic fluid, or blood components will facilitate the reliable diagnosis of currently undiagnosable disorders such as phenylketonuria due to phenylalanine hydroxylase deficiency (see Chap. 11).

4. ISOLATION OF FETAL CELLS FROM THE MATERNAL CIRCULATION

Because fetal blood cells, including nucleated erythrocytes and lymphocytes, have been detected in maternal blood after 14 weeks gestation, methods have been sought to selectively isolate the fetal cells for prenatal diagnostic studies. Using a fluorescence-activated cell sorter and fluorescent-tagged antifetal antibodies (e.g., anti-newborn lymphocyte or anti-Y antibodies), fetal lymphocytes have been selectively isolated from maternal cells (Chap. 10). This approach has been used to isolate fetal lymphocytes for chromosome analysis and has potential application for the diagnosis of metabolic disorders expressed in fetal erythrocytes and/or lymphocytes (see Chap. 7). However, adequate numbers of cells must be obtained to permit the detection of chromosomal mosaicism and heterozygosity for X-linked traits.

5. SOMATIC CELL HYBRIDIZATION FOR DIFFERENTIATED GENE EXPRESSION

The expression of human tissue-specific or differentiated gene functions in somatic cell hybrids of human amniocytes and rat hepatoma lines (Rankin and Darlington, 1979) suggested that such human genes might be expressed by fetal amniotic cells after hybridization with an appropriate rodent line. For example, amniotic cells from a fetus at risk for a liver-specific function, like α_1-antitrypsin deficiency or phenylalanine hydroxylase deficiency, might be induced to express the gene product by this technique. If such differentiated functions can be readily expressed and quantitated efficiently, this sophisticated approach may permit the prenatal diagnosis of a number of disorders that cannot be diagnosed by current methods (see Chap. 11).

6. GENETIC DIAGNOSIS USING RECOMBINANT DNA TECHNIQUES

The advent of recombinant DNA technology already has had a remarkable impact on the prenatal diagnosis of the hemoglobinopathies using cultured and uncultured amniotic cells (see Chap. 12). Methods for the isolation of pure mRNAs for the α- and β-globins have permitted the *in vitro* synthesis of radioactive complementary DNA (cDNA) for the respective globin. The cDNA probes can be used to detect normal, defective, or deleted α- or β-globin genes in leukocytes or cultured fibroblasts by the use of molecular hybridization (cot curves) or by gene-mapping techniques using restriction endonucleases (Alter, 1979; see Chap. 12). Using these methods, the various α-thalassemia states, $\delta\beta$-thalassemias and β°-thalassemia, which result from the respective deletion of α-, β-, and δ-, and β-globin genes, can be detected in cultured amniotic cells from at-risk fetuses (Kan *et al.*, 1976; Orkin *et al.*, 1978, 1979). These molecular techniques have been used recently for the prenatal diagnosis of β°-thalassemia in conjunction with a prospective genetic-screening program to identify at-risk couples in Sardinia (Kan *et al.*, 1980).

Restriction endonuclease (Hpa I) mapping of the β-globin gene revealed that an unusually high percentage of individuals with the sickle cell mutation had a 13 kilobase DNA fragment that contained their β-globin gene, whereas the β-globin gene from normal individuals was usually found in a 7.0 or 7.6 kilobase segment (Kan and Dozy, 1978). When peripheral leukocytes from both the mother and father of a fetus at risk for sickle cell disease are shown to be heterozygous for the 13 kilobase fragment, the prenatal diagnosis can be accomplished by restriction endonuclease studies of the cultured amniotic cells. In this way, sickle cell disease can be diagnosed without performing the higher-risk fetoscopy and fetal blood aspiration procedures. Similarly, a DNA polymorphism in the β-globin gene for one form of β°-thalassemia has been identified and used for prenatal diagnosis (Kan *et al.*, 1980).

The application of these molecular techniques for the prenatal diagnosis of the hemoglobinopathies was possible because highly purified mRNA molecules for the α- and β-globin chains could be isolated from thalassemic reticulocytes. Extension of these methods to the diagnosis of other inborn errors has been limited by the technologic difficulty of isolating the respective normal mRNA, which usually represents less than 1% of the total cellular mRNA. The availability of monospecific antibodies or the amino acid sequence is requisite for the immunoprecipitation of the specific mRNA or for the construction of an oligonucleotide probe for mRNA hybridization and isolation, respectively. For many enzyme-deficiency diseases, the normal enzyme has not been purified to homogeneity or in sufficient amounts to permit antibody production or amino acid sequencing. When improved methods are developed to isolate the mRNA molecules, which occur in only a few copies per cell, then cDNA probes can be made. Once these probes are available, it will be possible to use gene mapping, or ultimately, DNA-sequencing techniques, to characterize the gene mutations using cultured amniotic cells. This approach may become the technique of choice in the future, provided the current technologic obstacles can be overcome.

III. Prenatal Metabolic Diagnosis: Current and Potential Methods

A. Disorders of Sphingolipid Metabolism (Table I)

The disorders of sphingolipid metabolism (Table I) are characterized by the lysosomal accumulation of particular substrates due to specific enzyme defects in the sequential hydrolysis of the glycosidic and lipid moieties of sphingolipids. Comprehensive reviews of the clinical, pathologic, and biochemical abnormalities in each of these diseases are available (Stanbury *et al.*, 1978; Bondy and

TABLE I

DISORDERS OF SPHINGOLIPID METABOLISM

Disorder	McKusick catalog no.	Enzyme defect	Method of diagnosis	Prenatal diagnosis[a]	Method of prenatal diagnosis
Farber disease	22800	Ceramidase	Dulaney et al. (1976); Moser (1978)	Feasible	Dulaney et al. (1976)
Fabry disease	30150	α-Galactosidase A	Desnick et al. (1973b)	Made	Reddy (1977)
Gaucher disease					
1	23080	Acid β-glucosidase	Peters et al. (1977); Wenger et al. (1978a)	Made	Kitagawa et al. (1978); Hakansson and Svennerholm (1979)
2	23096	Acid β-glucosidase	Peters et al. (1977); Wenger et al. (1978a)	Made	Schneider et al. (1972); Hakansson and Svennerholm (1979)
3	23100	Acid β-glucosidase	Peters et al. (1977); Wenger et al. (1978a)	Made	Kitagawa et al. (1978)
Krabbe	24520	Galactocerebroside: β-galactosidase	Suzuki (1977)	Made	Suzuki et al. (1971)
G$_{M1}$-Gangliosidosis					
Infantile	23050	G$_{M1}$-ganglioside: β-galactosidase	Ho and O'Brien (1971)	Made	Booth et al. (1973); Lowden et al. (1973)
Juvenile	23060	G$_{M1}$-ganglioside: β-galactosidase	Lowden et al. (1974)	Feasible	Booth et al. (1973); Lowden et al. (1973)
Adult	23065	G$_{M1}$-ganglioside: β-galactosidase	Stevenson et al. (1978)	Feasible	Booth et al. (1973); Lowden et al. (1973)

(continued)

TABLE I (*continued*)

Disorder	McKusick catalog no.	Enzyme defect	Method of diagnosis	Prenatal diagnosis[a]	Method of prenatal diagnosis
G_{M2}-Gangliosidosis Tay-Sachs disease	27280	β-Hexosaminidase A	Kaback (1972)	Made	Dance *et al.* (1970); O'Brien *et al.* (1971); Rattazzi and Davidson (1972)
Juvenile	27277	β-Hexosaminidase A	Suzuki and Suzuki (1970)	Feasible	Dance *et al.* (1970); O'Brien *et al.* (1971); Rattazzi and Davidson (1972)
Adult	23073	β-Hexosaminidase A	Willner *et al.* (1981)	Feasible	Dance *et al.* (1970); O'Brien *et al.* (1971); Rattazzi and Davidson (1972)
Sandhoff disease Infantile	26880	β-Hexosaminidase A and B	Sandhoff *et al.* (1968); Ikonne *et al.* (1975)	Made	Desnick *et al.* (1973a)
Juvenile	26875	β-Hexosaminidase A and B	Wood and MacDougall (1976)	Feasible	Desnick *et al.* (1973a)
G_{M2}-Gangliosidosis AB variant	27275	β-Hexosaminidase activator	Conzelman and Sandhoff (1978)	Feasible	

106

Mucolipidosis IV	25265	Ganglioside neuraminidase (α-2,8)	Bach et al. (1975); Merin et al. (1975); Livni and Legum (1976)	Feasible	Bach et al. (1975, 1980)
Nieman-Pick disease					
Type A	25720	Sphingomyelinase	Wenger (1977); Gatt et al. (1978)	Made	Patrick et al. (1977); Wenger (1977)
Type B	25720	Sphingomyelinase	Callahan et al. (1975)	Feasible	Patrick et al. (1977); Wenger (1977)
Type C	25720	Sphingomyelinase	Callahan and Khalil (1975)	Feasible	Patrick et al. (1977); Wenger (1977)
Type D	25725	Sphingomyelinase (?)	Rao and Spence (1977)	Not possible	
Type E	25725	Sphingomyelinase (?)		Not possible	
Metachromatic leukodystrophy Infantile Juvenile Adult	25010	Arylsulfatase A	Potter et al. (1972); Dulaney and Moser (1977); Farrell et al. (1979)	Made	Potter et al. (1972); Leroy et al. (1973)
Metachromatic leukodystrophy	—	Galactocerebroside sulfate sulfatase activator	Fischer and Jatzkewitz (1975)	Feasible	
Multiple sulfatase deficiency	27220	Arylsulfatase A, B, C and steroid sulfatase	Eto et al. (1974); Fiddler et al. (1979); Fluharty et al. (1979)	Feasible	

[a] Explanation of terms:

Made—Prenatal diagnosis has been accomplished and confirmed.

Feasible—Methods are currently available or current techniques could be adapted for the prenatal diagnosis.

Plausible—Various strategies can or theoretically could be employed, on an experimental basis, and their use evaluated for prenatal diagnosis.

Not possible—Primary defect is not defined, secondary metabolic effects cannot presently be assessed, or technical difficulties must be overcome before the prenatal diagnosis is feasible.

Rosenberg, 1980). Table I references the methods used for the enzymatic diagnosis of affected individuals and for the prenatal diagnosis of each disease.

In most of these disorders, the prenatal diagnosis has been made by the demonstration of the enzymatic defect in cultured amniotic cells. To date, several hundred at-risk pregnancies for this group of disorders have been prenatally monitored. Fetuses diagnosed as affected and terminated have been confirmed by pathologic and enzymatic studies of affected tissues and fluids. However, certain of these disorders require further discussion related to potential pitfalls in their prenatal diagnosis.

1. G_{M2}-GANGLIOSIDOSIS

a. Tay-Sachs Disease. Tay-Sachs disease (β-hexosaminidase A deficiency) is the prototype disorder for prospective carrier detection and prenatal diagnosis of inherited metabolic diseases. Since the initiation of carrier screening in 1970, over 312,000 persons (primarily Ashkenazi Jews) have been tested for Tay-Sachs carrier status, and over 12,760 carriers have been identified, including more than 265 carrier couples. Over 800 at-risk pregnancies have been monitored for Tay-Sachs disease, and 175 fetuses with Tay-Sachs disease have been detected. Of the monitored pregnancies, over 250 were in families identified prospectively by carrier screening (Kaback, 1981, personal communication). The extensive experience with Tay-Sachs screening and prevention has demonstrated the effectiveness of this prototype program (Kaback *et al.,* 1977a,b). In addition, the potential pitfalls have been identified, which should prove instructive for future screening and prevention of other disorders that occur in high frequency among certain ethnic or demographic groups.

Optimal Prenatal Detection. Prenatal diagnostic studies should be based on the demonstration of deficient β-hexosaminidase A activity in cultured fibroblasts (Lowden *et al.,* 1977). The diagnosis should be confirmed by the electrophoretic demonstration of the enzymatic deficiency. Although cell-free amniotic fluid and uncultured amniocytes may be used for a preliminary indication, the definitive diagnosis should be based on the studies of cultured amniotic cells.

Heterozygote Identification. Heterozygosity for β-hexosaminidase A deficiency can be reliably predicted in over 97% of tested individuals by the demonstration of intermediate levels of enzymatic activity in serum or plasma (Kaback 1972). Significantly, pregnancy, the use of oral contraceptives or certain other drugs, and diabetes mellitus may alter the plasma or serum levels and lead to false-positive results (Kaback, 1972; Delvin *et al.,* 1974). Because many couples are screened for carrier status during pregnancy, the β-hexosaminidase assay should be performed in isolated peripheral blood leukocytes (Lowden *et al.,* 1977) and/or tears (Desnick *et al.,* 1977), which will give reliable assay results and avoid unnecessary amniocenteses and psychologic trauma to the family.

b. β-Hexosaminidase A Variants. Since the identification of deficient β-hexosaminidase A activity as the primary defect in Tay-Sachs disease (Okada and O'Brien, 1969), several other β-hexosaminidase A deficient variants have been described. These include juvenile-onset G_{M2}-gangliosidosis (Okada *et al.*, 1970; Suzuki and Suzuki, 1970; Brett *et al.*, 1973), later-onset disorders termed chronic and adult G_{M2}-gangliosidoses (Navon *et al.*, 1973, 1980; Rapin *et al.*, 1976; Yaffe *et al.*, 1979; Grabowski *et al.*, 1980a,b; Willner *et al.*, 1981), and β-hexosaminidase A deficiency in asymptomatic adults (Vidgoff *et al.*, 1973; O'Brien *et al.*, 1978; Thomas, 1981, personal communication). The chronic and adult G_{M2}-gangliosidosis variants have been reported in Ashkenazi Jewish individuals with onset of neurologic manifestations (ataxia, dysarthria, muscle weakness, and in some families, dementia) in childhood, adolescence, or adult life. Standard artificial substrate assays of β-hexosaminidase A activity in cultured fibroblasts (and presumably cultured amniotic cells) cannot differentiate the chronic or adult variants from infantile Tay-Sachs disease, or more importantly, from the apparently healthy individuals who have β-hexosaminidase A deficiency. Therefore, Kaback (1981) estimated that 1 in 20 affected fetuses detected in pregnancies of couples identified by carrier screening may have a variant β-hexosaminidase A deficiency other than classic Tay-Sachs disease. Further studies of the G_{M2}-ganglioside-cleaving activity in fibroblasts may provide a means to discriminate among these variants. However, because heterozygotes for these β-hexosaminidase A deficiency variants are enzymatically indistinguishable from classic Tay-Sachs disease, the phenotype of β-hexosaminidase A-deficient fetuses of carrier couples (identified by screening) cannot be predicted with certainty.

c. AB Variant. Recently, patients with the AB variant of G_{M2}-gangliosidosis have been recognized (Sandhoff *et al.*, 1968, 1971). The infantile disorder presents with a phenotype similar to infantile Sandhoff disease. In this disease, the activities of both β-hexosaminidases A and B are elevated when determined with artificial substrates, whereas hydrolytic activity toward the natural substrate is totally deficient in the absence of a specific activator molecule (Conzelman and Sandhoff, 1978). The prenatal diagnosis of this rare disease is possible by the determination of β-hexosaminidase A and B activities with natural substrate in the presence and absence of the specific purified activator or by quantitative immunologic determination of the activator molecule in cultured amniotic cells.

2. GAUCHER DISEASE

a. Genetic Heterogeneity. Gaucher disease (deficient acid β-glucosidase) is a phenotypically heterogeneous disorder with three major subtypes, each inherited as a distinct autosomal recessive trait. Type 1 disease has a predilection for Ashkenazi Jewish individuals (gene frequency $\simeq 0.02$) and is characterized by reticuloendothelial deposition of glucosyl ceramide and no neurologic involvement. Great variation in the severity of the clinical manifestations (i.e., hepatosplenomegaly and bony abnormalities) has been observed between and within families. For example, severely involved children with massive splenomegaly by 6 to 10 years as well as asymptomatic individuals in the eighth decade of life have been described (Beutler, 1977; Brady, 1978). In contrast to the variable expressivity characteristic of Type 1 disease, the clinical course of Type 2, the neurologic form, is constant. Affected individuals present with failure to thrive and neurologic involvement at 4 to 8 months of life. The neurologic involvement is progressive, and death usually occurs by 2 years of age. Type 2 disease is extremely rare, and there is no ethnic or demographic predilection. Type 3 disease is characterized by onset in childhood of both reticuloendothelial and neurologic manifestations. Type 3 disease is primarily limited to a genetic isolate located north of the Arctic Circle in Norbotten, Sweden (Dreborg et al., 1980). Individuals affected with this subtype usually expire from disease complications in the second or third decade of life.

Enzymatic diagnosis of individuals with each subtype has revealed the presence of residual acid β-glucosidase activity. Using the artificial substrate, 4-methylumbelliferyl-β-D-glucopyranoside, to assay acid β-glucosidase in cultured skin fibroblasts—the most reliable enzyme source because only the acid isozyme is expressed (Shafit-Zagardo et al., 1980)—Type 1 homozygotes have approximately 15–30% of mean normal activity, whereas the Type 2 and Type 3 homozygotes have about 5–10% and 10–15% of mean normal activity, respectively.

b. Heterozygote Detection. Efforts to identify heterozygotes for Type 1 disease among individuals of Ashkenazi Jewish ancestry ($2pq \simeq 1/25$) on a mass-screening basis have been precluded due to the inability to reliably detect heterozygous levels of acid β-glucosidase in sources other than cultured fibroblasts (Peters et al., 1977; Wenger et al., 1978a,b; Wenger and Olson, 1981). The major problem is the occurrence of a neutral β-glucosidase activity that also hydrolyzes the artificial substrate in all tissues, except cultured fibroblasts. Even though "reliable assays" have been developed in individual laboratories (Brady et al., 1965; Beutler and Kuhl, 1970; Wenger et al., 1978a,b; Peters et al., 1979), the enzymatic data obtained are not comparable among investigators (Peters et al., 1979). Thus at present each laboratory must establish an assay procedure with adequate numbers of normal, obligate heterozygote and homozygote control values. Current efforts are directed toward the development of an assay using the natural substrate that will be easily adapted for large-scale heterozygote screening using isolated leukocytes. If such an assay can reliably distinguish heterozygotes for Type 1 disease, then this assay can be performed in conjunction with Tay-Sachs heterozygote screening in approved centers.

c. Prenatal Diagnosis. The prenatal diagnosis of fetuses affected with Type 2 disease is straightforward and has been made using cultured amniotic cells in several centers (Schneider *et al.*, 1972; Kitagawa *et al.*, 1978; Desnick and Reddy, unpublished results). The prenatal diagnosis of Types 1 and 3 diseases are more difficult due to the presence of significant amounts of residual activity in affected homozygotes. Therefore, extreme care must be used to maximize the enzymatic discrimination of affected homozygotes from heterozygous carriers. This is particularly true for the diagnosis of Type 1 disease where the residual activity may approach that found in some heterozygous individuals. Particular attention must be directed to (1) the enzymatic assay conditions; (2) the use of adequate numbers of control amniotic cell lines, particularly from a homozygote and obligate heterozygote from the family at risk; and (3) the rigorous control of the culture conditions and degree of confluency. Moreover, the level of residual activity may vary 3- to 5-fold in amniocytes of affected fetuses, and 2- to 3-fold in normal (nonheterozygote) amniocytes, depending on the culture conditions, composition of the media (Beutler *et al.*, 1971; Hakansson, 1979; Hakansson and Svennerholm, 1979), and degree of confluency (Heukels-Dully and Niermeyer, 1976). This variation in β-glucosidase activity in amniocytes may not be significant for the prenatal diagnosis of the Type 2 and Type 3 disease because the level of residual activity is exceedingly low (Hakansson, 1979). However, in Type 1 Gaucher, the residual activity in fibroblasts (and presumably amniocytes) may overlap with the obligate heterozygote range depending on the assay conditions (especially pH) and culture media (Beutler *et al.*, 1971. When monospecific anti-β-glucosidase antibodies are available, the levels of CRIM-specific activity should abrogate problems with the assay based on activity alone.

Finally, certain ethical considerations are involved in the prenatal diagnosis of Type 1 Gaucher disease. As noted above, this subtype is characterized by marked variation in the clinical severity of the disease, even among affected individuals of Ashkenazi Jewish ancestry from the same family. Therefore, it is not possible to predict the clinical course of the disease in an affected fetus by the experience of other family members or relatives. Until disease severity can be correlated with specific metabolic or genetic factors, or until efficacious therapy is developed, many at-risk families may be faced with difficult decisions concerning prenatal diagnosis and selective abortion of affected fetuses. Also, it should be noted that therapeutic enzyme-replacement endeavors have not proved clinically effective to date (Brady *et al.*, 1974, 1980; Beutler *et al.*, 1980; Gregoriadis *et al.*, 1980).

3. METACHROMATIC LEUKODYSTROPHY

a. Genetic Heterogeneity. Several subtypes of metachromatic leukodystrophy have been identified. The infantile, late-infantile or juvenile, and adult-onset forms are all severe neurodegenerative diseases resulting from the deficiency of arylsulfatase A (i.e., cerebroside sulfatase) activity (Moser, 1978). Recently, a variant with the phenotype of the infantile disease was discovered in which the arylsulfatase A activity was normal when assayed with artificial substrates including p-nitrocatechol-sulfate and 4-methylumbelliferyl-sulfate (Shapiro *et al.*, 1979). Studies have suggested that an activator protein for the enzyme (Fischer and Jatzkewitz, 1975) was defective, analogous to the defect in the AB variant of G_{M2}-gangliosidosis (Conzelman and Sandhoff, 1978).

b. Heterozygote Identification—The Pseudoallele. It is essential that all obligate heterozygotes for metachromatic leukodystrophy be evaluated enzymatically. Although most have half-normal levels of arylsulfatase A activity, several obligate heterozygotes recently have been described with as low levels of leukocyte and fibroblast activity as affected homozygotes (Dubois *et al.*, 1975). These individuals have no clinical findings, normal urinary sulfatide excretion, and normal nerve-conduction velocities (Lott *et al.*, 1976), but apparently have a "pseudoallele" whose gene product does not hydrolyze the artificial substrates for arylsulfatase A. The occurrence of the pseudogene together with the mutant gene for the natural substrate is responsible for the deficient levels of arylsufatase A and the low levels of cerebroside sulfatase activity in these obligate heterozygotes. Therefore, at-risk couples for the recurrence of metachromatic leukodystrophy in future offspring must be tested to document their heterozygous state and to determine if they also have the pseudoallele. When the pseudoallele has been identified in a family at risk, the prenatal diagnosis of an affected homozygote detected by the use of an artificial substrate must be confirmed by radiolabeled cerebroside sulfate-loading and clearance studies (Fluharty *et al.*, 1978).

Another potential pitfall in the diagnosis of metachromatic leukodystrophy involves the prenatal diagnosis of the variant due to the deficiency of the cerebroside sulfatase-activator activity (Fischer and Jatzkewitz, 1975). This diagnosis should be suspected in individuals with the disease phenotype who have normal arylsulfatase activity toward the artificial substrates. Although the prenatal diagnosis of an activator-defective variant has not been attempted, it should be possible by the cerebroside sulfate-loading and clearance studies just noted (Fluharty *et al.*, 1978), in combination with natural substrate assays in the presence and absence of the purified activator or with heat-treated cell extracts.

B.   Disorders of Neutral Lipid Metabolism (Table II)

The disorders of neutral lipid metabolism are a heterogeneous group characterized by the accumulation of cholesterol, cholesterol esters, sterols, and unsaturated fatty acids in the cytoplasm of cells or in the plasma. The detailed clinical, pathologic, and biochemical findings in these diseases have been reviewed (Stanbury *et al.*, 1978).

1.   TYPE II HYPERCHOLESTEROLEMIA

Familial hypercholesterolemia is an autosomal dominant trait that results from the deficiency of cell-surface receptors for low-density lipoproteins (LDL)

TABLE II

DISORDERS OF NEUTRAL LIPID METABOLISM

Disorder	McKusick catalog no.	Enzyme defect	Method of diagnosis	Prenatal diagnosis[a]	Method of prenatal diagnosis
Type II hypercholesterolemia	14440	Low-density-lipoprotein receptor deficiency	Brown and Goldstein (1974)	Made	Brown et al. (1979)
Wolman disease	27800	Acid lipase	Young and Patrick (1970)	Made	Patrick et al. (1977)
Cholesterol ester-storage disease	21500	Acid cholesteryl hydrolase	Fredrickson et al. (1972)	Feasible	See Section III,B,2
Cerebrotendinous xanthomatosis	21370	?	Setoguchi et al. (1974)	Plausible	See Section III,B,3
Lecithin: cholesterol acyltransferase deficiency	24590	Lecithin: cholesterol acyltransferase	Stokke and Norum (1971)	Plausible	See Section III,B,4
Refsum disease	26650	Phytanic acid α-hydrolase	Herndon et al. (1969); Steinberg (1978)	Feasible	Herndon et al. (1969)
Type IV X-linked ichthyosis	30810	Steroid sulfatase	Shapiro et al. (1979)	Feasible	Epstein and Leventhal (1981)
Adrenoleukodystrophy	30010	Long-chain fatty acid	Kawamura et al. (1978)	Made	Moser et al. (1982)

[a] Explanation of terms:

Made—Prenatal diagnosis has been accomplished and confirmed.

Feasible—Methods are currently available or current techniques could be adapted for the prenatal diagnosis.

Plausible—Various strategies can or theoretically could be employed, on an experimental basis, and their use evaluated for prenatal diagnosis.

Not possible—Primary defect is not defined, secondary metabolic effects cannot presently be assessed, or technical difficulties must be overcome before the prenatal diagnosis is feasible.

(Goldstein and Brown, 1974; Brown and Goldstein, 1974). Because the LDL–cholesterol complex cannot be internalized normally, the receptor abnormality leads to derepression of the synthesis of 3-hydroxy-3-methylglutaryl-coenzyme A (HMG-CoA) reductase, the crucial enzyme in cellular cholesterol biosynthesis. The subsequent extracellular accumulation and intracellular overproduction of cholesterol leads to premature atherosclerosis and myocardial infarction in heterozygotes (often by age 35) and in homozygotes during childhood or adolescence (Stone *et al.*, 1974; Brown and Goldstein, 1976).

The homozygous and heterozygous states can be diagnosed in cultured fibroblasts by the deficient LDL binding and internalization or by the lack of HMG-CoA reductase suppression following the addition of LDL–cholesterol (Goldstein and Brown, 1974). The most reliable method of diagnosis is the direct demonstration of the receptor defect by quantitative [^{125}I]LDL binding and uptake studies. This assay requires the stimultanous addition of [^{125}I]LDL and [^{14}C]oleate to assess both the surface binding and the rate of cholesterol esterification to radiolabeled cholesterol–oleate. In addition, the cell-associated [^{125}I]LDL and the kinetics of free ^{125}I by cells after LDL internalization are determined. More indirectly, the suppression of HMG-CoA reductase activity can be assessed at varying concentrations of LDL in the culture media (Goldstein and Brown, 1974). These assays require significant expertise and adequate numbers of control studies in normal, heterozygous, and homozygous fibroblasts and amniotic cells. These assays have been successfully used to diagnose a homozygous fetus prenatally using cultured amniotic fluid cells (Brown *et al.*, 1979). They also could be used to diagnose heterozygous fetuses.

2.   Cholesterol Ester-Storage Diseases

Cholesterol ester-storage disease (CESD) and Wolman disease are thought to be allelic mutations of the enzyme responsible for cholesterol ester hydrolysis (acid lipase) (Fredrickson and Ferrans, 1978). The prenatal diagnosis of Wolman disease has been made in cultured amniotic cells (Patrick *et al.*, 1976). Extension of this assay to families at risk for a fetus with CESD should permit the reliable prenatal diagnosis.

3.   Cerebrotendinous Xanthomatosis

Although presently undefined, the primary defect in this rare neurodegenerative disease may be due to an enzymatic defect in the biosynthesis of chenodeoxycholic acid (Setoguchi *et al.*, 1974). However, the synthetic pathway for chenodeoxycholic acid is restricted to the liver (Setoguchi *et al.*, 1974). Thus a more generalized disorder of cholestanol metabolism must be elucidated to account for the systemic and central nervous system accumulation of cholestanol.

Because plasma cholestanol levels are elevated in affected adults, the prenatal diagnosis of this disease may be possible by the determination of fetal blood cholestanol levels (Salen, 1971), provided that increased plasma levels are documented first in affected infants. Until such data are available or the basic defect is demonstrated in cultured fibroblasts, the prenatal diagnosis of cerebrotendinous xanthomatosis is not possible.

4. LECITHIN: CHOLESTEROL ACYLTRANSFERASE (LCAT) DEFICIENCY

Although the enzymatic activity is not expressed in cultured fibroblasts or amniotic cells, two methods for the prenatal diagnosis of primary LCAT deficiency appear feasible by fetal blood sampling. They include (1) the measurement of plasma LCAT activity and (2) the determination of the cholesterol ester content in fetal plasma. Alternatively, if proteinuria, albuminuria, and α-migrating proteinuria (Gjone, 1974) can be documented shortly after birth in affected individuals, an indication of LCAT deficiency might be possible by the determination of these proteins or α-fetoprotein in the amniotic fluid of at-risk fetuses.

5. REFSUM DISEASE

The prenatal diagnosis of Refsum disease, phytanic acid-storage disease, should be feasible in cultured amniotic cells because the enzymatic defect in phytanic acid α-oxidation has been demonstrated in cultured fibroblasts (Herndon et al., 1969). A prerequisite for the determination of the enzymatic deficiency is the addition of another lipid, e.g., radiolabeled palmitate (Steinberg, 1978), so the incorporation of phytanic acid into cellular lipids can be compared to that of a control whose metabolism is unaffected by the enzymatic block (Herndon et al., 1969; Steinberg, 1978).

6. ADRENOLEUKODYSTROPHY

Adrenoleukodystrophy is an X-linked disorder in which neurodegeneration and adrenal insufficiency account for the major clinical and pathologic findings (Schaumberg et al., 1975). Although the basic enzymatic defect has not been defined, a consistent abnormality of long-chain fatty acid metabolism in cerebral and adrenal cholesterol esters, sphingomyelin, and gangliosides has been described (Igarishi et al., 1976; Menkes and Corbo, 1977; Kawamura et al., 1978). The expression of this abnormality as an excess of abnormally long free fatty acids in cultured fibroblasts from affected individuals has permitted the prenatal diagnosis of a homozygote with this disease (Moser et al., 1982).

Similar analyses of long-chain fatty acids in plasma indicate that screening of at-risk families may identify potential heterozygotes (Ropers *et al.*, 1977; Moser *et al.*, 1981) and that fibroblast-cloning studies can be used to confirm the screening results.

C.   Disorders of Glycoprotein Metabolism (Table III)

The abnormalities in this group of disorders result from defects in the degradation or processing of asparagine-linked glycoprotein oligosaccharide moieties. The particular compounds stored in lysosomes are due to a specific defective glycosidase activity or, in the mucolipidoses, due to a presumed defect in the processing of the glycoprotein in the oligosaccharide moiety. Reviews of the clinical, pathologic, and biochemical abnormalities in these disorders are available (Stanbury *et al.*, 1978; Bondy and Rosenberg, 1980).

1.   ASPARTYLGLUCOSAMINURIA

The primary defect of 4-L-aspartylglucosamine amino hydrolase activity has been documented in a variety of tissues from affected individuals including cultured skin fibroblasts (Aula *et al.*, 1973, 1976). A concomitant accumulation of 2-acetamido-1-(β-L-aspartamide, 1,2-dideoxy-β-D-glucose) in tissues and the excretion of several larger glycoasparagines containing sialic acid, galactose, and mannose in urine have been found (Palo *et al.*, 1973). The latter compounds presumably result from the partial degradation of glycoprotein oligosaccharides. Although the prenatal diagnosis has not been accomplished, it should be feasible by use of the natural substrate assay in cultured amniotic cells. In addition, the presence of the characteristic urinary oligosaccharides in the amniotic fluid, detected by thin-layer chromatography or high-performance liquid chromatography, may provide a rapid preliminary diagnosis of at-risk fetuses.

2.   FUCOSIDOSIS

The first attempts to diagnose α-L-fucosidase deficiency prenatally poignantly illustrate the need for standardization of tissue-culture techniques and proper controls for prenatal monitoring. Matsuda *et al.* (1975) found 30% of normal fibroblast activity in a primary epithelial cell culture derived from the amniotic fluid and predicted a heterozygous fetus. Unfortunately, a twin pregnancy was not detected, and following delivery, both twins were found to be affected. Although the precise reason for the error is not known, several factors may be involved: (1) higher α-L-fucosidase activity in epithelioid cells than in fibroblast controls (Butterworth and Guy, 1977); (2) the lack of sufficient normal, heterozygous, and homozygous control values; (3) the lack of standardization in passage number (Poenareo *et al.*, 1976); and (4) the possible failure to control

TABLE III

DISORDERS OF GLYCOPROTEIN METABOLISM

Disorder	McKusick catalog no.	Enzyme defect	Method of diagnosis	Prenatal diagnosis[a]	Method of prenatal diagnosis
Aspartylglucosaminuria	20840	N-aspartyl-β-glucosaminidase	Aula et al. (1973, 1976)	Feasible	Aula et al. (1976)
Fucosidosis	23000	α-L-Fucosidase	Beratis et al. (1975a, 1977)	Made	Robinson and Thorpe (1974); Galjaard (1980)
Mannosidosis	24850	Acidic α-mannosidase	Desnick et al. (1976)	Feasible	Galjaard (1980)
Sialidosis					
Infantile, juvenile	25655	(2,3) or (2,6) α-N-acetylneur-aminidase (glycoprotein)	Cantz et al. (1977); Wenger et al. (1978b)	Feasible	Mueller and Wenger (1981)
Adult	—	(2,3) or (2,6) α-N-acetylneur-aminidase (glycoprotein)	Kobayashi et al. (1979)	Feasible	
Galactosialidosis	—	α-N-acetylneuraminidase and β-galactosidase	Wenger et al. (1978b)	Made	Kleijer et al. (1979); Grabowski and Desnick, 1981, unpublished results
Mucolipidosis					
II	25250	UDP-GlcNAc: Glycoprotein GlcNAc-1-phosphotransferase	Hasilik et al. (1981); Reitman et al. (1981)	Made	Huijing et al. (1973); Aula et al. (1975)
III	25260	UDP-GlcNAc: Glycoprotein GlcNAc-1-phosphotransferase	Reitman et al. (1981)	Feasible	See Section III,C,5

[a] Explanation of terms:

Made—Prenatal diagnosis has been accomplished and confirmed.

Feasible—Methods are currently available or current techniques could be adapted for the prenatal diagnosis.

Plausible—Various strategies can or theoretically could be employed, on an experimental basis, and their use evaluated for prenatal diagnosis.

Not possible—Primary defect is not defined, secondary metabolic effects cannot presently be assessed, or technical difficulties must be overcome before the prenatal diagnosis is feasible.

the degree of cell confluency (Galjaard, 1980). To date, one successful prenatal diagnosis of fucosidosis has been reported and confirmed (Galjaard, 1980).

3. MANNOSIDOSIS

The primary defect in mannosidosis, acidic α-mannosidase activity, can be detected in a variety of tissues and in cultured fibroblasts using the artificial substrate, 4-methylumbelliferyl-α-D-mannopyranoside (Desnick *et al.*, 1976; Grabowski *et al.*, 1980a). Although the prenatal diagnosis of mannosidosis has not been accomplished, the presence of the defect in cultured amniotic cells should prove diagnostic. Only cultured amniotic cells should be assayed, because Hultberg and Masson (1977) found normal levels of an acidic α-mannosidase activity in the culture media from α-mannosidase-deficient fibroblasts, suggesting that the level of amniotic fluid enzyme activity may provide erroneous information. The enzymatic diagnosis should be confirmed by electrophoresis or anion-exchange chromatography of the α-mannosidase isozymes in the cultured amniotic cells. In addition, the ability to easily detect and quantitate the urinary oligosaccharides in mannosidosis (Matsuura *et al.*, 1981) suggests that amniotic fluid analysis of these compounds may be a useful adjunct for the rapid preliminary prenatal diagnosis of this disease.

4. SIALIDOSIS

The term sialidosis refers to a heterogeneous group of disorders characterized by the recessively inherited deficiency of α-N-acetylneuraminidase activity toward $\alpha(2,3)$ or $\alpha(2,6)$ sialyl linkages in glycoproteins (O'Brien, 1978). Several different phenotypes resulting from the primary deficiency of α-neuraminidase activity have been described (Lowden and O'Brien, 1979). The term sialidosis includes those disorders in which the only deficient enzymatic activity is α-neuraminidase. Galactosialidosis is the designation for those patients with a primary neuraminidase deficiency and a secondary decrease in the activity of β-galactosidase. Large quantities of sialyloligosaccharides are excreted in the urine of patients with both disorders. Infantile-, juvenile-, and adult-onset variants have been reported in both sialidosis and galactosialidosis, indicating the genetic heterogeneity within these entities. Homozygotes for sialidosis typically present with decreasing visual activity, myoclonus, or both. Macular cherry-red spots are present, and intelligence is usually not impaired. Patients with galactosialidosis have the above findings, and, in addition, they typically have dysostosis multiplex, corneal clouding, hepatosplenomegaly, umbilical hernias, sensorineural hearing loss, and low normal to moderately retarded intelligence. The β-galactosidase deficiency is usually of variable degree, being totally absent in plasma or leukocytes and diminished in other tissue sources (Wenger *et al.*, 1978a). In addition, β-galactosidase activity in obligate heterozygotes is normal, distinguishing this disease from primary β-galactosidase deficiency, G_{M1}-gangliosidosis. In contrast, neuraminidase activity is profoundly deficient in fresh, unfrozen tissue sources from homozygotes and is reportedly present in half-normal levels in obligate heterozygotes (Wenger *et al.*, 1978a). In addition, two other lysosomal storage disorders involving sialic acid metabolism have been described. However, neither is due to deficient α-neuraminidase activity. Salla disease appears to be a lysosomal storage disease in which large quantities of sialic acid-rich materials are found in tissue lysosomes (Aula *et al.*, 1979a; Virtanen *et al.*, 1980). To date, the disease has only been reported in patients of Finnish ancestry. The disease, which presents a phenotype similar to aspartylglucosaminuria, is transmitted as an autosomal recessive trait; the nature of the enzymatic defect is unknown. Recently a new disorder characterized by the generalized accumulation of free sialic acid has been reported (Horwitz *et al.*, 1981). The single affected patient had hepatomegaly, ascites, and apparently no skeletal abnormalities. The nature of the metabolic defect is currently under investigation.

The prenatal diagnosis of sialidosis (mucolipidosis Type I) has been attempted recently by the demonstration of α-neuraminidase deficiency in cultured amniotic cells (Mueller and Wenger, 1981). The studies demonstrated the fetus to have active α-neuraminidase activity, and the diagnosis of a normal individual was confirmed after birth. Characterization of the amniotic fluid sialyloligosaccharides was consistent with a normal diagnosis. Thus the prenatal diagnosis of this group of disorders can be made in at-risk pregnancies. The use of amniotic fluid sialyloligosaccharides may prove useful, provided the range of levels in gestation-matched normal fluids are determined.

The prenatal diagnosis of galactosialidosis (combined α-neuraminidase and β-galactosidase deficiencies) has been accomplished in two pregnancies (Kleijer *et al.*, 1979; Grabowski and Desnick, 1981, unpublished observation). The first was performed in a couple known to be at risk for a child with neuraminidase deficiency (Kleijer *et al.*, 1979). The second was performed in a couple with a child previously diagnosed as having G_{M1}-gangliosidosis (β-galactosidase deficiency). However, neither parent proved to be heterozygous for β-galactosidase deficiency in the latter family. The prenatal diagnosis of an affected fetus was confirmed by the demonstration of deficient β-galactosidase activity (5% of normal) in frozen fetal liver tissue.

The accumulated storage compounds in tissues of patients with sialidosis and galactosialidosis have been partially characterized and are the sialylated oligosaccharide side-chains of asparagine-linked glycoproteins (O'Brien, 1978). Because similar sialylated oligosaccharides are excreted in the urine, amniotic fluid oligosaccharide content in at-risk pregnancies should be evaluated to determine the usefulness of this simple procedure as a rapid preliminary indication of the prenatal diagnosis of the other defects of sialic acid metabolism. To date, the prenatal diagnosis of Salla disease has not been performed. In the absence of a specific enzymatic defect, pregnancies at risk for Salla disease might be detected by the bound sialic acid levels in amniotic fluid, whereas future pregnancies in the single family with the disorder characterized by the generalized accumulation of free sialic acid might be monitored by the levels of the unbound compound in amniotic fluid.

5. MUCOLIPIDOSES II AND III

The diagnosis of mucolipidosis II or III in suspected patients is confirmed by demonstration of elevated lysosomal hydrolase activities in plasma or the media from cultured fibroblasts and by the intracellular deficiency of multiple lysosomal hydrolases (Leroy *et al.*, 1972). The deficient intracellular activities are not found in liver, brain, spleen, or kidney of affected individuals (Leroy *et al.*, 1973).

Because the primary defects in mucolipidoses II and III were unknown, the prenatal diagnosis has been accomplished by demonstrating the elevation of selected lysosomal hydrolase activities in amniotic fluid and their deficiencies in cultured amniotic cells (Huijing *et al.*, 1973; Aula *et al.*, 1975). Approximately 30 pregnancies at risk for mucolipidosis II and one for mucolipidosis III have been monitored in this way (Galjaard, 1980). Recently the deficient activity of UDP-GlcNAc: glycoprotein GlcNAc-1-phosphotransferase in cultured fibroblasts of mucolipidoses II and III has been demonstrated (Hasilik *et al.*, 1981; Reitman *et al.*, 1981). This defect appears to be the primary lesion, providing a direct assay for the prenatal diagnosis. In addition, half-normal levels of this enzyme activity have been demonstrated in obligate heterozygotes for mucolipidoses II and III (S. Kornfeld, 1981, personal communication). Another method to confirm the diagnosis of these disorders involves the recent studies of Hasilik and Neufeld (1980) on the biosynthesis of lysosomal enzymes in cultured fibroblasts. These studies demonstrated the lack of ^{32}P incorporation into various lysosomal enzymes synthesized in mucolipidosis II cells. Application of this technique using cultured amniotic cells may prove useful for prenatal diagnostic studies.

D. Disorders of Mucopolysaccharide Metabolism (Table IV)

The clinical, pathologic, and biochemical aspects of these disorders have been comprehensively reviewed (McKusick, 1972; McKusick *et al.*, 1978). Prior to the identification of the specific enzymatic defects in each of the mucopolysaccharidoses (MPS), the prenatal diagnoses were accomplished by quantitation of $^{35}SO_4$ uptake and clearance in cultured amniocytes from at-risk fetuses for MPS

I-H, II, III A, III B, and VI (Neufeld and Cantz, 1973). Although these studies are still useful for confirmatory diagnosis, most investigators rely on the determination of the specific enzymatic activity for each disorder in cultured amniotic cells (McKusick *et al.*, 1978). The largest experience has been with MPS I-H (Hurler disease); more than 100 at-risk pregnancies have been monitored by the determination of α-L-iduronidase activity in cultured amniotic cells (Galjaard, 1980). The diagnosis of the MPS I-H/S (Hurler–Scheie compound) is also possible by this assay. More than 60 pregnancies at risk for MPS II (Hunter disease) have been monitored using the iduronate sulfatase assay in cultured amniocytes and/or amniotic fluid (Liebaers and Neufeld, 1976; Liebaers *et al.*, 1977). Because MPS II is inherited as an X-linked recessive trait, the sex of the fetus is first determined cytogenetically.

The MPS III phenotype (Sanfilippo disease) has been shown to result from four different enzymatic defects (Kresse *et al.*, 1980). The prenatal diagnoses of MPS III A (heparan sulfatase deficiency) and MPS III B (α-N-acetylglucosaminidase deficiency) have been accomplished by the demonstration of the specific enzymatic defects in cultured amniotic cells (Harper *et al.*, 1974; Greenwood *et al.*, 1978; Galjaard, 1980). The prenatal diagnoses of the two recently described disorders, MPS III C [deficient acetyl-CoA:α-glucosaminide N-acetyltransferase (Klein *et al.*, 1978)] and MPS III D [deficient N-acetylglucosamine 6-sulfate sulfatase (Kresse *et al.*, 1980)], also are possible by demonstration of the enzymatic lesions.

The prenatal diagnosis of MPS IV has been reported by the demonstration of deficient galactosamine-6-sulfate sulfatase (von Figura *et al.*, 1982). The prenatal diagnosis of MPS VI (Maroteaux–Lamy disease; deficient arylsulfatase B) has been accomplished by direct arylsulfatase B assay (Kleijer *et al.*, 1976; Fluharty, 1981; Van Dyke *et al.*, 1981) and by the chromatographic separation and quantitation of arylsulfatases A and B in cultured amniotic cells. The pitfalls in the interpretation of residual arylsulfatase B activity have been emphasized (Van Dyke *et al.*, 1981). The diagnosis of an affected fetus with MPS VII (deficient β-glucoronidase) also has been reported (Glaser and Sly, 1973). Except for MPS I-H, MPS I-S/H, MPS III B, VI, and VII, the diagnostic enzyme assays for the other mucopolysaccharidoses are performed in only a few laboratories worldwide. Therefore, the prenatal diagnosis of MPS II, III A, III C, III D, and IV should be performed by these experienced investigators.

E.   Disorders of Carbohydrate Metabolism (Table V)

The galactosemias and the glycogen-storage diseases are the most common inborn errors of carbohydrate metabolism. The extensive literature on the clinical, pathologic, and biochemical abnormalities in these diseases and their variants have been reviewed (Howell, 1978; Segal, 1978).

TABLE IV

Disorders of Mucopolysaccharide Metabolism

Disorder	McKusick catalog no.	Enzyme defect	Method of diagnosis	Prenatal diagnosis[a]	Method of prenatal diagnosis
MPS I-H	25280	α-L-Iduronidase	Matalon and Dorfman (1972); Kelly and Taylor (1976)	Made	Hall and Neufeld (1978)
MPS I-S	25280	α-L-Iduronidase	Liem and Hooghwinkel (1975)	Feasible	Hall and Neufeld (1978)
MPS I-S/H	25280	α-L-Iduronidase		Feasible	Hall and Neufeld (1978)
MPS II Severe	30990	α-L-Iduronate sulfatase	Lim et al. (1974); Liebaers and Neufeld (1976)	Made	Liebaers et al. (1977)
Mild	30990	α-L-Iduronate sulfatase	Lim et al. (1974); Liebaers and Neufeld (1976)	Feasible	Liebaers et al. (1977)

MPS III					
A	25290	Heparan N-sulfatase	Kresse and Neufeld (1972); Kresse (1973)	Made	Kresse and Neufeld (1972); Greenwood et al. (1978)
B	25292	N-acetyl-α-D-glucosaminidase	O'Brien (1972); von Figura and Kresse (1973)	Made	O'Brien (1972); von Figura and Kresse (1973)
C	25293	Acetyl CoA: α-glucosaminide N-acetyltransferase	Klein et al. (1978)	Feasible	
D	—	N-acetylglucosamine 6-sulfate sulfatase	Kresse et al. (1980)	Feasible	
MPS IV	25300	Hexosamine-6-sulfatase	Matalon et al. (1974a)	Made	von Figura et al. (1982)
MPS IV B	25301	β-Galactosidase	Arbisser et al. (1977)	Feasible	
MPS VI	25320	N-acetylgalactosamine sulfatase	Matalon et al. (1974b); Beratis et al. (1975a,b)	Made	Kleijer et al. (1976)
MPS VII	25322	β-Glucuronidase	Hall et al. (1973); Sly et al. (1973)	Made	Glaser and Sly (1973)

[a] Explanation of terms:

Made—Prenatal diagnosis has been accomplished and confirmed.

Feasible—Methods are currently available or current techniques could be adapted for the prenatal diagnosis.

Plausible—Various strategies can or theoretically could be employed, on an experimental basis, and their use evaluated for prenatal diagnosis.

Not possible—Primary defect is not defined, secondary metabolic effects cannot presently be assessed, or technical difficulties must be overcome before the prenatal diagnosis is feasible.

TABLE V

DISORDERS OF CARBOHYDRATE METABOLISM

Disorder	McKusick catalog no.	Enzyme defect	Method of diagnosis	Prenatal diagnosis[a]	Method of prenatal diagnosis
Galactosemia	23040	Galactose-1-phos-phate-uridyl trans-ferase	Krooth and Weinburg (1961); Segal (1978)	Made	Nadler (1968); Ng et al. (1977)
Galactosemia	23020	Galactokinase	Pickering and Howell (1972)	Feasible	Ng et al. (1977)
Glycogen-storage disease					
Type I	23220	Glucose-1-phosphatase	Steinitz (1967); Van Hoof et al. (1972)	Feasible	See Section III,E,2
Type II	23230	Acid maltase (α-1,4-glucosidase)	Seilver et al. (1973); Beratis et al. (1978)	Made	Galjaard (1980)
Type III	23240	Amylo-1,6-glucosidase	Huijing (1975); Howell (1978)	Plausible	Justice et al. (1970)

Type IV	23250	α-1,4-Glucan:α1,4-glucan-6-glucosyl-transferase (branching enzyme)	Brown and Brown (1966); Howell et al. (1971)	Made	Howell et al. (1971); Hsu and Hirschhorn (1974)
Type V	23260	Muscle phosphorylase	Schmid et al. (1959); Pearson et al. (1961)	Plausible	See Section III,E,2
Type VI	23270	Hepatic phosphorylase	Williams and Field (1963); Hers and van Hoof (1968)	Plausible	See Section III,E,2
Type VII	23280	Muscle phosphofructo-kinase	Tauri et al. (1965, 1969)	Plausible	See Section III,E,2
Type VIII	30600	Hepatic phosphorylase kinase	Huijing (1967); Huijing and Sandberg (1970)	Plausible	See Section III,E,2

[a] Explanation of terms:

Made—Prenatal diagnosis has been accomplished and confirmed.

Feasible—Methods are currently available or current techniques could be adapted for the prenatal diagnosis.

Plausible—Various strategies can or theoretically could be employed, on an experimental basis, and their use evaluated for prenatal diagnosis.

Not possible—Primary defect is not defined, secondary metabolic effects cannot presently be assessed, or technical difficulties must be overcome before the prenatal diagnosis is feasible.

1. GALACTOSEMIA

Since the first report by Nadler (1968), the prenatal diagnosis of classical galactosemia, complete galactose-1-phosphate-uridyl transferase deficiency, has been performed in over 50 cases by enzyme assay in cultured amniotic cells (Galjaard, 1980). Particular attention should be paid to the assay conditions because two false negatives have been reported, presumably due to maternal cell contamination (Milunsky, 1979).

Once an affected fetus is detected, several options are available to the parents: (1) elective termination of pregnancy, (2) institution of prenatal maternal dietary galactose restriction, and (3) early institution of dietary therapy in the affected newborn. Although dietary galactose restriction in these patients has resulted in normal mental and physical development, a higher frequency of learning disabilities, behavioral disorders, and lower mean I.Q. values have been reported in longitudinal studies of homozygotes maintained on dietary therapy (Fishler *et al.*, 1972). However, comparative studies of dietary therapy instituted at birth, prior to the onset of the severe metabolic consequences, and later therapeutic intervention are necessary to determine whether the observed brain dysfunction is a component of the disease or a consequence of galactose-induced severe neonatal metabolic disease. The presence of congenital cataracts in some affected homozygotes and the greatly elevated levels of amniotic fluid galactitol (Allen *et al.*, 1980), a toxic galactose metabolite, support the prenatal onset of the metabolic abnormalities. Thus maternal restriction of galactose intake and amniotic fluid monitoring of galactitol levels in a prenatally diagnosed homozygote may offer a more effective therapy of this disease.

2. GLYCOGEN-STORAGE DISEASES

Of the 10 glycogen-storage diseases (Howell, 1978), only Types II, III, and IV express their respective enzymatic defects in cultured skin fibroblasts and are potentially diagnosable *in utero* using current technology. Defective phosphorylase kinase in Type VIII has also been demonstrated in cultured fibroblasts from some homozygotes (Migeon and Huijing, 1974), and the enzyme assay in cultured amniotic cells should allow for the prenatal diagnosis in at-risk families. The remaining types of glycogen-storage disease express the enzymatic defect in specialized tissues, liver, muscle, and/or blood cells (Howell, 1978). The prenatal diagnostic methods for glycogen-storage disease Types II, III, and IV are referenced in Table V.

The specific enzymatic defects in Types I, VI, and VII have been demonstrated in platelets (Negishi *et al.*, 1974), leukocytes (Ockerman *et al.*, 1966), and erythrocytes (Tauri *et al.*, 1969), respectively. These findings suggest that fetal blood may provide sources for the prenatal diagnosis of at-risk fetuses.

However, the timing of fetal expression of the specific glycogenolytic enzymes is not known, and the presently available assay procedures may require larger sample sizes than can presently be obtained by current fetal blood aspiration methods. The determination of secondary blood abnormalities, such as elevations of lipids and uric acid usually associated with Type I, would probably not be possible in fetal blood because of the direct shunting of blood around the liver by the ductus venosus.

Because muscle and erythrocyte phosphofructokinase are immunologically identical (Tauri *et al.*, 1969), and because Layzer *et al.* (1967) demonstrated the absence of CRIM in a patient with Type VIII, radioimmunoassay of phosphofructokinase in fetal erythrocytes from an at-risk pregnancy in CRIM-negative families may provide a more sensitive and reliable determination of the fetal genetic status. For Type V, intrauterine muscle biopsy may be the only potentially plausible approach unless the defect can be demonstrated in fibroblasts or blood-formed elements.

F.   Urea Cycle Disorders (Table VI)

Of the five urea cycle disorders, only heterozygotes for citrullinemia and affected homozygotes for argininosuccinic acidemia have been prenatally diagnosed by determination of the specific enzymatic defect in cultured amniotic cells (Goodman *et al.*, 1973; Roerdink *et al.*, 1973; Tedesco and Mellman, 1975; Fleisher *et al.*, 1979; Rassin *et al.*, 1979). The lack of detectable carbamyl phosphate synthetase (CPS), ornithine carbamyltransferase (OCT), and arginase activities in cultured fibroblasts or amniotic cells (Shih, 1978) has precluded the prenatal diagnosis of these disorders in amniotic fluid cells. However, the advent of fetal blood sampling under fetoscopic observation and the detection of CPS and arginase activity in blood cells (Terheggen *et al.*, 1969; Wolfe and Gatfield, 1975) indicates the potential of detecting these defects prenatally. Indeed, the rationale for this experimental approach is derived from the detection of CPS deficiency in leukocytes (Gatfield *et al.*, 1975) and arginase deficiency in erythrocytes (Terheggen *et al.*, 1969) of affected individuals. Although the fetal blood sample size is small, the use of specific antienzyme antibodies may permit the use of sensitive immunologic assays of the respective enzyme in fetal blood cells (Nakane and Pierce, 1967). For example, the immunologic approach would be particularly relevant to the X-linked CRIM-negative OCT deficiencies (McReynolds *et al.*, 1977).

OCT is expressed in liver only, and recently OCT deficiency in a male fetus was demonstrated following an intrauterine liver biopsy performed during fetoscopy (Rodeck, 1981, personal communication).

In addition to the specific enzymatic determination in argininosuccinic aciduria and OCT deficiency, the quantitation of amniotic fluid or maternal uri-

TABLE VI

DISORDERS OF THE UREA CYCLE CONSTITUENTS

Disorder	McKusick catalog no.	Enzyme defect	Method of diagnosis	Prenatal diagnosis[a]	Method of prenatal diagnosis
Congenital hyperammonemia CPS Deficiency	23730	Carbamyl phosphate synthetase	Jones (1971); Gelehrter and Snodgrass (1974); Wolfe and Gatfield (1975)	Plausible	See Section III,F
OCT Deficiency	31125	Ornithine carbamyl-transferase	Sunshine et al. (1972); Campbell et al. (1973); Aylesworth et al. (1975); Wolfe and Gatfield (1975)	Made	Rodeck 1981, personal communication; See Section III,F
Citrullinemia	21570	Argininosuccinate synthetase	Roerdink et al. (1973); Tedesco and Mellman (1975)	Feasible	Roerdink et al. (1973); Christensen et al. (1981)
Argininosuccinic acidemia	20790	Argininosuccinic acid lyase	Tomlinson and Westall (1964); Glick et al. (1976)	Made	Goodman et al. (1973); Fleisher et al. (1979)
Hyperargininemia	20780	Arginase	Tomlinson and Westall (1964); Cederbaum et al. (1977)	Feasible	See Section III,F
Hyperornithinemia Type I	—	Ornithine decarboxylase	Shih (1978)	Feasible	See Section III,F
Type II	25887	Ornithine Aminotransferase	Shih (1978); Valle et al. (1980a)	Feasible	See Section III,F

[a] Explanation of terms:
Made—Prenatal diagnosis has been accomplished and confirmed.
Feasible—Methods are currently available or current techniques could be adapted for the prenatal diagnosis.
Plausible—Various strategies can or theoretically could be employed, on an experimental basis, and their use evaluated for prenatal diagnosis.
Not possible—Primary defect is not defined, secondary metabolic effects cannot presently be assessed, or technical difficulties must be overcome before the prenatal diagnosis is feasible.

nary metabolites may provide useful adjuncts for the prenatal diagnosis. Increased levels of argininosuccinic acid in these sources as well as in fetal tissues have been documented in affected fetuses with argininosuccinic acid lyase deficiency (Goodman *et al.*, 1973; Fleisher *et al.*, 1979; Rassin *et al.*, 1979). Presumably, the argininosuccinate produced by the enzyme-deficient fetus is rapidly excreted by the pregnant heterozygote. Similarly, the abnormal amounts of the pyrimidine by-product, orotic acid, should be evaluated in amniotic fluid and/or maternal urine in pregnancies at risk for OCT deficiency. Similar approaches to CPS and arginase deficiency are unlikely to be of diagnostic use, because consistently abnormal quantities of metabolites other than ammonia and arginine, respectively, have not been observed in these disorders (Rosenberg and Scriver, 1980).

The prenatal diagnoses of the two well-defined hyperornithinemias are possible because the enzymatic defects have been demonstrated in cultured skin fibroblasts of affected individuals (Shih, 1978). The prenatal diagnosis of ornithine aminotransferase deficiency may prove particularly useful for the immediate institution of arginine restriction (and B_6 supplementation, if responsive) in affected newborns to prevent the development of gyrate atrophy of the choroid and retina (Valle *et al.*, 1980a,b).

G.   Disorders of Branched-Chain Amino Acids (Table VII)

The clinical, pathologic, biochemical, and therapeutic aspects of maple-syrup urine disease, valinemia, isovaleric acidemia, and β-methylcrotonic acidemia have been reviewed (Dancis and Levitz, 1978). The prenatal diagnosis for each of these diseases is possible because the specific enzymatic defects are expressed in cultured fibroblasts (see Table VII). To date, the prenatal diagnosis of maple-syrup urine disease has been undertaken in approximately 50 at-risk pregnancies (Wendel *et al.*, 1973; Galjaard, 1980). Both affected (Wendel *et al.*, 1973; Cox *et al.*, 1978), and unaffected (Dancis, 1972) fetuses have been detected and confirmed.

H.   Disorders of Methylmalonate and Propionate Metabolism (Table VIII)

1.   THE METHYLMALONIC ACIDEMIAS

The discovery of the different defects in the genetic variants of methylmalonic acidemia (MMA) lead to increased understanding of this metabolic pathway, including the function of vitamin B_{12} and the pivotal role of propionate and methylmalonate in human lipid and protein metabolism (for review, see Rosen-

TABLE VII

BRANCHED-CHAIN AMINO ACID DISORDERS

Disorder	McKusick catalog no.	Enzyme defect	Method of diagnosis	Prenatal diagnosis[a]	Method of prenatal diagnosis
Maple-syrup urine disease	24860	Branched-chain ketoacid de-carboxylase	Dancis et al. (1963); Danner and Elsas (1975)	Made	Wendel et al. (1973); Cox et al. (1978)
Valinemia	27710	Valine transaminase	Wada et al. (1963); Dancis et al. (1967)	Feasible	Dancis et al. (1967)
Isovaleric acidemia	24350	Isovaleryl-CoA dehydrogenase	Tanaka et al. (1966); Shih et al. (1973)	Made	Blaskovics (1978)
β-Methylcrotonic acidemia	21020	β-Methylcrotonic carboxylase	Finne et al. (1976); Dancis (1978)	Feasible	Finne et al. (1976)

[a] Explanation of terms:
Made—Prenatal diagnosis has been accomplished and confirmed.
Feasible—Methods are currently available or that current techniques could be adapted for the prenatal diagnosis.
Plausible—Various strategies can or theoretically could be employed, on an experimental basis, and their use evaluated for prenatal diagnosis.
Not possible—Primary defect is not defined, secondary metabolic effects cannot presently be assessed, or technical difficulties must be overcome before the prenatal diagnosis is feasible.

TABLE VIII

Disorders of Propionate and Methylmalonate Metabolism

Disorder	McKusick catalog no.	Enzyme defect	Method of diagnosis	Prenatal diagnosis[a]	Method of prenatal diagnosis
Methylmalonic acidemia	25100	Methylmalonyl-CoA mutase	Stokke et al. (1967); Rosenberg et al. (1968); Rosenberg (1978); Willard et al. (1979)	Made	Morrow et al. (1970); Gompertz et al. (1974)
	25110	Adenosylcobalamin synthesis deficiency	Rosenberg et al. (1969)	Made	Ampola et al. (1975); Mahoney et al. (1975)
	25112	Methylmalonyl-CoA racemase	Kang et al. (1972)	Feasible	
	—	Methylcobalamin methyltransferase	Mudd et al. (1969); Goodman et al. (1970); Levy et al. (1970)	Feasible	
α-Methylacetoacetic acidemia	20375	β-Ketothiolase	Hillman and Keating (1974)	Feasible	
Propionic acidemia	23200	Propionyl-CoA carboxylase	Hsia et al. (1971); Rosenberg (1978); Wolf and Tuck (1979)	Made	Gompertz et al. (1973); Hill and Goodman (1974)
Multiple carboxylase deficiency	23605	Holocarboxylase synthetase	Barlett and Gompertz (1976); Weyler et al. (1977); Saunders et al. (1979); Theone et al. (1979)	Feasible	Section III,H,3

[a] Explanation of terms:
Made—Prenatal diagnosis has been accomplished and confirmed.
Feasible—Methods are currently available or current techniques could be adapted for the prenatal diagnosis.
Plausible—Various strategies can or theoretically could be employed, on an experimental basis, and their use evaluated for prenatal diagnosis.
Not possible—Primary defect is not defined, secondary metabolic effects cannot presently be assessed, or technical difficulties must be overcome before the prenatal diagnosis is feasible.

berg, 1978). In four of these genetic variants, the block in the conversion of propionyl-CoA to succinyl-CoA results in the accumulation of methylmalonic acid in blood, urine, and other tissues with resultant ketoacidosis. The fifth variant results from defective adenosylcobalamin and methylcobalamin synthesis and is characterized by the accumulation of methylmalonate and homocystine (Mudd *et al.*, 1969; Goodman *et al.*, 1970). The prenatal diagnosis of several MMA variants has been accomplished by quantitation of midtrimester amniotic fluid MMA (Morrow *et al.*, 1970, Ampola *et al.*, 1975), by the demonstration of deficient methylmalonyl-coenzyme A (MM-CoA) mutase activity or decreased propionate oxidation, and by absent intracellular adenosylcobalamin—cob(III) or (II)alamin reductase deficiency (Ampola *et al.*, 1975).

The first attempt of ''intrauterine therapy'' for an inborn error of metabolism was made by Ampola *et al.* (1975). These investigators instituted maternal vitamin B_{12} supplementation during the final 2 months of gestation of a fetus affected with a cobalamin reductase form of MMA. Maternal urinary MMA, which had been elevated, decreased during B_{12} therapy. After an uneventful pregnancy, labor, and delivery, dietary restriction and B_{12} supplementation has maintained normal growth and development in this child. However, without demonstration of prenatal damage due to MMA, the superiority of this form of ''prenatal therapy'' to the prompt postdelivery institution of conventional therapies remains to be determined (Rosenberg, 1978).

The prenatal diagnosis of MM-CoA racemase deficiency and defective adenosylcobalamin and methylcobalamin synthesis have not been reported. However, the demonstration of defective propionate to succinate conversion and abnormal cobalamin metabolism in cultured fibroblasts (Rosenberg, 1978; Rosenberg *et al.*, 1975) from affected individuals make their prenatal diagnosis possible in families at risk for these defects.

2. PROPIONIC ACIDEMIA

The clinical and biochemical aspects of propionyl-CoA carboxylase deficiency have been reviewed (Rosenberg, 1978). The prenatal diagnosis of an affected fetus was confirmed after birth of a child who later died from ketoacidosis at 1 year of age (Gompertz *et al.*, 1973). At least eight other pregnancies have been monitored by the determination of the enzymatic activity in cultured amniotic cells (Galjaard, 1980).

Recently, Sweetman *et al.* (1979) and Buchanan *et al.* (1980) demonstrated the value of amniotic fluid methylcitrate levels in the prenatal diagnosis of this disease. The level of propionyl-CoA carboxylase was normal in cultured amniotic cells from an at-risk pregnancy. However, methylcitrate, an abnormal metabolite present in the urine of affected individuals, was present in the amniotic fluid. An affected female was delivered and confirmed by enzymologic techniques. Further studies on the amniotic cell culture revealed overgrowth by maternal cells. Thus the detection of abnormal metabolites may provide important diagnostic information for this and other disorders.

3. MULTIPLE CARBOXYLASE DEFICIENCY

This disorder of biotin metabolism results in propionic acidemia, lactic acidosis, and β-methylcrotonic acidemia (Bartlett and Gompertz, 1976; Weyler *et al.*, 1977). The phenotype of affected individuals is similar to that in propionic acidemia and results from defects in either biotin transport or the holocarboxylase synthetase complex required for propionyl-CoA, β-methylcrotonyl-CoA, and pyruvate carboxylase activities (Theone *et al.*, 1979; McKeon *et al.*, 1980). Cultured fibroblasts from affected individuals with either defect demonstrate defective carboxylase activities only when cultured in biotin-deficient media (Weyler *et al.*, 1977). Thus the prenatal diagnosis is potentially possible using amniotic cells cultured under the appropriate conditions. A specific assay for the primary defect of biotin transport or holocarboxylase synthetase would provide a more accurate prenatal diagnosis than the determination of the associated carboxylase defects. To date, the prenatal diagnosis of combined carboxylase deficiency has not been reported. However, Roth (1981, personal communication) instituted oral maternal biotin supplementation (10 mg/day) in an at-risk pregnancy at 34 weeks' gestation. At term, healthy dizygotic twins were delivered. Subsequently, biochemical analyses of cultured fibroblasts from the twins revealed one affected and one unaffected twin. Cord blood had a 7-fold increase in biotin levels as compared to normal control cord blood. No untoward effects of biotin were observed in either twin or the mother. These studies suggest that biotin supplementation for prenatal therapy in at-risk pregnancies may prevent the life-threatening metabolic sequelae of this disease.

I. Disorders of Dibasic Amino Acid Metabolism (Table IX)

The disorders of dibasic amino acid metabolism are rare autosomal recessive disorders whose clinical spectrum and biochemical features have not been completely defined (Goodman *et al.*, 1975; Ghadimi, 1978). All these disorders appear to be associated with severe mental retardation, although two patients with one form of persistent hyperlysinemia reportedly had normal intellects (Woody *et al.*, 1966). The genetic heterogeneity of these disorders is indicated by the phenotypic and biochemical diversity of the hyperlysinemias and the glutaric acidemias. The studies of Goodman *et al.* (1975) and Rhead and Tanaka (1979), which demonstrated two different enzymatic defects in glutaric acidemia, indicate the need to characterize the specific molecular defect(s) in probands before attempting the prenatal diagnosis. At this time, the prenatal

TABLE IX

DISORDERS OF DIBASIC AMINO ACID METABOLISM

Disorder	McKusick catalog no.	Enzyme defect	Method of diagnosis	Prenatal diagnosis[a]	Method of prenatal diagnosis
Hyperlysinemia	23870	Lysine-ketoglutarate reductase	Dancis et al. (1969a,b)	Feasible	See Section III,I
Glutaric acidemia					
Type I	23167	Glutaryl-CoA dehydrogenase	Goodman et al. (1975)	Made	Goodman et al. (1979)
Type II	23167	Electrontransfer flavoprotein?	Rhead and Tanaka (1979)	Feasible	
Saccharopinuria	26870	Saccharopine dehydrogenase	Simell et al. (1973)	Feasible	

[a] Explanation of terms:

Made—Prenatal diagnosis has been accomplished and confirmed.

Feasible—Methods are currently available or current techniques could be adapted for the prenatal diagnosis.

Plausible—Various strategies can or theoretically could be employed, on an experimental basis, and their use evaluated for prenatal diagnosis.

Not possible—Primary defect is not defined, secondary metabolic effects cannot presently be assessed, or technical difficulties must be overcome before the prenatal diagnosis is feasible.

diagnosis for these diseases appears possible by the determination of the appropriate defective enzyme in cultured amniocytes, and indeed, Goodman *et al.* (1975) have accurately diagnosed an affected fetus with glutaric acidemia, Type I.

J. The Hyperphenylalaninemias (Table X)

To date, several enzymatic defects have been described that result in hyperphenylalaninemia (Tourian and Sidbury, 1978; Rosenberg and Scriver, 1980). Because the defect in Types IV, V, and VI are expressed in cultured fibroblasts, these disorders should be prenatally diagnosable in cultured amniotic cells by determination of the specific enzymatic activity (see Table X). Until the primary enzymatic defect in Type IX (hereditary tyrosinemia)—fumarylacetoacetase (Lindblad *et al.*, 1977)—is confirmed and shown to be expressed in fibroblasts, the prenatal diagnosis of this disease may be feasible only by enzymatic assay of intrauterine-biopsied liver or by the determination of succinylacetone and δ-aminolevulinate levels in amniotic fluid. Therefore, this discussion will focus on approaches to the prenatal diagnosis of the most common hyperphenylalaninemia, phenylalanine hydroxylase deficiency.

Type I, or classical phenylketonuria, has been the prototype for the retrospective mass screening, diagnosis, and dietary treatment of an inborn error of metabolism. Controlled studies have demonstrated that early institution of dietary phenylalanine restriction can prevent the occurrence of the profound mental retardation usually observed in untreated patients. However, the long-term outcome of early dietary therapy has not been fully assessed.

To date, human phenylalanine hydroxylase activity has been detected only in hepatic and renal tissue (Woo *et al.*, 1974). Thus approaches to the prenatal diagnosis could include (1) amniotic fluid phenylalanine levels, (2) fetal liver biopsy for direct enzyme assay, and/or (3) somatic cell hybridization studies to induce amniotic cell enzyme expression.

Blood phenylalanine levels in newborns with phenylketonuria are normal prior to the establishment of adequate protein intake (Kennedy *et al.*, 1976; Tourian and Sidbury, 1978), presumably due to the rapid and efficient maternal placental exchange of phenylalanine. Therefore, the phenylalanine levels are likely to be normal in amniotic fluid or fetal blood. To date, amniotic fluid or fetal blood levels of phenylalanine and tyrosine have not been determined in subsequent pregnancies of at-risk couples. Thus the usefulness of these sources remains a matter for speculation.

Intrauterine hepatic biopsy under fetoscopic visualization may provide a plausible approach to the prenatal diagnosis. The rationale is derived from Raiha's studies (1973), which demonstrated the presence of normal levels of phenylalanine hydroxylase by 7 weeks gestation in human fetal liver. The feasi-

TABLE X

HYPERPHENYLALANINEMIAS

Disorder	McKusick catalog no.	Enzyme defect	Method of diagnosis	Prenatal diagnosis[a]	Method of prenatal diagnosis
Type I	26160	Phenylalanine hydroxylase	Friedman et al. (1973); Bartholome et al. (1975)	Plausible	See Section III,J
Type II	26158	Low phenylalanine hydroxylase	Justice et al. (1967)	Plausible	See Section III,J
Type IV	—	Phenylalanine transaminase (?)	Auerbach et al. (1963); Rosenberg and Scriver (1980)	(?)	
Type V	26163	Dihydropteridine reductase	Kaufman et al. (1975)	Feasible	See Section III,J
Type VI	26164	Dihydropteridine reductase kinetic abnormality	Tourian and Sidbury (1978)	Feasible	See Section III,J
Type IX (tyrosinemia)	27670	Fumarylacetoacetase	Scriver (1967); Lindblad et al. (1977)	Feasible	See Section III,J
Type X (Hereditary tyrosinemia, Oregon type)	27660	Cytosolic tyrosine aminotransferase	de Groot (1980)	Feasible	See Section III,J

[a] Explanation of terms:

Made—Prenatal diagnosis has been accomplished and confirmed.

Feasible—Methods are currently available or current techniques could be adapted for the prenatal diagnosis.

Plausible—Various strategies can or theoretically could be employed, on an experimental basis, and their use evaluated for prenatal diagnosis.

Not possible—Primary defect is not defined, secondary metabolic effects cannot presently be assessed, or technical difficulties must be overcome before the prenatal diagnosis is feasible.

bility of intrauterine hepatic biopsy has been demonstrated for the prenatal diagnosis of ornithine carbamyltransferase deficiency (Rodeck, 1981, personal communication). However, the risk of this invasive and experimental procedure may be such as to dissuade many at-risk couples, because the disease is treatable.

Induction of liver-specific enzymes and other proteins has been accomplished by the fusion of rodent hepatoma cell lines with cultured human amniotic cells (see Chap. 11). For example, after fusion, expression of human phenylalanine hydroxylase may be detectable in rat hepatoma–human fibroblast clones. Indeed, the use of the rat hepatoma cell line H4-II-E-C3 or MH_1C_1 in these fusion studies may facilitate enzyme expression, because steroids or N^6-$O^{2'}$-dibutyryl-3'5'-cyclic adenosine monophosphate stimulate phenylalanine hydroxylase synthesis 3-fold in these cell lines (Haggerty et al., 1973)—potentially providing an intracellular milieu for human enzyme expression. The rat and human enzyme activities could be distinguished by electrophoretic and/or isoelectric-focusing systems (Tourian, 1976), and the synthesis of the normal or mutant human phenylalanine hydroxylase could be monitored by activity and immunologic techniques. Because rat and human phenylalanine hydroxylase share some antigenic determinants (Friedman et al., 1972), this system could be monitored by selecting a specific anti-human phenylalanine hydroxylase monoclonal antibody that has no cross-reactivity with the rat hepatoma isozyme.

K.   Disorders of Sulfur Amino Acid Metabolism (Table XI)

The inborn errors of sulfur amino acid metabolism constitute a heterogeneous group of disorders in which the phenotypes range from asymptomatic to severe physical and mental abnormalities. Current reviews of the clinical, pathologic, and biochemical aspects of these disorders are available (Mudd and Levy, 1978). This discussion will focus on the improvement in the prenatal diagnostic techniques for the homocystinurias, because the other disorders of sulfur amino acid metabolism in which the enzymatic defect has been defined in cultured fibroblasts can be prenatally diagnosed in cultured amniotic cells. The prenatal diagnosis of cystathionuria, although possible, is of doubtful significance, because this enzymatic deficiency is not associated with any consistent clinical sequelae (Mudd and Levy, 1978).

1.   CYSTATHIONINE β-SYNTHASE DEFICIENCY

The basic defect in classical homocystinuria is the deficiency of cystathionine β-synthase activity (Gaull et al., 1969; Mudd and Levy, 1978), which results in homocystinemia, methioninemia, hypocystinemia, and the accumulation of homocysteine–cysteine mixed disulfide in body fluids and tissues (for review, Mudd and Levy, 1978). At least two different allelic mutations of cystathionine

TABLE XI

Disorders of Sulfur Amino Acid Metabolism

Disorder	McKusick catalog no.	Enzyme defect	Method of diagnosis	Prenatal diagnosis[a]	Method of prenatal diagnosis
Homocystinuria	23620	Cystathionine β-synthase	Gaull et al. (1969); Fleisher et al. (1973)	Feasible	Fleisher et al. (1974)
Homocystinuria	23625	N(5,10) Methylene tetrahydrofolate reductase	Wong et al. (1977)	Feasible	See Section III,K,2
Cystinosis	21980	Unknown	States et al. (1974); Schneider et al. (1978)	Made	Schulman et al. (1970); Schneider et al. (1974)
Cystathionuria	21950	γ-Cystathionase	Bittles and Carson (1974); Tallan et al. (1971)	Feasible	See Section III,K
β-Mercapto-lactate cysteine disulfiduria	24965	β-Mercaptopyruvate sulfotransferase (?)	Ampola et al. (1969)	Not possible	
Pyroglutamic aciduria	26613	Glutathione synthase	Wellner et al. (1974)	Feasible	
Sulfocystinuria	27230	Sulfite oxidase	Irreverre et al. (1967)	Feasible	

[a] Explanation of terms:

Made—Prenatal diagnosis has been accomplished and confirmed.

Feasible—Methods are currently available or current techniques could be adapted for the prenatal diagnosis.

Plausible—Various strategies can or theoretically could be employed, on an experimental basis, and their use evaluated for prenatal diagnosis.

Not possible—Primary defect is not defined, secondary metabolic effects cannot presently be assessed, or technical difficulties must be overcome before the prenatal diagnosis is feasible.

β-synthase, one pyridoxine-responsive and the other nonresponsive, occur in the population in approximately equal numbers (Mudd and Levy, 1978). The tissues of individuals with the pyridoxine-responsive mutation are CRIM-positive for the enzyme, whereas nonresponsive forms are both CRIM-positive and CRIM-negative. The differential *in vivo* responsiveness in CRIM-positive homocystinurics can be predicted by determination of the K_m of cystathionine β-synthase for pyridoxal phosphate in fibroblasts cultured in pyridoxine-deficient medium. The K_m for pyridoxal phosphate was 2–4 times normal in the responsive mutations, whereas the K_m was 16–23 times normal in the nonresponsive mutations (Lipson et al., 1980). Other nonresponders were CRIM-negative as determined with antibody to normal human cystathionine β-synthase (Skovby et al., 1980). Thus the presence of residual enzymatic activity, the K_m for pyridoxal-5'-phosphate, and/or the presence of CRIM in amniotic cells may correlate with future therapeutic response to pyridoxine supplementation.

Unaffected individuals have been correctly predicted by the assay of cystathionine β-synthase activity in cultured amniotic cells (Gaull et al., 1969; Fleisher et al., 1974). To date, no affected fetus has been detected. However, care must be exercised in establishing control ranges for cystathionine β-synthase, because cultured fetal fibroblasts and amniotic cells have significantly higher enzymatic activity than adult fibroblast cell lines (Fleisher et al., 1974). The long delay time needed to grow the large numbers of cells required for this enzymatic assay suggests that more sensitive immunologic approaches requiring less cells should be developed.

2. $N(5,10)$ METHYLENE TETRAHYDROFOLATE REDUCTASE DEFICIENCY

This rare autosomal recessive enzymatic defect presents as a syndrome similar to classic homocystinuria (Mudd and Levy, 1978). Thus it is imperative to establish the precise enzymatic defect in patients with homocystinuria. The ability to detect the enzymatic defect in cultured fibroblasts from affected homozygotes (Wong et al., 1977) makes possible the prenatal diagnosis of affected fetuses.

L.   Other Disorders of Amino Acid Metabolism (Table XII)

Except for nonketotic hyperglycinemia and hyperprolinemia Type I, the primary defects in these diseases have been demonstrated in cultured fibroblasts and presumably are present in fibroblastic amniocytes from affected fetuses (see Table XII). Consequently, these enzymopathies should be prenatally diagnosable by determination of the specific enzymatic defect in cultured amniotic cells from at-risk pregnancies. Alternative approaches will be required for the specific diagnosis of the other disorders because the basic biochemical defects are expressed only in specialized tissues.

TABLE XII

OTHER DISORDERS OF AMINO ACID METABOLISM

Disorder	McKusick catalog no.	Enzyme defect	Method of diagnosis	Prenatal diagnosis[a]	Method of prenatal diagnosis
Histidinemia	23580	Histidase	La Du et al. (1963); Zannoni and La Du (1963)	Feasible	See Section III,L
Nonketotic hyperglycinemia	23830	Glycine decarboxylation	Perry et al. (1975); Rosenberg and Scriver (1980)	Made	See Addendum
Hyperprolinemia					
Type I	23950	Proline oxidase	Efron (1965)	Plausible	See Section III,L,2
Type II	23951	δ-1-Pyrroline-5-carboxylate dehydrogenase	Valle et al. (1974)	Feasible	
Defective folate absorption	26395	Prolidase	Powell et al. (1974)	Feasible	
	22905	?	Rowe (1978)	Not possible	
Dihydrofolate reductase deficiency	24925	Dihydrofolate reductase	Tauro et al. (1976)	Feasible	
Formiminotransferase deficiency	22910	Formiminotransferase	Rowe (1978)	Feasible	

[a] Explanation of terms:

Made—Prenatal diganosis has been accomplished and confirmed.

Feasible—Methods are currently available or current techniques could be adapted for the prenatal diagnosis.

Plausible—Various strategies can or theoretically could be employed, on an experimental basis, and their use evaluated for prenatal diagnosis.

Not possible—Primary defect is not defined, secondary metabolic effects cannot presently be assessed, or technical difficulties must be overcome before the prenatal diagnosis is feasible.

1. NONKETOTIC HYPERGLYCINEMIA

Nonketotic hyperglycinemia is thought to result from the defective decarboxylation of glycine in liver and brain (Perry *et al.*, 1975; Rosenberg and Scriver, 1980). Although the primary defect has not been demonstrated in cultured fibroblasts, recent studies indicate defective glycine-transport kinetics in cultured fibroblasts derived from affected homozygotes (Revsin and Morrow, 1976; Feneant *et al.*, 1980). Because these determinations were performed on confluent fibroblasts grown on coverslips, the procedure may be directly applicable to the prenatal diagnosis of this disease. However, the kinetic differences between normal and affected cell lines, although statistically significant, are small, and adequate numbers of positive and negative control samples are required to make accurate diagnostic predictions.

A more direct approach would be a fetal hepatic biopsy with direct determination of glycine decarboxylation. At present, the timing of fetal liver expression of the glycine-decarboxylation system has not been determined. In addition, the obscure nature of the fundamental defect in this disease (CRIM status, residual enzyme characterization, genetic heterogeneity) requires greater understanding before other meaningful approaches can be developed for the prenatal diagnosis of nonketotic hyperglycinemia.

2. HYPERPROLINEMIA TYPE I

Proline oxidase, the biochemical defect in hyperprolinemia Type I, is expressed primarily in hepatocytes (Efron, 1965), and no activity of this enzyme is detectable in normal cultured fibroblasts (see note 8 in Valle *et al.*, 1974). Thus fetal hepatic biopsy and/or hepatoma-fibroblast hybrid techniques may provide the only presently available approaches for the prenatal diagnosis of this disorder. However, the lack of a definite association between renal and/or neurologic pathology and proline oxidase deficiency (Scriver, 1978) indicates that this disorder may be benign. The clinical spectrum and genetic heterogeneity of this disorder must be more clearly defined in order to determine if prenatal diagnosis is of value.

M. Immunodeficiency and Complement Disorders (Table XIII)

The clinical, pathologic, and immunologic aspects of the disorders of immune competence have been recently reviewed (Bergsma *et al.*, 1975; Rosen, 1981). Of these disorders, acatalasemia, severe combined immunodeficiency disease (associated with adenosine deaminase deficiency), and purine nucleoside phosphorylase deficiency (a T-cell immune defect), express the enzymatic defect in cultured skin fibroblasts (Krooth *et al.*, 1962; Hirschhorn *et al.*, 1976; Stoop *et*

TABLE XIII

Disorders of Immune Competence

Disorder	McKusick catalog no.	Enzyme defect	Method of diagnosis	Prenatal diagnosis[a]	Method of prenatal diagnosis
Acatalasemia	20020	Catalase deficiency	Krooth et al. (1962); Ogata et al. (1974)	Feasible	See Section III,M
Severe combined immunodeficiency	24275	Adenosine deaminase	Hirschhorn et al. (1976)	Made	Hirschhorn et al. (1975)
T-Cell immune defect	16405	Nucleoside phosphorylase	Stoop et al. (1977)	Feasible	See Section III,M,1
X-Linked agammaglobulinemia	30040	?	Gayl-Peczalska et al. (1973)	Plausible	See Section III,M,2
Disorders of complement metabolism	21695	C1r	Klemperer (1969); de Bracco et al. (1974); Gibson et al. (1976)	Plausible	
	21700	C2		Plausible	
	12070	C3	Ballow et al. (1975); Einstein et al. (1977)	Plausible	
	12080	C4	Rosenfeld et al. (1969); Ochs et al. (1977)	Plausible	
	12090	C5	Rosenfeld et al. (1976)	Plausible	
	21705	C6	Leddy et al. (1974)	Plausible	
	21707	C7	Delage et al. (1977)	Plausible	
	12095	C8	Peterson et al. (1976)	Plausible	
Angioneurotic edema	10610	C1′ Inhibitor	Johnson et al. (1971)	Plausible	

[a] Explanation of terms:
Made—Prenatal diagnosis has been accomplished and confirmed.
Feasible—Methods are currently available or current techniques could be adapted for the prenatal diagnosis.
Plausible—Various strategies can or theoretically could be employed, on an experimental basis, and their use evaluated for prenatal diagnosis.
Not possible—Primary defect is not defined, secondary metabolic effects cannot presently be assessed, or technical difficulties must be overcome before the prenatal diagnosis is feasible.

al., 1977). To date, only severe combined immunodeficiency disease associated with adenosine deaminase deficiency has been prenatally diagnosed by demonstration of the defect in cultured amniocytes from at-risk pregnancies (Hirschhorn *et al.*, 1975). In families with severe combined immunodeficiency with normal adenosine deaminase activity, the prenatal diagnosis could be made by the assessment of B- and T-cell function in fetal blood. The prenatal diagnosis of acatalasemia and purine nucleoside phosphorylase deficiency should be readily accomplished in a similar fashion. The remaining disorders (see Table XIII) are defects in the synthesis or function of various blood constituents (e.g., immunoglobulin and complement components), which are normally expressed in specialized tissues (B cells, intestine and/or liver) and secreted into the blood. Approaches for the prenatal diagnosis of these disorders are discussed below.

1.   X-Linked Agammaglobulinemia

Although the primary defect in X-linked agammaglobulinemia is unknown, the blood of patients lacks both B-cell lymphocytes and the major subclasses of immunoglobulins (IgM, IgG, and IgA) (Lawton *et al.*, 1975). Normal human fetuses produce B-cell lymphocytes with membrane-bound IgM, IgG, and IgA by 9 to 11 weeks gestation, and normal adult levels of each of these immunoglobulins are produced in B-lymphocytes by 14 weeks gestation (Lawton *et al.*, 1972). Paradoxically, serum immunoglobulin levels are virtually absent until 6 to 9 months gestation (Cooper and Lawton, 1972). Because affected males completely lack B-lymphocytes (IgM, IgG, and IgA classes), this cellular deficiency and the associated immunoglobulin deficiencies could be detected in fetal blood obtained from an affected male fetus at 14 to 16 weeks gestation. Care must be taken to characterize the B-cell deficiency in the index case prior to prenatal studies. Thus the prenatal diagnosis of this X-linked disease should be possible even though the basic defect is unknown.

2.   Disorders of Complement

The complement system involves the specific interaction of more than 20 individual plasma proteins to maintain normal host-defense mechanisms (Colten *et al.*, 1981). Inherited defects of individual complement components result in clinical manifestations including immune-complex diseases with vasculitis and lupus-like syndromes (Clr, Clq, C4, and C2), recurrent bacterial infections (C3 or C3b inhibitor), recurrent infections due to Neisserian organisms (C5, C6, C7, and C8), or hereditary angioneurotic edema (C1′ inhibitor) (Alper and Rosen, 1976; Thompson *et al.*, 1980; Colten *et al.*, 1981). Certain of these disorders are treatable with appropriate antibiotic prophylaxis or androgen therapy (for angioneurotic edema).

Although the clinical severity of several of these disorders is not clear (particularly C1r, C1s, C1q deficiencies), the prenatal diagnosis of complement deficiencies is feasible by determination of the specific complement component in fetal blood; or for C2 and C4 deficiencies, by HLA-antigen segregation in cultured amniotic cells. The presence of total serum complement activity and the individual complement components have been demonstrated in fetal serum. Thus the complement-deficiency disorders, including C1′ esterase-inhibitor deficiency, should be detectable prenatally by the immunologic measurement of individual complement components in fetal sera (Colten and Rosen, 1973; Ruddy and Austen, 1978).

An alternative approach for the diagnosis of C2 and C4 deficiencies is based on the close linkage of C2, C4, and the HLA complex on chromosome 6 (Dupont et al., 1977). Based on HLA studies of the parents, grandparents, and an affected sibling, Pollack et al. (1979) prenatally diagnosed a heterozygote for C4 deficiency by HLA analysis of the antigens present on the cultured amniotic cells. The HLA-linkage approach for the prenatal diagnosis of these disorders requires the HLA genotypes of both parents and the affected individual in order to identify an affected fetus. Prenatal diagnosis by this technique would be precluded in families where one parent is homozygous for a particular antigen.

N.   Disorders of Steroid Metabolism (Table XIV)

The disorders of steroid metabolism include the defects in steroid hormone synthesis and those due to the lack of end-organ responsiveness (e.g., receptor defective) to certain steroid hormones. Examples of the former group are the congenital adrenal hyperplasia (CAH) syndromes; the latter group includes the androgen-resistance syndromes. The clinical and biochemical defects in these disorders have been thoroughly reviewed (Bongiovanni, 1978; Wilson and MacDonald, 1978; Griffin and Wilson, 1980).

Because defective dihydrotestosterone binding or deficient 5α-reductase activity, the primary defects in two of the androgen-resistance syndromes, are detectable only in cultured fibroblasts from genital skin (Griffin et al., 1981), these disorders are not currently prenatally diagnosable in cultured amniotic cells or biopsied fetal skin. Investigation of methods designed to up-regulate the androgen-receptor activity in nongenital fibroblasts, perhaps by exposure to dihydrotestosterone (Pinsky, 1981, personal communication), may permit the diagnosis of these disorders in the future.

As discussed in Section I, CAH Type III (21-hydroxylase deficiency) has been prenatally diagnosed by HLA-linkage studies in cultured fibroblasts and amniotic cells from at-risk families (Pollack et al., 1979). This approach is useful in those families with at least one affected child and in which neither parent is homozygous for an HLA antigen. Misdiagnoses could result from a recombination event

TABLE XIV

DISORDERS OF STEROID METABOLISM

Disorder	McKusick catalog no.	Enzyme defect	Method of diagnosis	Prenatal diagnosis[a]	Method of prenatal diagnosis
Congenital adrenal hyperplasia					
Type I	20171	20, 22 Desmolase	Degenhart et al. (1972)	Plausible	See Section III,N
Type II	20181	3β-Steroid dehydrogenase	Bongiovanni (1962)	Plausible	See Section III,N
Type III	20191	21-Hydroxylase	Bongiovanni et al. (1978)	Made	Pollack et al. (1979)
Type IV	20201	11-Hydroxylase	Thistlethwaite et al. (1975)	Plausible	See Section III,N
Type V	21211	17-Hydroxylase	Biglieri et al. (1966)	Plausible	See Section III,N
Type VI	—	17, 20 Desmolase	Zuchman et al. (1972)	Plausible	See Section III,N
Complete testicular feminization	31370	Dihydrotestosterone-binding protein	Gehring and Tomkins (1974); Amrhein et al. (1976); Griffin et al. (1976)	Not possible	See Section III,N
Incomplete male pseudo-hermaphroditism					
Type I	31380	Dihydrotestosterone-binding protein (?)	Perez-Palacios et al. (1975)	Not possible	See Section III,N
Type II	26460	Testosterone 5α-reductase	Imperato-McGinley et al. (1974); Griffin et al. (1981)	Not possible	See Section III,N

[a] Explanation of terms:

Made—Prenatal diagnosis has been accomplished and confirmed.

Feasible—Methods are currently available or current techniques could be adapted for the prenatal diagnosis.

Plausible—Various strategies can or theoretically could be employed, on an experimental basis, and their use evaluated for prenatal diagnosis.

Not possible—Primary defect is not defined, secondary metabolic effects cannot presently be assessed, or technical difficulties must be overcome before the prenatal diagnosis is feasible.

between the HLA and the 21-hydroxylase loci; however, these loci are closely linked and the probability of recombination is low. Rosenmann *et al.* (1980) have demonstrated the usefulness of amniotic fluid 17-hydroxyprogesterone as an adjunct for the prenatal diagnosis prior to 26 weeks of gestation. In addition, more than 15 other steroid metabolites have been detected in the urine of 21-hydroxylase-deficient patients (Bongiovanni, 1978), but none have been quantitated in amniotic fluid of normal or at-risk pregnancies. This is especially relevant in that the major urinary metabolites in affected infants are 11-keto pregnanetriol and Δ^5-16-hydroxy-21-methylpregnene derivatives (Bongiovanni *et al.*, 1959; Reynolds, 1963). Thus these studies may be useful for later gestational determination or confirmation of the genetic status of at-risk fetuses.

The remaining five forms of CAH are not known to be HLA linked, and, indeed, Type V is not (Mantero *et al.*, 1980). In addition, none of the specific steroid hormone biosynthetic enzymes are expressed in fibroblasts or in tissues other than the adrenal gland and/or gonads (Bongiovanni, 1978). Therefore, indirect approaches to the prenatal diagnosis of CAH Types I–VI, including the evaluation of amniotic fluid for characteristic abnormal steroids that accumulate prior to the enzymatic block, may be of value for the prenatal diagnosis of these diseases. Indeed, the lack of urinary 17-ketosteroids and C_{19}-steroids in Types I and IV (Prader and Gurtner, 1955; Zuchman *et al.*, 1972) and the presence of only Δ^5-3β-OH steroids in Type II (Bongiovanni, 1962), indicate that the pattern of amniotic fluid steroids may be diagnostically useful, but the variable levels of these steroids in amniotic fluid at different gestational ages must be fully assessed prior to their implementation.

An alternative and highly speculative approach to the prenatal diagnosis of the enzymatic defects in CAH syndromes would include enzymatic analyses of hybrids of steroid-producing (cortisol) adrenal cortical carcinoma cells and amniotic fibroblasts. Theoretically, these hybrids may express human adrenal gland specific functions including the enzymes in cortisol biosynthesis; expression of the human CAH gene could be determined by CRIM-specific activity.

O.   Disorders of Collagen Metabolism (Table XV)

1.   EHLERS–DANLOS SYNDROMES

The biochemical defects in four of the eight types of Ehlers–Danlos (ED) syndrome (Table XV) have been identified (Bornstein and Byers, 1980). The specific metabolic defect in each of the recessively inherited ED syndromes is expressed in cultured skin fibroblasts from affected individuals (Table XV). The defective enzymatic activity can be determined in Types V and VI, whereas deficient product in Type IV B and accumulated precursor in Type VII can be

TABLE XV

DISORDERS OF COLLAGEN METABOLISM

Disorder	McKusick catalog no.	Defect	Method of diagnosis	Prenatal diagnosis[a]	Method of prenatal diagnosis
Ehlers–Danlos syndromes					
Type I	13000	Type I collagen	Bornstein and Byers (1980)	Plausible	See Section III,O,1
Type II	13000	Type I collagen	Bornstein and Byers (1980)	Plausible	See Section III,O,1
Type III	13000	Type I collagen	Bornstein and Byers (1980)	Plausible	See Section III,O,1
Type IV A	13005	Unknown	Byers et al. (1979)	Plausible	See Section III,O,1
Type IV B	22535	Absent Type III procollagen	Pope et al. (1975); Gay et al. (1976)	Feasible	See Section III,O,1
Type V	30520	Lysyl oxidase	Di Ferrante et al. (1975a,b)	Feasible	See Section III,O,1
Type VI	22540	Collagen lysyl hydroxylase	Pinnell et al. (1972); Quinn and Krane (1976)	Feasible	See Section III,O,1
Type VII	22541	Procollagen protease	Lichtenstein et al. (1973a,b)	Feasible	See Section III,O,1
Marfan syndrome	15470	Extracellular matrix	Matalon and Dorfman (1969); Lamberg and Dorfman (1973); Priest et al. (1973)	Plausible	See Section III,O,2
Osteogenesis imperfecta	25940	Abnormal Type I collagen	Bornstein and Byers (1980)	Made	Byers et al. (1981)

[a] Explanation of terms:

Made—Prenatal diagnosis has been accomplished and confirmed.

Feasible—Methods are currently available or current techniques could be adapted for the prenatal diagnosis.

Plausible—Various strategies can or theoretically could be employed, on an experimental basis, and their use evaluated for prenatal diagnosis.

Not possible—Primary defect is not defined, secondary metabolic effects cannot presently be assessed, or technical difficulties must be overcome before the prenatal diagnosis is feasible.

demonstrated by immunologic (Steinmann *et al.*, 1980), peptide fragment (Pope *et al.*, 1975), and/or amino acid composition (Lichtenstein *et al.*, 1973a,b) studies in specialized laboratories. However, these sophisticated biochemical techniques have revealed biochemical heterogeneity within each type of ED syndrome (Byers *et al.*, 1979). Therefore, even though the prenatal diagnosis of these diseases may be possible in cultured amniotic cells, the specific nature of the defect in the affected proband must be characterized prior to amniocentesis.

The basic defects in ED Types I, II, and III are likely to involve abnormalities of Type I collagen (Bornstein and Byers, 1980). Until the specific defects are elucidated, fetal skin biopsy for ultrastructural analysis (Vogel *et al.*, 1976) may provide the only method for prenatal diagnosis of these disorders. However, the risks of complications to both an affected mother and a potentially affected fetus, including fetoscopic induced labor, scar formation, and abnormal healing at the amnion entry site, must be thoroughly assessed prior to undertaking these studies.

2.   MARFAN SYNDROME

The connective-tissue abnormalities in Marfan syndrome, including cutaneous, cardiovascular, and ligamentous laxity, led investigators to postulate a primary defect in collagen metabolism in this disease (McKusick, 1972). To date, evidence to indicate an abnormality in collagen amino acid composition is lacking (Bornstein and Byers, 1980). Indeed, the similarities to the collagen cross-linking abnormalities caused by homocysteine (Kang and Trelstad, 1973; Siegel, 1977) suggest that the primary defect in Marfan syndrome may result from defective extracellular matrix–collagen associations or from abnormal post-translational modification of collagen (Bornstein and Byers, 1980).

Matalon and Dorfman (1969) first reported the abnormally high synthesis and secretion of hyaluronic acid by cultured skin fibroblasts from affected individuals. Confirmatory observations (Lamberg and Dorfman, 1973; Priest *et al.*, 1973) indicate that determination of this abnormality in cultured amniocytes may provide one approach to the prenatal diagnosis. However, until the basic defect in this disease is identified, the prenatal diagnosis must rely on determinations of secondary phenomena with the attendant interpretive problems and pitfalls.

3.   OSTEOGENESIS IMPERFECTA

The clinical spectrum of the osteogenesis imperfecta (OI) syndromes (for review see Bornstein and Byers, 1980) are exceeded only by the plethora of biochemical findings associated with these diseases. Unfortunately, many of the reported collagen abnormalities have been impossible to compare because the phenotypes of the affected individuals have not been fully defined. For example, Peltonen *et al.* (1980a,b) demonstrated an abnormal mannose content in Type I and III collagen carboxyl-terminal moieties and the resulting slower secretion of Type I procollagen in fibroblasts. This abnormal collagen was more prone to aggregation, which presumably resulted in less functional collagen. More recently, Byers *et al.* (1981) reported the presence of abnormal peptide fragments of Type I collagen in fibroblasts from severe congenital OI. These findings have been directly applied to the prenatal diagnosis of OI in cultured amniocytes (Byers *et al.*, 1981). In addition to the biochemical analyses, ultrasound and radiographic studies may confirm the diagnosis.

P. Disorders of Purine and Pyrimidine Metabolism (Table XVI)

1. GOUT

Two enzymatic defects, hypoxanthine-guanine phosphoribosyl transferase (HGPRT) and 5-phospho-D-ribosyl-1-pyrophosphate synthetase (PPRP), have been shown to result in primary gout (Wyngaarden and Kelly, 1978). Each defect results in the massive overproduction of uric acid, albeit by different pathophysiologic mechanisms. Partial HGPRT deficiency leads to decreased negative-feedback control of the rate-limiting enzyme in purine biosynthesis, amidophosphoribosyltransferase, and disruption of the purine-salvage pathway. More severe HGPRT deficiency results in the Lesch–Nyhan syndrome (see next section). Uric acid overproduction also results from mutations of PPRP synthetase. One mutation decreases the K_m of this enzyme (Becker *et al.*, 1973), whereas the other results in resistance to feedback inhibition by ADP and GDP (Zoref *et al.*, 1975) and overproduction of PPRP (Seegmiller, 1980). These disorders are distinguished from multifactorial forms of gout by their earlier symptomatic presentation and more severe uric acid overproduction. Only 1% of all primary gout is due to HGPRT deficiency, and only four families have been described with increased PPRP synthetase activity, uric acid overproduction, and gout (Becker *et al.*, 1973). The clinical, pathologic, and biochemical aspects of gout are the subject of recent exhaustive reviews (Wyngaarden and Kelly, 1978; Seegmiller, 1980).

Because the defects in these disorders are detectable in cultured fibroblasts, the prenatal diagnosis of these disorders, specifically partial HGPRT deficiency, is possible in cultured amniotic cells. Prenatal monitoring of PPRP synthetase abnormalities requires prior characterization of the mutant enzymatic activity in affected hemizygotes from the same family. Because the enzyme deficiency may result from a kinetic or allosteric defect, the level of CRIM-specific activity

TABLE XVI

DISORDERS OF PURINE AND PYRIMIDINE METABOLISM

Disorder	McKusick catalog no.	Enzyme defect	Method of diagnosis	Prenatal diagnosis[a]	Method of prenatal diagnosis
Gout	31185	5-Phospho-D-ribosyl-1-pyro-phosphate synthetase	Becker et al. (1973); Zoref et al. (1975)	Feasible	See Section III,P,1
Gout	30800	Partial hypoxanthine-guanine-phosphoribosyltransferase deficiency	Kelley and Wyngaarden (1978)	Feasible	See Section III,P,1
Lesch–Nyhan syndrome	30800	Complete hypoxanthine-guanine-phosphoribosyl transferase deficiency	Henderson et al. (1974)	Made	Fujimoto et al. (1968); Halley and Heukels-Dully (1977)
APRT deficiency	—	Adenine phosphoribosyl-transferase	Seegmiller (1980)	Feasible	See Section III,P,3
Hereditary xanthinuria	27830	Xanthine oxidase	Sperling et al. (1971)	(?)	
Hereditary orotic acidemia					
Type I	25890	Orotate phosphoribosyltrans-ferase and orotodine 5'-phosphate decarboxylase	Worthy et al. (1974)	Feasible	See Section III,P,4
Type II	25892	Orotidine 5'-phosphate decar-boxylase	Fox et al. (1969)	Feasible	See Section III,P,4

[a] Explanation of terms:

Made—Prenatal diagnosis has been accomplished and confirmed.

Feasible—Methods are currently available or current techniques could be adapted for the prenatal diagnosis.

Plausible—Various strategies can or theoretically could be employed, on an experimental basis, and their use evaluated for prenatal diagnosis.

Not possible—Primary defect is not defined, secondary metabolic effects cannot presently be assessed, or technical difficulties must be overcome before the prenatal diagnosis is feasible.

and/or the K_m (phosphate) and the K_i (ADP and GDP) must be characterized in at-risk and normal control amniotic cells and in the fibroblasts of affected hemizygotes.

2. LESCH–NYHAN SYNDROME

Approximately 50 at-risk pregnancies for Lesch–Nyhan Syndrome (Wyngaarden and Kelly, 1978) have been accurately monitored by the determination of HGPRT activity in cultured amniotic cells (Galjaard, 1980). In affected hemizygotes, the demonstration of severely deficient HGPRT activity is sufficient for the prenatal diagnosis, even though at least two different mutations have been described: one with normal levels of CRIM and the other with CRIM levels corresponding to the amount of residual activity (Ghangas and Milman, 1975; Upchurch et al., 1975). The use of these immunologic techniques should increase the accuracy and sensitivity of this diagnosis.

3. ADENINE PHOSPHORIBOSYLTRANSFERASE (APRT) DEFICIENCY

This enzymatic defect has been demonstrated in cultured skin fibroblasts from four homozygous affected individuals with renal calculi consisting of 2,8-dihydroxyadenine (Seegmiller, 1980). Treatment with allopurinol and a low-purine diet eliminates stone formation. The clear association of clinical abnormalities, other than urinary stones, with APRT deficiency must await the description of further families. The prenatal diagnosis of this abnormality is possible by enzymatic assay in cultured amniotic cells.

4. HEREDITARY OROTIC ACIDEMIA

The primary defect in hereditary orotic acidemia results in the deficiency of two enzymatic activities, orotate phosphoribosyl transferase (OPRT) and orotidine-5′-phosphate decarboxylase (OPDC), which have sequential action in orotate metabolism (Worthy et al., 1974). Based on the occurrence of these two enzymes in a complex, Kelly and Smith (1978) postulated that a structural mutation in one enzyme could disrupt the enzyme complex, resulting in loss of both enzymatic activities. However, one patient with Type II orotic acidemia had isolated OPDC deficiency, indicating that this pathologic mechanism was unlikely. Several other mechanisms have been postulated, including a mutation affecting the coordinate expression of both enzymes and a mutation in a single subunit common to both (Seegmiller, 1980).

The activities of both OPRT and OPDC in affected homozygotes are undetectable in leukocytes or erythrocytes, whereas cultured fibroblasts have residual activity of about 2–5% of mean normal values (Rogers et al., 1968). Thus the prenatal diagnosis may be accomplished by determination of both OPRT and OPDC activities in cultured amniocytes.

Q.   Disorders of DNA Repair and Chromosomal Breakage (Table XVII)

1.   XERODERMA PIGMENTOSUM

Xeroderma pigmentosum, an autosomal recessive trait, has been shown to result from defective repair of ultraviolet light-induced DNA damage (Cleaver and Trosko, 1970). Seven complementation groups have been identified, indicating the genetic heterogeneity in this phenotype. To date, the primary enzymatic defects have not been identified, but appear to be associated with a reduced ability to excise UV-induced cyclobutane pyrimidine dimers (Setlow *et al.*, 1969; Cleaver and Trosko, 1970). Because seven complementation groups (Galjaard, 1980) of xeroderma pigmentosum have been described, this excision process requires the interaction of at least seven different genes.

The prenatal diagnosis of this disease has been accomplished by demonstrating defective DNA repair after UV irradiation and [³H]thymidine incorporation into short-term amniotic cell cultures (Ramsey *et al.*, 1974; Lehmann *et al.*, 1977). Similarly, unaffected fetuses in at-risk pregnancies have been identified and confirmed after birth (Halley *et al.*, 1979). The accuracy of prenatal diagnosis is critically dependent on the expertise of the laboratory, the amniotic cell type assayed (Halley *et al.*, 1979), and characterization of the specific mutation (level of residual DNA-repair activity) in cultured fibroblasts from the index case.

2.   ATAXIA TELANGIECTASIA

Cerebellar ataxia, ocular and cutaneous telangiectases, frequent and severe pulmonary infections, and a high incidence of neoplasia characterize the clinical course of this progressive disease. Although the primary defect in ataxia telangiectasia (AT) is unknown, an abnormality in the repair of γ-radiation-induced DNA damage has been demonstrated in cultured fibroblasts from affected individuals of some families (Paterson *et al.*, 1976; Painter and Young, 1980). Two interrelated abnormalities induced by γ-irradiation of AT fibroblasts can be measured: (1) decreased repair replication and (2) a decreased rate of loss of γ-endonuclease sites (Paterson *et al.*, 1976). In contrast to xeroderma pigmentosum, DNA-repair mechanisms in AT are normal following ultraviolet irradiation (Lehmann *et al.*, 1977). Recent studies indicate that the defect in AT may result from the loss of the normal control of replicon initiation, similar to the abnormalities induced by caffeine treatment in normal cells (Painter and Young,

TABLE XVII

DISORDERS OF DNA REPAIR AND CHROMOSOMAL BREAKAGE

Disorder	McKusick catalog no.	Enzyme defect	Method of diagnosis	Prenatal diagnosis[a]	Method of prenatal diagnosis
Xeroderma pigmentosum	27871–27874	Defective DNA repair (UV damage)	Setlow et al. (1969); Cleaver and Trosko (1970)	Made	Ramsey et al. (1974); Halley et al. (1979)
Ataxia telangiectasia	20890	Defective DNA repair (γ-radiation damage)	Paterson et al. (1976); Paterson (1978)	Feasible	See Section III,Q,2
Fanconi anemia	22765	?	Latt et al. (1975); Auerbach et al. (1981)	Made	Auerbach et al. (1981)
Bloom syndrome	21090	?	Chaganti et al. (1977); German et al. (1977)	Feasible	See Section III,Q,4
Cockayne syndrome	21640	?			

[a] Explanation of terms:

Made—Prenatal diagnosis has been accomplished and confirmed.

Feasible—Methods are currently available or current techniques could be adapted for the prenatal diagnosis.

Plausible—Various strategies can or theoretically could be employed, on an experimental basis, and their use evaluated for prenatal diagnosis.

Not possible—Primary defect is not defined, secondary metabolic effects cannot presently be assessed, or technical difficulties must be overcome before the prenatal diagnosis is feasible.

1980). The presence of at least two complementation groups in AT with differing rates of γ-irradiation-induced DNA repair and loss of γ-endonuclease sites (Paterson *et al.*, 1976) indicate the genetic heterogeneity of the basic defect in AT.

The prenatal diagnosis has recently been accomplished by the demonstration of induced chromosome aberrations in normal lymphocytes incubated in the amniotic fluid from an at-risk fetus (Shaham *et al.*, 1980). Cultured amniotic fluid cells from at-risk fetuses should be studied cytogenetically because translocations involving 14q may occur constitutionally, and increased chromosomal abnormalities may be induced *in vitro* by ionizing radiation and radiomimetic agents. In addition, studies of cell survival after γ-irradiation of cultured amniocytes may provide diagnostic information. Because of the genetic heterogeneity, the rate of DNA repair and loss of γ-endonuclease sites in fibroblasts of the proband should be characterized prior to an attempted prenatal diagnosis. Demonstration of diminished *in vitro* cellular immune responses of fetal lymphocytes and/or absent to low secretory IgA and serum IgE might also support the diagnosis.

A useful adjunct to the prenatal diagnosis may be the level of α-fetoprotein in amniotic fluid—or, more diagnostic, in fetal serum. Waldmann and McIntire (1972) found a 2- to 10-fold elevation in serum α-fetoprotein in affected AT patients. This abnormality may be reflected in elevated amniotic fluid or maternal serum α-fetoprotein levels and warrants investigation in at-risk families.

3. FANCONI ANEMIA

Fanconi anemia is a rare autosomal recessive trait characterized by pancytopenia, various congenital abnormalities (e.g., radial aplasia), and spontaneous chromosome instability. There is variability in the phenotypic expression of the disease, and the diagnosis may be difficult in homozygotes with only pancytopenia. In most patients, an increased frequency of spontaneous chromosomal breakage has been observed in peripheral lymphocytes and cultured skin fibroblasts (Swift and Hirschhorn, 1966; Bushkell *et al.*, 1976; Latt *et al.*, 1980).

Recently, cytogenetic methods have been developed to identify affected homozygotes and heterozygous carriers for Fanconi anemia based on an increased number of chromosomal breaks induced by diepoxybutane, a bifunctional alkylating agent (Auerbach and Wolman, 1976, 1978) or by mitomycin (Cervenka *et al.*, 1981). The diepoxybutane technique has been used successfully to identify affected fetuses by the effect of the clastogenic agent on the chromosomes in cultured amniotic cells (Auerbach *et al.*, 1979, 1981). The prenatal diagnoses of five at-risk fetuses were confirmed after the birth of normal infants or by the finding of congenital anomalies in aborted fetuses, and/or increased chromosomal breakage in fetal fibroblasts that were exposed to the clastogen (Auerbach *et al.*, 1981).

4. BLOOM SYNDROME

Bloom syndrome is a rare autosomal recessive trait characterized by dwarfism, hypogammaglobulinemia, focal dermal hypoplasia, sensitivity to sunlight, and a high incidence of malignancies (Gorlin *et al.*, 1976). Multiple nonspecific chromosomal breaks and exchanges (particularly between homologous chromosomes) are observed in the lymphocytes and fibroblasts of affected individuals. A useful diagnostic adjunct to the clinical manifestations is the presence of increased sister chromatic exchange (SCE) in peripheral blood leukocytes (Chaganti *et al.*, 1977). In contrast to Fanconi anemia, the increased number of SCEs in Bloom syndrome is present constitutionally and is enhanced by the use of ethylmethane sulfonate (German *et al.*, 1977). In addition, the chromatid exchange in this disorder is primarily between homologous chromosomes, whereas nonhomologous exchange is more frequent in Fanconi anemia (German *et al.*, 1977). Because an increased frequency of SCEs is present in cultured fibroblasts from Bloom syndrome patients (Tice *et al.*, 1978), the frequency of SCEs with or without mutagenic agents should provide a useful technique for the prenatal diagnosis of this disease (Shiriashi and Sandberg, 1978).

5. COCKAYNE SYNDROME

Cockayne syndrome is an autosomal recessively inherited cachetic dwarfism characterized by mental retardation, intracranial calcifications, progressive cerebellar deficits, retinitis pigmentosum, and photosensitivity (Pattidson *et al.*, 1963). Although the basic biochemical defect in this disease is unknown, Schmickel *et al.* (1975) demonstrated a defect in the repair of ultraviolet-induced DNA damage in cultured fibroblasts from two Cockayne patients. Because this defect is similar to that observed in xeroderma pigmentosum, the prenatal diagnosis is possible by the approach outlined in Section III,Q,1.

R. Disorders of Heme Biosynthesis—The Porphyrias (Table XVIII)

The porphyrias are a diverse family of disorders due to the deficiency of specific enzymes in the heme-biosynthetic pathway (Meyer and Schmid, 1978). These diseases can be differentiated on the basis of their clinical manifestations, metabolic defects, and modes of inheritance. The specific enzymatic defect in each of these disorders has been identified during the past decade, although the availability of these assays is limited to a few centers (see Table XVIII). The hepatic or "acute" porphyrias can be life-threatening, whereas the erythropoietic porphyrias can scar and deform affected individuals. On the other hand, early diagnosis and avoidance of precipitating factors (certain drugs, steroids, starvation, etc.) that exacerbate the hepatic porphyrias, and the avoidance of sunlight

TABLE XVIII

DISORDERS OF HEME BIOSYNTHESIS—THE PORPHYRIAS

Disorder	McKusick catalog no.	Enzyme defect	Method of diagnosis	Prenatal diagnosis[a]	Method of prenatal diagnosis
Congenital erythropoietic porphyria	26370	Uroporphyrinogen III cosynthase	Romeo and Levin (1969); Romeo et al. (1970)	Made	Nitowsky et al. (1978); Deyback et al. (1980); Kaiser (1980)
δ-Aminolevulinate dehydratase deficiency	—	δ-Aminolevulinate dehydratase	Doss et al. (1979)	Feasible	
Acute intermittent porphyria	17600	Porphobilinogen deaminase	Sassa et al. (1975); Anderson and Desnick (1980, 1981)	Made	Sassa et al. (1975); Anderson and Desnick (1981)
Hereditary coproporphyria	12130	Coproporphyrinogen III oxidase	Elder et al. (1977); Grandchamp and Nordmann (1977)	Feasible	
Variegate porphyria	17620	Protoporphyrinogen oxidase	Brenner and Bloomer (1980)	Feasible	
Porphyria cutanea tarda	17610	Uroporphyrinogen decarboxylase	Kurshner et al. (1976)	Feasible	
Protoporphyria	17700	Ferrochelatase	Bonkowsky et al. (1975)	Feasible	

[a] Explanation of terms:

Made—Prenatal diagnosis has been accomplished and confirmed.

Feasible—Methods are currently available or current techniques could be adapted for the prenatal diagnosis.

Plausible—Various strategies can or theoretically could be employed, on an experimental basis, and their use evaluated for prenatal diagnosis.

Not Possible—Primary defect is not defined, secondary metabolic effects cannot presently be assessed, or technical difficulties must be overcome before the prenatal diagnosis is feasible.

for the photosensitive porphyrias, will minimize the expression and severity of these disorders.

The hepatic porphyrias include acute intermittent porphyria, variegate porphyria, coproporphyria, porphyria cutanea tarda, and the newly described δ-aminolevulinate dehydratase deficiency (Doss *et al.*, 1979). The hepatic porphyrias are inherited as autosomal dominant traits with the exception of the latter, which is transmitted as an autosomal recessive disease. Of these disorders, only acute intermittent porphyria has been prenatally diagnosed by the demonstration of half-normal porphobilinogen deaminase (also known as uroporphyrinogen I synthase) levels in cultured amniotic cells (Sassa *et al.*, 1975). Although this is a sensitive assay, prenatal diagnosis is difficult because the porphobilinogen deaminase activity in cultured normal fibroblasts and amniotic cells is very low. For families in which the defective enzyme is CRIM-positive (Anderson and Desnick, 1981), determination of CRIM-specific activity should improve the sensitivity of the assay. In addition, the levels of the precursor and substrate, δ-aminolevulinic acid and porphobilinogen, should be determined in cell-free amniotic fluid to assess whether they are increased in affected pregnancies.

The prenatal diagnoses of variegate porphyria, coproporphyria, and porphyria cutanea tarda are all possible, but difficult because the specific enzyme assays are cumbersome to perform and require specially synthesized substrates. The amniotic fluid uroporphyrin and coproporphyrin levels (and ratios) may be useful in these three hepatic porphyrias (Goodlin and Schwartz, 1962).

The erythropoietic porphyrias, congenital erythropoietic porphyria and protoporphyria, are both prenatally detectable. Fetuses with congenital erythropoietic porphyria have been diagnosed by the demonstration of increased porphyrins (uroporphyrinogen I) in the amniotic fluid, which appeared reddish brown or chocolate brown in color (Nitowsky *et al.*, 1978; Kaiser, 1980). Deybach *et al.* (1980) were able to exclude the diagnosis in two at-risk fetuses by the demonstration of normal uroporphyrinogen III cosynthase activity in cultured amniotic cells. The recent development of improved assays for uroporphyrinogen III cosynthase (Jordan *et al.*, 1980) should permit the enzymatic diagnosis in cultured amniotic cells. Because protoporphyria is a disorder primarily limited to relatively mild cutaneous manifestations, prenatal diagnosis may not be warranted. However, recent reports of progressive liver disease leading to fatal cirrhosis in patients with protoporphyria may alter the concept of the disorder to a more severe disease (Meyer and Schmid, 1978). If future evaluation of patients with protoporphyria indicates that progressive liver disease is a common feature, and if the hepatic involvement is not treatable, then prenatal diagnosis may be considered more seriously. The diagnosis could be made by the demonstration of half-normal ferrochelatase activity in cultured amniotic cells (Bonkowsky *et al.*, 1975) and supported by the finding of increased erythrocyte protoporphyrin levels in fetal blood.

S. Disorders of Metal Metabolism (Table XIX)

1. MENKES DISEASE

The basic defect in this X-linked neurodegenerative disease results in the abnormal accumulation of intracellular copper in fibroblasts and intestinal cells of affected hemizygotes. By exploiting this finding, Horn (1976) was able to perform the first prenatal diagnosis of Menkes disease. Since that time, more than 50 at-risk male fetuses have been reliably monitored (Galjaard, 1980) by determining the copper content of amniotic cells by atomic-absorption spectrometry (Goka et al., 1976) or by determining ^{64}Cu incorporation into cultured amniocytes (Horn, 1976; LaBadie et al., 1980). Recent evidence of increased constitutive levels of metallothionein in Menkes disease fibroblasts (Labadie et al., 1981) suggests that quantitative determination of metallothionein (by ^{35}S-uptake studies or by immunologic quantitation) may provide another diagnostic method for the prenatal diagnosis of this disease.

2. HEMOCHROMATOSIS

Idiopathic hemochromatosis results from an inherited abnormality in an intracellular iron-carrier protein, which leads to increased gastrointestinal iron absorption and the subsequent development of cirrhosis and diabetes mellitus due to tissue iron deposition (Pollycove, 1978). The pathophysiology, biochemistry, and genetics of this disease have been recently reviewed (Pollycove, 1978; Simon et al., 1980).

The inheritance of this disease and the potential for prenatal diagnosis remained unclear until Simon et al. (1975) established the association of idiopathic hemochromatosis with the HLA-A3 locus. Subsequent studies (Walters et al., 1975; Shewan et al., 1976; Simon et al., 1976; Fauchet et al., 1977) on 384 unrelated patients with hemochromatosis established this highly significant concordance. Moreover, HLA-A3 was not associated with the secondary hemochromatoses in patients with alcoholic liver disease (Simon et al., 1977a). Simon et al. (1977b) also found 21 of 27 hemochromatosis siblings to be homozygous for the same HLA-A and B loci. In summary, these and other data (Simon et al., 1980) indicated the autosomal recessive inheritance of idiopathic hemochromatosis and the ability to diagnose this disease prenatally by amniocyte HLA typing. Lack of complete concordance of shared haplotypes between sibs with hemochromatosis (Simon et al., 1977b, 1980) suggested that the linkage of the HLA region and the gene(s) for hemochromatosis may not be close, and therefore subject to recombination events. Thus approximately 10–20% of fetuses who have no antigens or only one in common with an affected sib will be

TABLE XIX

DISORDERS OF METAL METABOLISM

Disorder	McKusick catalog no.	Enzyme defect	Method of diagnosis	Prenatal diagnosis[a]	Method of prenatal diagnosis
Menkes disease	30940	Intracellular copper accumulation	LaBadie *et al.* (1980)	Made	Horn (1976)
Hemochromatosis	14160	Abnormal intracellular iron binding	Pollycove (1978)	Feasible	See Section III,S,2

[a] Explanation of terms:

Made—Prenatal diagnosis has been accomplished and confirmed.

Feasible—Methods are currently available or current techniques could be adapted for the prenatal diagnosis.

Plausible—Various strategies can or theoretically could be employed, on an experimental basis, and their use evaluated for prenatal diagnosis.

Not possible—Primary defect is not defined, secondary metabolic effects cannot presently be assessed, or technical difficulties must be overcome before the prenatal diagnosis is feasible.

misdiagnosed as normal. Conversely, less than 8% of fetuses who share both haplotypes with an affected sibling will be misdiagnosed as affected (see Table 5, in Simon *et al.*, 1980). Until the basic defect in idiopathic hemochromatosis is identified, the HLA association remains the only method for the prenatal diagnosis of this disease.

T. α_1-Antitrypsin Deficiency and Cystic Fibrosis

1. α_1-ANTITRYPSIN DEFICIENCY

The association of α_1-antitrypsin deficiency (particularly the PiZZ phenotype) and cirrhosis in childhood (Sharp *et al.*, 1969) or pulmonary emphysema in adults (Laurell and Erickson, 1963) is well known. Because the development of pulmonary emphysema occurs during the fifth or sixth decades of life and because only about 10% of the PiZZ homozygotes develop severe liver disease (O'Brien *et al.*, 1978; Sveger, 1978), it is likely that the prenatal diagnosis will be considered only in families that have had a previous child with α_1-antitrypsin deficiency and cirrhosis. The prenatal diagnosis can be made using amniotic fluid because it contains only fetal α_1-antitrypsin (Kaiser *et al.*, 1974; Evans *et al.*, 1975; O'Brien *et al.*, 1978). Recently, an at-risk fetus was monitored in one such family by the determination of the amniotic fluid Pi type, trypsin-inhibitory capacity, and level of α_1-antitrypsin (Roth *et al.*, 1980). On the basis of these studies, the Pi type of the fetus was MZ and the diagnosis was confirmed at birth.

2. CYSTIC FIBROSIS

Cystic fibrosis is one of the most frequently inherited metabolic diseases. Unfortunately, efforts to develop a specific test for the reliable prenatal diagnosis of this disease have been precluded by the elusiveness of the primary metabolic defect. Although attempts have been made to extend findings in cultured skin fibroblasts for the prenatal diagnosis of this disorder (Danes and Bearn, 1966; Beratis *et al.*, 1973; Bowman *et al.*, 1973; Holsi and Vogt, 1977; Breslow *et al.*, 1978), these methods have not proved reliable (Davis and di Sant'Agnese, 1980). Recently, Nadler and Walsh (1980) have developed a predictive test for the intrauterine diagnosis of this disease by the extension of their previous demonstration of arginine esterase deficiency in the plasma and saliva of affected individuals (Rao and Nadler, 1975). They established methods to determine the serine protease activity using quantitative and qualitative measurements of the 4-methylumbelliferyl-guanidinobenzoate (MUGB) reactive proteases in amniotic fluid (Walsh *et al.*, 1980; Nadler and Walsh, 1980). With these methods, pregnancies for cystic fibrosis have been monitored and the prediction in the majority of cases has been confirmed after delivery (Nadler and Walsh, 1980; Harris *et al.*, 1981). False negatives also have occurred, possibly due to the genetic heterogeneity within the phenotype (Harris *et al.*, 1981). Further refinement and evaluation of this procedure must occur before this experimental technique can be considered reliable. If this or other methods are proven accurate, and a screening test to identify carriers of the cystic fibrosis gene(s) is developed (see Manson and Brock, 1980), it is likely that the antenatal detection of this disease will become the most requested prenatal metabolic diagnosis (Sklower and Desnick, 1979).

IV.   Prospectus

The past 20 years have witnessed a remarkable increase in the recognition, delineation, and understanding of inherited metabolic diseases. The specific enzymatic, receptor, or transport defects in an ever-increasing number of these disorders have been identified; the characterization of these defects has made us aware of the extensive heterogeneity within a given "phenotype" that has been revealed by differences at the biochemical and/or genetic level. Although effective therapies have not been developed for most, the knowledge of the specific metabolic aberration has led to the rapid implementation of prenatal diagnosis for many of these disorders. Indeed, the ability to monitor an at-risk pregnancy and determine the health of the fetus has provided many families with the opportunity to have only normal offspring. The increasing demand for prenatal diagnosis reflects the importance and acceptance of this service by families at high risk for these tragic and often devastating diseases.

This article has emphasized the present advances, special considerations, and future directions for prenatal metabolic diagnosis. What can we expect in the future? First, for the many disorders in search of a specific metabolic etiology, we can anticipate that intensive research efforts will lead to the elucidation of their primary defects. Because many of these defects will be expressed in cultured fibroblasts, the extension for prenatal diagnosis should be straightforward. For these and those disorders in which the specific defects are already known, future diagnoses will be based on both functional and immunologic assays. In this way, the enzymatic activity and the level of enzyme protein (CRIM) will be simultaneously determined to ensure reliable diagnoses. In addition, the sensitive immunologic techiques may not require as many cultured amniocytes, thus increasing the rapidity of the diagnosis.

For those disorders in which the defect is tissue-specific, newer strategies will be employed to demonstrate the metabolic lesion. These will include the use of (1) somatic cell genetic techniques to achieve expression of the differentiated function in hybrid cells; (2) linkage analyses to identify closely linked genes that are expressed in cultured amniocytes; and (3) recombinant DNA techniques to characterize the integrity and sequence of the specified gene in amniocytes.

It is also anticipated that the rapid advances in molecular biology and in the delineation of the human gene map will increase our diagnostic armamentarium dramatically. For example, the ability to characterize the restriction map of a given gene should not only identify the mechanism by which the gene function or expression has been deranged, but in addition should provide diagnostic capabilities by the demonstration of gene deletions (e.g., α-thalassemia), altered mRNA translation ($\beta°$-thalassemia), abnormal restriction maps (e.g., Hemoglobin Arab), or unique DNA polymorphisms (e.g., sickle cell disease). As noted, the molecular characterization of the erythrocyte-specific gene product, hemoglobin, has already previewed the newer methods for prenatal diagnosis using amniocytes, thus precluding the need to perform fetal blood aspiration with its attendant morbidity and mortality. It is likely that prenatal diagnoses currently made by assaying a specific enzymatic activity in cultured amniocytes will be accomplished, either in conjunction with the activity (function) assay or solely by DNA techniques to assess gene structure and/or expression.

Efforts will also be directed to decreasing the psychologically burdensome period between amniocentesis and diagnosis. The development of microtechniques for the assay of various enzymes in a few or even single cells is already a reality. The extension of these techniques, particularly using sensitive immunoassays, should make the diagnosis more rapid. In addition, the determination of CRIM-specific activity may resolve the problems associated with enzymes whose activities are a function of cell density and tissue-culture conditions. Furthermore, it may be possible to use uncultured cells for CRIM-specific assays as well as for DNA analyses. If safer, simpler methods for fetal blood aspiration are developed, many disorders might be more rapidly diagnosed using fetal blood components rather than waiting for adequate numbers of cultured amniotic cells.

Finally, it is also likely that the elucidation of the precise nature of the biochemical and genetic defects within individual families will provide important information for the family and the physician. For example, an increased understanding of B_{12} and biotin metabolism and function has resulted in trials of ''prenatal therapy'' for certain forms of methylmalonic acidemia and multiple carboxylase deficiency, respectively. Indeed, the precise identification of the defects in some disorders will lead to the development of specific (but not proven) therapies, thereby confronting families with another major consideration when an affected fetus is diagnosed.

Concomitant with the advances in the elucidation and prenatal diagnosis of inherited metabolic diseases, ancillary programs must be expanded for the identification of affected individuals, heterozygote detection, counseling of at-risk families, and education of professionals and the lay public. Metabolic screening of newborns should incorporate new technology to identify affected newborns for referrals to specialized centers for confirmatory testing, management, and counseling for specific diseases. Heterozygote-detection programs should be developed for at-risk family members and populations in which the gene is prevalent, so that prospective counseling and prenatal diagnosis can be made available. Educational programs should be designed to increase the awareness of physicians and the public of the availability of prenatal diagnosis. Most importantly, genetic counseling and support programs for at-risk families should be expanded. The implementation of these newer diagnostic techniques, together with the expansion and regionalization of specialized centers for prenatal metabolic diagnosis and counseling, should provide an important asset to the many families who request these services.

ACKNOWLEDGMENTS

The authors are indebted to Drs. L. Fleisher, G. Gaull, M. M. Cohen, and N. Gusman for their critical review of portions of the manuscript, and to Mrs. L. Lugo for her expert clerical skills in the preparation of the manuscript.

REFERENCES

Allen, S. T., Gillett, M., Holton, J. B., King, G. S., and Pettit, B. R. (1980). *Lancet* **1,** 603.
Alper, C. A., and Rosen, F. S. (1976). *Adv. Hum. Genet.* **7,** 141–188.
Alter, B. P. (1979). *J. Pediatr.* **95,** 501–513.
Amihein, J. A., Meyer, W. J., Jones, H. W., and Migeon, C. J. (1976). *Proc. Natl. Acad. Sci. U.S.A.* **73,** 891–894.
Ampola, M. G., Efron, M. L., Bixby, E. M., and Meshorer, E. (1969). *Am. J. Dis. Child.* **117,** 66–70.
Ampola, M. G., Mahoney, M. J., Nakamura, E., and Tanaka, K. (1975). *N. Engl. J. Med.* **293,** 313–317.
Anderson, P. A., and Desnick, R. J. (1980). *J. Biol. Chem.* **255,** 1993–1999.
Anderson, P. A., and Desnick, R. J. (1981). *J. Clin. Invest.* **68,** 1–12.
Arbisser, A. I., Donnely, K. A., Scott, C. I., DiFerrante, N. M., Singh, J., Stevenson, R. E., Aylesworth, A. S., and Howell, R. R. (1977). *Am. J. Med. Genet.* **1,** 195–205.
Auerbach, A. D., and Wolman, S. R. (1976). *Nature* **261,** 494–496.
Auerbach, A. D., and Wolman, S. R. (1978). *Nature* **271,** 69–71.
Auerbach, V. H., DiGeorge, A. M., Brigham, M. P., and Dobbs, J. M. (1963). *J. Pediatr.* **6,** 938–943.
Auerbach, A. D., Warburton, D., and Bloom, A. D. (1979). *Am. J. Hum. Genet.* **31,** 77–84.
Auerbach, A. D., Adler, B., and Chaganti, R. S. K. (1981). *Pediatrics* **67,** 128–136.
Aula, P., Nanto, V., Laipio, M. L., and Autio, S. (1973). *Clin. Genet.* **4,** 297–300.
Aula, P., Rapola, J., Autio, S., Raivio, S., and Karjalainen, O. (1975). *J. Pediatr.* **87,** 221–226.
Aula, P., Raivio, K., and Autio, S. (1976). *Pediatr. Res.* **10,** 625–629.

Aula, P., Autio, S., Raivio, K. O., Rapola, J., Thoden, C- J., Koskela, S- L., and Yamashina, I. (1979a). *Arch. Neurol.* **36**, 88–94.

Aula, P., Karjalainen, O., Teramo, K., Vaara, L., and Seppala, M. (1979b). *Ann. Clin. Res.* **11**, 156–163.

Aylesworth, A. S., Swisher, C. N., and Kirkman, H. N. (1975). *Am. J. Hum. Genet.* **27**, 15A.

Bach, G., Cohen, M., and Kohn, G. (1975). *Biochem. Biophys. Res. Commun.* **66**, 1483–1490.

Bach, G., Zeigler, M., and Kohn, M. (1980). *Clin. Chim. Acta* **106**, 121–128.

Ballow, M., Shira, J. E., Harden, L., Yang, S. Y., and Day, N. K. (1975). *J. Clin. Invest.* **56**, 703–713.

Bartholome, K., Lutz, P., and Bickel, H. (1975). *Pediatr. Res.* **9**, 899–903.

Bartlett, K., and Gompertz, D. (1976). *Lancet* **2**, 804–805.

Becker, M. A., Kostel, P. J., Meyer, L. J., and Seegmiller, J. E. (1973). *Proc. Natl. Acad. Sci. U.S.A.* **70**, 2749–2752.

Benzie, R. J., and Doran, T. A. (1975). *Am. J. Obstet. Gynecol.* **121**, 460–464.

Beratis, N. G., Conover, J. H., Conrad, E. J., Bonforte, R. J., and Hirschhorn, K. (1973). *Pediatr. Res.* **7**, 958–962.

Beratis, N. G., Turner, B. M., Weiss, R., and Hirschhorn, K. (1975a). *Pediatr. Res.* **9**, 475–480.

Beratis, N. G., Turner, B. M., and Hirschhorn, K. (1975b). *J. Pediatr.* **87**, 1193–1198.

Beratis, N. G., Turner, B. G., LaBadie, G. U., and Hirschhorn, K. (1977). *Pediatr. Res.* **11**, 862–866.

Beratis, N. G., LaBadie, G. U., and Hirschhorn, K. (1978). *Pediatr. Res.* **62**, 1264–1274.

Bergsma, D., Good, R. A., Finstad, J., and Paul, N. W. (1975) "Immunodeficiency in Man and Animals, Birth Defects Original Article Series (XI)." Sinauer Associates, Sunderland, Mass.

Beutler, E. (1977). *J.A.M.A.* **237**, 2529.

Beutler, E., and Kuhl, W. (1970). *J. Lab. Clin. Med.* **76**, 747–754.

Beutler, E., Kuhl, W., Trinidad, F., Teplitz, R., and Nadler, H. (1971). *Am. J. Hum. Genet.* **23**, 62–66.

Beutler, E., Dale, G. L., and Kuhl, W. (1980). *In* "Enzyme Therapy in Genetic Diseases: 2" (R. J. Desnick, ed.), pp. 383–392. Alan R. Liss, New York.

Biglieri, E. G., Herron, M. A., and Buist, N. (1966). *J. Clin. Invest.* **45**, 1946–1954.

Bittles, A. H., and Carson, N. A. J. (1974). *J. Med. Genet.* **11**, 121–122.

Blaskovics, M. E. (1978). *J. Inher. Metab. Dis.* **1**, 9–11.

Bondy, P. K., and Rosenberg, L. E. (1980). "Metabolic Control and Disease." Saunders, Philadelphia.

Bongiovanni, A. M. (1962). *J. Clin. Invest.* **41**, 2086–2092.

Bongiovanni, A. M. (1978). *In* "The Metabolic Basis of Inherited Disease," 4th Edition (J. B. Stanbury, J. B. Wyngaarden, and D. S. Fredrickson, eds.), pp. 868–893. McGraw-Hill, New York.

Bongiovanni, A. M., Ebertein, W. R., Smith, J. D., and McPadden, A. J. (1959). *J. Clin. Endocrinol.* **19**, 1608–1617.

Bonkowsky, H. L., Bloomer, J. R., Ebert, P. S., and Mahoney, M. J. (1975). *J. Clin. Invest.* **56**, 1139–1148.

Booth, C. W., Gerbie, A. B., and Nadler, H. L. (1973). *Pediatrics* **52**, 521–524.

Bornstein, P., and Byers, P. H. (1980). *In* "Metabolic Control and Disease" (P. K. Bondy and L. E. Rosenberg, eds.), pp. 1089–1153. Saunders, Philadelphia.

Borregaard, N., Bang, J., Berthelsen, J. G., Johansen, K. S., Koch, C., Philip, J., Rasmussen, K., Schwartz, M., Therkelsen, A. J., and Valerius, N. H. (1982). *Lancet* **1**, 114.

Bowman, B. H., Lockhart, L. H., Herzberg, V. L., Barnett, D. R., and Kramer, J. (1973). *J. Clin. Genet.* **4**, 461–466.

Brady, R. O. (1978). *In* "The Metabolic Basis of Inherited Disease," 4th Edition (J. B. Stanbury, J. B. Wyngaarden, and D. S. Fredrickson, eds.), pp. 731–746. McGraw-Hill, New York.

Brady, R. O., Gal, A. E., Kanfer, J. N., and Bradley, R. M. (1965). *J. Biol. Chem.* **240,** 3766–3770.

Brady, R. O., Pentchev, P. G., Gal, A. E., Hibbert, S. R., and Dekaban, A. S. (1974). *N. Engl. J. Med.* **291,** 989–994.

Brady, R. O., Barringer, J. A., Gal, A. E., Pentchev, P. G., and Furbish, F. S. (1980). *In* "Enzyme Therapy in Genetic Disease: 2" (R. J. Desnick, ed.), pp. 361–368. Alan R. Liss, New York.

Brenner, D. A., and Bloomer, J. R. (1980). *N. Engl. J. Med.* **302,** 765–769.

Breslow, J. L., Epstein, J., Fontaine, J. H., and Forbes, G. B. (1978). *Science* **201,** 180–181.

Brett, E. M., Ellis, R. B., Haas, L., Ikonne, J. U., Lake, B. D., Patrick, A. D., and Stephens, R. (1973). *Arch. Dis. Child.* **48,** 775–785.

Brown, B. I., and Brown, D. H. (1966). *Proc. Natl. Acad. Sci. U.S.A.* **56,** 725–729.

Brown, D. M., and Dent, P. B. (1971). *Pediatr. Res.* **5,** 181–191.

Brown, M. S., and Goldstein, J. L. (1974). *Science* **185,** 161–163.

Brown, M. S., and Goldstein, J. L. (1976). *Science* **191,** 150–154.

Brown, M. S., Goldstein, J. L., VandenBerghe, K., Fryns, J. P., Kovanen, P. T., Eeckels, R., VandenBerghe, H., and Carriman, J. J. (1979). *Lancet* **1,** 526–529.

Buchanan, P. D., Kahler, S. G., Sweetman, L., and Nyhan, W. L. (1980). *Clin. Genet.* **18,** 177–183.

Bushkell, L. L., Kersey, J. H., and Cervenka, J. (1976). *Clin. Genet.* **9,** 583–590.

Butterworth, J., and Guy, G. J. (1977). *Clin. Genet.* **12,** 297–302.

Byers, P. H., Holbrook, K. A., McGillivray, B., Macloed, P. M., and Lowry, R. B. (1979). *Hum. Genet.* **47,** 141–150.

Byers, P. H., Barsh, G. S., Peterson, K. E., Phillips, J. H., Shapiro, J., Holbrook, K. A., Levin, L. S., and Rowe, D. W. (1981). *Pediatr. Res.* **15,** 559–567.

Callahan, J. W., and Khalil, M. (1975). *Pediatr. Res.* **9,** 914–918.

Callahan, J. W., Khalil, M., and Philippart, M. (1975). *Pediatr. Res.* **9,** 908–913.

Cameron, A. H. (1980). *N. Engl. J. Med.* **303,** 22–24.

Campbell, A. G. M., Rosenberg, L. E., Snodgrass, P. J., and Nuzum, C. T. (1973). *N. Engl. J. Med.* **228,** 7–11.

Cantz, M., Gehler, I., and Spranger, J. W. (1977). *Biochem. Biophys. Res. Commun.* **74,** 732–738.

Cederbaum, S. P., Shaw, K. N. F., and Valente, M. (1977). *J. Pediatr.* **90,** 569–573.

Cervenka, J., Arthur, D., and Yasis, C. (1981). *Pediatrics* **67,** 119–127.

Chaganti, R. S. K., Schonberg, S., and German, J. (1977). *Proc. Natl. Acad. Sci. U.S.A.* **71,** 4508–4512.

Christensen, E., Brandt, N. J., Philip, J., and Kennaway, N. G. (1980). *J. Inher. Metab. Dis.* **3,** 73–75.

Christomanou, H., Cap, C., and Sandhoff, K. (1978). *Klin. Wochenschr.* **56,** 1133–1135.

Cleaver, J. E., and Trosko, J. E. (1970). *Photochem. Photobiol.* **11,** 547–555.

Colten, H. R., and Rosen, F. S. (1973). *In* "Immunologic Disorders in Infants and Children" (R. E. Stiehm and V. A. Fulginiti, eds.), pp. 99–106. Saunders, Philadelphia.

Colten, H. R., Alper, C. A., and Rosen, F. S. (1981). *N. Engl. J. Med.* **304,** 653–656.

Conzelman, E., and Sandhoff, K. (1978). *Proc. Natl. Acad. Sci. U.S.A.* **75,** 3979–3983.

Cooper, M. D., and Lawton, A. R. (1972). *Am. J. Pathol.* **69,** 513–523.

Cox, R. P., Hutzler, J., and Dancis, J. (1978). *Lancet* **2,** 212.

Dance, N., Price, R. G., and Robinson, D. (1970). *Biochim. Biophys. Acta* **222,** 662–664.

Dancis, J. (1972). *In* "Antenatal Diagnosis" (A. Dorfman, ed.), pp. 123–125. Univ. of Chicago Press, Chicago.

Dancis, J., and Levitz, M. (1978). *In* "The Metabolic Basis of Inherited Disease," 4th Edition (J. B. Stanbury, J. B. Wyngaarden, and D. S. Fredrickson eds.), pp. 397–410. McGraw-Hill, New York.

Dancis, J., Hutzler, J., and Levitz, M. (1963). *Pediatrics* **32,** 234–240.

Dancis, J., Hutzler, J., Toda, Y., Wada, Y., Morikawa, T., and Arakawa, T. (1967). *Pediatrics* **39**, 813.

Dancis, J., Hutzler, J., and Cox, R. P. (1969a). *Biochem. Med.* **2**, 407.

Dancis, J., Hutzler, J., Cox, R. P., and Woody, N. C. (1969b). *J. Clin. Invest.* **48**, 1447–1452.

Danes, B. S., and Bearn, A. G. (1966). *J. Exp. Med.* **123**, 1–7.

Danner, D. J., and Elsas, L. J. (1975). *Biochem. Med.* **13**, 7–22.

Darsee, R. J., Heymsfiedd, B. S., and Nutter, O. D. (1979). *N. Engl. J. Med.* **300**, 877–882.

Davidson, R. G., and Rattazzi, M. C. (1972). *Clin. Chem.* **18**, 179–187.

Davis, P. B., and di Sant'Agnese, P. A. (1980). *Pediatr. Res.* **14**, 83–87.

de Bracco, M. E., Windhorst, D., Stroud, R. M., and Moncada, B. (1974). *Clin. Exp. Immunol.* **16**, 183–190.

Degenhart, H. J., Visser, H. K. A., Boon, H., and O'Doherty, N. J. (1972). *Acta Endocrinol.* **71**, 512–518.

de Groot, G. W. (1980). *Pediatr. Res.* **14**, 7–14.

Delage, J. M., Bergeron, P., Simard, J., Lehner-Netsch, G., and Prochazka, E. (1977). *J. Clin. Invest.* **60**, 1061–1069.

Delvin, E., Pottier, A., Scriver, C. R., and Gold, R. J. M. (1974). *Clin. Chem. Acta* **53**, 135–143.

Desnick, R. J. (1981). *In* "Genetic Issues in Pediatrics, Perinatology, and Obstetrical Practice" (M. M. Kaback, ed.), pp. 525–566. Year Book Medical Publishers, Inc., Chicago.

Desnick, R. J. and Grabowski, G. A. (1981). *In* "Advances in Human Genetics" (H. Harris and K. Hirschhorn, eds.), pp. 281–369. Plenum, New York.

Desnick, R. J., Krivit, W., and Sharp, H. L. (1973a). *Biochem. Biophys. Res. Commun.* **51**, 20–26.

Desnick, R. J., Allen, K. Y., Desnick, S. J., Raman, M. K., Bernlohr, R. W., and Krivit, W. (1973b). *J. Lab. Clin. Med.* **81**, 157–164.

Desnick, R. J., Sharp, H. L., Grabowski, G. A., Brunning, R. D., Quie, P. G., Sung, J. H., Gorlin, R. J., and Ikonne, J. U. (1976). *Pediatr. Res.* **10**, 985–996.

Desnick, R. J., Truex, J. H., and Goldberg, J. D. (1977). *In* "Tay-Sachs Disease: Screening and Prevention" (M. M. Kaback, D. L. Rimoin, and J. S. O'Brien, eds.), pp. 245–266. Alan R. Liss, New York.

Deybach, J. C., Grandchamp, B., Grelier, M., Nordmann, Y., Boué, J., Boué, A. A., and de Barranger, N. (1980). *Hum. Genet.* **53**, 217–221.

Di Ferranti, N., Leachman, R. D., Angelini, P., Donnelly, P. V., Francis, G., and Almazan, A. (1975a). *Connect. Tissue Res.* **3**, 49–53.

Di Ferranti, N., Leachman, R. D., Angelini, P., Donnelly, R. V., Francis, G., Almazan, A., Segni, G., Franzblau, C., and Jordan, R. E. (1975b). *Birth Defects* **11**(6), pp. 31–37.

Doss, M., von Tiepermann, R., Schneider, J., and Schmid, H. (1979). *Klin. Wochenschr.* **57**, 1123–1127.

Dreborg, S., Erikson, A., and Hagberg, B. (1980). *Eur. J. Pediatr.* **133**, 107–118.

Dubois, G., Turpin, J. C., and Baumann, N. (1975). *N. Engl. J. Med.* **293**, 302–308.

Dulaney, J. T., and Moser, H. W. (1977). *In* "Practical Enzymology of the Sphingolipidoses" (R. H. Glew and S. P. Peters, eds.), pp. 137–171. Alan R. Liss, New York.

Dulaney, J. T., Milunsky, A., Sidbury, J. B., Hobolth, N., and Moser, H. W. (1976). *J. Pediatr.* **89**, 59–61.

Dupont, B., Smithwick, E. M., Oberfield, S. E., Lee, T. D., and Levine, L. S. (1977). *Lancet* **2**, 1309–1312.

Efron, M. L. (1965). *N. Engl. J. Med.* **272**, 1243–1254.

Einstein, L. P., Hanson, P. J., Ballow, M., Davis, A. E., III, Davis, J. S., Alper, C. A., Rosen, F. S., and Colten, H. R. (1977). *J. Clin. Invest.* **60**, 963–969.

Elder, G., Evans, J. O., Thomas, N., Cox, R., Brodie, M. J., Goldberg, A., and Nicholson, D. C. (1977). *Lancet* **2**, 1217–1219.

Epstein, E. H., and Leventhal, M. E. (1981). *J. Clin. Invest.* **67,** 1257–1262.

Eto, Y., Rampini, S., Wiesmann, U., and Herschkowitz, M. N. (1974). *J. Neurochem.* **23,** 1161–1170.

Evans, H. E., Glass, L., and Mardl, J. (1975). *Biol. Neonate* **27,** 232–236.

Evans, H. J., Hamerton, J. L., Klinger, H. P., and McKusick, V. A., eds. (1979). *Cytogenet. Cell Genet.* **25,** 1–236.

Fairweather, D. V. I., Modell, B., Berdoukas, V., Alter, B. P., Nathan, D. G., Loukopoulos, D., Wood, W., Glegg, J. B., and Weatherall, D. J. (1978). *Br. Med. J.* **1,** 350–353.

Fairweather, D. V. I., Ward, R. H. T., and Modell, B. (1980). *Br. J. Obstet. Gynaecol.* **87,** 87–99.

Farrell, D. F., McMartin, M. P., and Clark, A. F. (1979). *Neurology* **29,** 16–20.

Fauchet, R., Simon, M., Genetet, B., Kerbaol, M., Bansard, J. Y., Genetet, N., and Bourel, M. (1977). *Tissue Antigens* **10,** 206–211.

Feneant, M., Moatti, N., Lemonnier, F., Maccaris, M., Gantier, C., Charpentier, C., and Lemonnier, A. (1980). *J. Inher. Metab. Dis.* **3**(3), 97–98.

Fenson, A. H., Benson, P. F., Rodeck, C. H., Cambell, S., and Gould, J. D. M. (1979). *Br. Med. J.* **1,** 21–22.

Fiddler, M. B., Vine, D., Shapira, E., and Nadler, H. L. (1979). *Nature* **282,** 98–100.

Fikrig, S. M., Smithnick, E. M., Suniharalingam, K., and Good, R. A. (1980). *Lancet* **1,** 18–19.

Finne, M. D. A., Cottrall, K., Seakins, J. W. T., and Snedelen, R. (1976). *Clin. Chim. Acta* **73,** 513–519.

Firshein, S. I., Hoyer, L. W., Lazarchick, J., Forget, B. G., Hobbins, J. C., Clyne, L. P., Pitlick, F. A., Muir, W. A., Merkatz, I. R., and Mahoney, M. J. (1979). *N. Engl. J. Med.* **300,** 937–941.

Fischer, G., and Jatzkewitz, H. (1975). *Hoppe Seylers Z. Physiol. Chem.* **356,** 605–613.

Fishler, K., Donnell, G. N., Bergen, W. R., and Koch, R. (1972). *Pediatrics* **50,** 412–419.

Fleisher, L. D., Tallan, H. H., Beratis, N. G., Hirschhorn, K., and Gaull, G. E. (1973). *Biochem. Biophys. Res. Commun.* **55,** 38–44.

Fleisher, L. D., Longhi, R. C., Tallan, H. H., Beratis, N. G., Hirschhorn, K., and Gaull, G. E. (1974). *J. Pediatr.* **85,** 677–680.

Fleisher, L. D., Rassin, D. K., Desnick, R. J., Salwen, H. R., Rogers, P., Bean, M., and Gaull, G. E. (1979). *Am. J. Hum. Genet.* **31,** 439–445.

Fletcher, J. C. (1979). *In* "Genetic Disorders and the Fetus" (A. Milunksy, ed.), pp. 621–635. Plenum, New York.

Fluharty, A. L. (1981). *In* "Lysosomes and Lysosomal Storage Diseases" (J. W. Callahan and J. A. Lowden, eds.), pp. 249–261. Raven Press, New York.

Fluharty, A. L., Stevens, R. L., and Kihara, H. (1978). *J. Pediatr.* **92,** 782–790.

Fluharty, A. L., Stevens, R. L., de la Flor, S. D., Shapiro, L. J., and Kihara, H. (1979). *Am. J. Hum. Genet.* **31,** 574–580.

Fox, A. M., O'Sullivan, W. J., and Firkin, B. G. (1969). *Am. J. Med.* **47,** 332–336.

Fredrickson, D. S., and Ferrans, V. J. (1978). *In* "The Metabolic Basis of Inherited Disease," 4th Edition (J. B. Stanbury, J. B. Wyngaarden, and D. S. Fredrickson, eds.), pp. 671–687. McGraw-Hill, New York.

Fredrickson, D. S., Sloan, H. R., Ferrans, V. J., and Demosky, S. R., Jr. (1972). *Trans. Assoc. Am. Physicians* **85,** 109–115.

Friedman, J. M. (1974). *Univ. Penn. Law Rev.* **123,** 92–156.

Friedman, P. A., Lloyd, J., and Kaufman, S. (1972). *Mol. Pharmacol.* **8,** 501–512.

Friedman, P. A., Fisher, D. B., Kang, E. S., and Kaufman, S. (1973). *Proc. Natl. Acad. Sci. U.S.A.* **70,** 552–556.

Fujimoto, W. Y., Seegmiller, J. E., Uhlendorf, B. W., and Jacobson, C. B. (1968). *Lancet* **1,** 511–512.

Galjaard, H. (1980). "Genetic Metabolic Diseases: Early Diagnosis and Prenatal Analysis." Elsevier-North Holland, Amsterdam.

Garcia-Castro, J. M., Isales-Forsythe, C. M., Levy, H., Shih, V. E., Lao-Velez, C. R., Gonzalez-Rios, C. M., and Reyes de Torres, L. C. (1982). *N. Engl. J. Med.* **306**, 79-81.

Gatfield, P. D., Taller, E., Wolfe, D. M., and Haust, M. D. (1975). *Pediatr. Res.* **9**, 488-493.

Gatt, S., Dinur, T., and Barenholtz, Y. (1978). *Biochim. Biophys. Acta* **530**, 503-507.

Gaull, G. E., Rassin, D., and Sturman, J. A. (1969). *Neuropaediatrie* **1**, 199-226.

Gay, S., Martin, G. R., Muller, P. K., Timpi, R., and Kuhn, K. (1976). *Proc. Natl. Acad. Sci. U.S.A.* **73**, 4037-4040.

Gayl-Peczalska, K. J., Park, B. H., Biggar, W. D., and Good, R. A. (1973). *J. Clin. Invest.* **52**, 919-923.

Gehring, U., and Tomkins, G. M. (1974). *Cell* **3**, 59-64.

Gelehrter, T. D., and Snodgrass, P. J. (1974). *N. Engl. J. Med.* **290**, 430-433.

German, J., Schonberg, S., Loue, E., and Chaganti, R. S. K. (1977). *Am. J. Hum. Genet.* **29**, 248-255.

Ghadimi, H. (1978). *In* "The Metabolic Basis of Inherited Disease," 4th Edition (J. B. Stanbury, J. B. Wyngaarden, and D. S. Fredrickson, eds.), pp. 387-396. McGraw-Hill, New York.

Ghangas, G. S., and Milman, G. (1975). *Proc. Natl. Acad. Sci. U.S.A.* **72**, 4147-4152.

Gibson, D. J., Glass, P., Carpenter, C. B., and Schur, P. H. (1976). *J. Immunol.* **116**, 1065-1071.

Gjone, E. (1974). *Scand. J. Clin. Lab. Invest.* **33**, (Suppl. 137), 73-95.

Glaser, J. H., and Sly, W. S. (1973). *J. Lab. Clin. Med.* **82**, 969-977.

Glick, N. R., Snodgrass, P. J., and Schafer, I. A. (1976). *Am. J. Hum. Genet.* **28**, 22-30.

Goka, T. J., Stevenson, R. E., Hefferan, P., and Howell, R. R. (1976). *Proc. Natl. Acad. Sci. U.S.A.* **73**, 604-606.

Golbus, M. S., Kan, Y. W., and Naglich-Craig, M. (1976). *Am. J. Obstet. Gynecol.* **124**, 653-654.

Golbus, M. S., Stephens, J. D., Mahoney, M. J., Hobbins, J. C., Haseltine, F. P., Caskey, C. T., and Banker, B. Q. (1979). *N. Engl. J. Med.* **300**, 860-861.

Golbus, M. S., Sagebiel, R. W., Filly, R. A., Gindhart, T. D., and Hall, J. G. (1980). *N. Engl. J. Med.* **302**, 93-95.

Goldstein, J. L., and Brown, M. S. (1974). *J. Biol. Chem.* **249**, 5153-5162.

Gompertz, D., Goodey, P. A., Thom, H., Russell, G., McLean, M. Q., Ferguson-Smith, M. E., and Ferguson-Smith, M. A. (1973). *Lancet* **1**, 1009-1010.

Gompertz, D., Goodey, P. A., Sauderbury, J. M., Charpentier, C., and Chignolle, A. (1974). *Pediatrics* **54**, 511-513.

Goodlin, R. D., and Schwartz, S. (1962). *Am. J. Obstet. Gynecol.* **84**, 808-815.

Goodman, S. I., Moe, P. G., Hammond, K. B., Mudd, S. H., and Uhlendorf, B. W. (1970). *Biochem. Med.* **4**, 500-506.

Goodman, S. I., Mace, J. W., Turner, B., and Garrett, W. I. (1973). *Clin. Genet.* **4**, 226-240.

Goodman, S. I., Markey, S. P., Moe, P. G., Miles, B. S., and Teng, C. C. (1975). *Biochem. Med.* **12**, 12-21.

Goodman, S. I., Wise, G., Halpern, B., Ryan, E., and Whelan, D. (1979). *Am. J. Hum. Genet.* **31**, 49A.

Gorlin, R. J., Pindborg, J. J., and Cohen, M. M., Jr. (1976). "Syndromes of the Head and Neck," 2nd Edition. McGraw-Hill, New York.

Grabowski, G. A., Walling, L., and Desnick, R. J. (1980a). *In* "Enzyme Therapy in Genetic Disease: 2" (R. J. Desnick, ed.), pp. 319-334. Alan R. Liss, New York.

Grabowski, G. A., Willner, J. P., Bender, A., Gordon, R. E., and Desnick, R. J. (1980b). *Pediatr. Res.* **14**, 632.

Grandchamp, B., and Nordmann, Y. (1977). *Biochem. Biophys. Res. Commun.* **74**, 1089-1095.

Greenwood, R. S., Hillman, R. E., Aeola, H., and Sly, W. R. (1978). *Clin. Genet.* **13**, 241-250.

Gregoriadis, G., Neerunjun, D., Meade, T. W., Goolamali, S. K., Weereratne, H., and Ball, G. (1980). *In* "Enzyme Therapy in Genetic Diseases: 2" (R. J. Desnick, ed.), pp. 383-392. Alan R. Liss, New York.

Griffin, J. E., and Wilson, J. D. (1980). *In* "Metabolic Control and Disease" (P. K. Bondy and L. E. Rosenberg, eds.), pp. 1535-1578. Saunders, Philadelphia.

Griffin, J. E., Punyashthiti, K., and Wilson, J. D. (1976). *J. Clin. Invest.* **57,** 1342-1351.

Griffin, J. E., Allman, D. R., Durrant, J. L., and Wilson, J. D. (1981). *J. Biol. Chem.* **256,** 3662-3666.

Grimes, D. A., Schultz, K. E., Cates, W., Jr., and Tyler, C. W., Jr. (1977). *N. Engl. J. Med.* **296,** 1141-1145.

Haggerty, D., Young, P. L., Popjak, G., and Carnes, W. H. (1973). *J. Biol. Chem.* **248,** 223-230.

Hakansson, G. (1979). Ph.D. Thesis, Univ. of Göteberg, Sweden.

Hakansson, G., and Svennerholm, L. (1979). *In* "Proceedings of the Third European Conference on Prenatal Diagnosis" (J. D. Marken, S. Stengel-Rutkowski, and E. Schwinger, eds.), pp. 301-304. Enke, Stuttgart, Federal Republic of Germany.

Hall, C., and Neufeld, E. F. (1978). *Arch. Biochem. Biophys.* **154,** 817-821.

Hall, C. W., Cantz, M., and Neufeld, E. F. (1973). *Arch. Biochem. Biophys.* **155,** 32-38.

Halley, D., and Heukels-Dully, M. J. (1977). *J. Med. Genet.* **14,** 100-102.

Halley, D. J., Keizer, W., Jaspers, N. G. J., Niermeyer, M. F., Kleijer, W. J., Boué, J., Boué, A., and Bootsma, D. (1979). *Clin. Genet.* **16,** 137-146.

Harper, P. S., Lawrence, K. M., Parkes, F. S., Wusteman, F. S., Kresse, H., von Figura, K., Ferguson-Smith, M. A., Duncan, D. M., Logan, R. W., Hall, F., and Whiteman, P. (1974). *J. Med. Genet.* **11,** 123-132.

Harris, C. J., Mesirow, K., Rembelski, P., and Nadler, H. L. (1981). *Pediatr. Res.* **15,** 562.

Hasilik, A., and Neufeld, E. F. (1980). *J. Biol. Chem.* **255,** 4937-4945.

Hasilik, A., Waheed, A., and von Figura, K. (1981). *Biochem. Biophys. Res. Commun.* **98,** 761-767.

Henderson, J. F., Frasser, J. H., and McCoy, E. E. (1974). *Clin. Biochem.* **7,** 339-358.

Herndon, J. H., Steinberg, D., Uhlendorf, B. W., and Fales, H. W. (1969). *J. Clin. Invest.* **48,** 1017-1032.

Hers, H. G., and van Hoof, F. (1968). *In* "Carbohydrate Metabolism and Its Disorders" (F. Dickens, P. J. Randle, and W. I. Whelam, eds.), p. 151. Academic Press, New York.

Heukels-Dully, M. J., and Niermeyer, M. F. (1976). *Exp. Cell. Res.* **97,** 304-312.

Hill, H. Z., and Goodman, S. I. (1974). *Clin. Genet.* **6,** 73-78.

Hillman, R., and Keating, J. P. (1974). *Pediatrics* **53,** 221-225.

Hirschhorn, R., Beratis, N. G., Rosen, F. S., Parkman, R., Stern, R., and Polman, S. (1975). *Lancet* **1,** 73-75.

Hirschhorn, R., Beratis, N., and Rosen, F. S. (1976). *Proc. Natl. Acad. Sci. U.S.A.* **73,** 213-217.

Ho, M. W., and O'Brien, J. S. (1971). *Clin. Chim. Acta* **32,** 443-450.

Hobbins, J. C. (1979). *Contemp. OB/GYN.* **13,** 143-152.

Hobbins, J. C., and Mahoney, M. J. (1974). *N. Engl. J. Med.* **290,** 1065-1067.

Hobbins, J. C., Mahoney, M. J., and Goldstein, L. A. (1974). *Am. J. Obstet. Gynecol.* **118,** 1069-1072.

Holmberg, L. (1980). *Acta Paediatr. Scand.* **69,** 809-813.

Holsi, P., and Vogt, E. (1977). *Hum. Genet.* **41,** 169-176.

Horn, N. (1976). *Lancet* **1,** 1156-1158.

Horwitz, A. L., Hancock, L., Dawson, G., and Thaler, M. M. (1981). *Pediatr. Res.* **15,** 593.

Howell, R. R. (1978). *In* "The Metabolic Basis of Inherited Disease," 4th Edition (J. B. Stanbury, J. B. Wyngaarden, and D. S. Fredrickson, eds.), pp. 137-159. McGraw-Hill, New York.

Howell, R. R., Kaback, M. M., and Brown, B. I. (1971). *J. Pediatr.* **78,** 638-642.

Hsia, L., Scully, K. J., and Rosenberg, L. E. (1971). *J. Clin. Invest.* **50,** 127-136.

Hsu, L., and Hirschhorn, K. (1974). *Life Sci.* **14,** 2311-2336.

Huijing, F. (1967). *Biochim. Biophys. Acta* **148,** 601-603.

Huijing, F. (1975). *Physiol. Rev.* **55,** 609-658.

Huijing, F., and Sandberg, D. H. (1970). *South Med. J.* **63,** 1482.

Huijing, F., Warren, R. J., and McLeod, A. G. W. (1973). *Clin. Chim. Acta* **44,** 453–455.

Hultberg, B., and Masson, P. K. (1977). *Biochim. Biophys. Acta* **481,** 573–577.

Igarishi, M., Schaumberg, H. H., Powers, J., Kishimoto, Y., Kolodny, E. H., and Suzuki, K. (1976). *J. Neurochem.* **26,** 851–860.

Ikonne, J. U., Rattazzi, M. C., and Desnick, R. J. (1975). *Am. J. Hum. Genet.* **27,** 639–650.

Imperato-McGinley, J., Guerrero, L., Gautier, T., and Peterson, R. E. (1974). *Science* **186,** 1213–1215.

Insley, J., Bird, G. W. G., and Harper, P. S. (1976). *Lancet* **1,** 806.

Irreverre, F., Mudd, S. H., Heiyer, W. D., and Laster, L. (1967). *Biochem. Med.* **1,** 187–196.

Jackson, J. F., Currier, R. D., Terasaki, P. J., and Morton, N. E. (1977). *N. Engl. J. Med.* **296,** 1138–1141.

Johnson, A. M., Alper, C. A., Rosen, F. S., and Craig, J. M. (1971). *Science* **173,** 553–554.

Jones, M. E. (1971). *Adv. Enzyme Regul.* **9,** 19–45.

Jordan, P. M., Nordlov, H., Burton, G., and Scott, A. I. (1980). *FEBS Lett.* **115,** 269–272.

Justice, P., O'Flynn, M. E., and Hsia, D. Y. (1967). *Lancet* **1,** 928–930.

Justice, P., Ryan, C., Hsia, D. Y., and Krimpotik, E. (1970). *Biochem. Biophys. Res. Commun.* **39,** 301–306.

Kaback, M. M. (1972). *In* "Methods in Enzymology" (V. Ginsburg, ed.), Vol. 28, pp. 862–867. Academic Press, New York.

Kaback, M. M. (1981). *In* "Lysosomes and Lysosomal Storage Diseases" (J. W. Callahan and J. A. Lowden, eds.), pp. 331–342. Raven Press, New York.

Kaback, M. M., Nathan, T. J., and Greenwald, S. (1977a). *In* "Tay-Sachs Disease: Screening and Prevention" (M. M. Kaback, D. L. Rimoin, and J. S. O'Brien, eds.), pp. 13–36. Alan R. Liss, New York.

Kaback, M. M., Rimoin, D. L., and O'Brien, J. S., eds. (1977b). "Tay-Sachs Disease: Screening and Prevention." Alan R. Liss, New York.

Kaiser, D., Rennert, O. M., Goedde, H. W., Benkman, H. G., Wuillod, H., Kehrli, P., and Sollberger, H. (1974). *Humangenetik* **25,** 241–250.

Kaiser, I. H. (1980). *Obstet. Gynecol.* **56,** 383–384.

Kan, Y. W., and Dozy, A. M. (1978). *Proc. Natl. Acad. Sci. U.S.A.* **75,** 5631.

Kan, Y. W., Valenti, C., Carazza, V., Guidotti, R., and Rieder, R. F. (1974). *Lancet* **1,** 79–80.

Kan, Y. W., Golbus, M. S., and Dozy, A. M. (1976). *N. Engl. J. Med.* **295,** 1165.

Kan, Y. W., Golbus, M. S., Trecartin, R. F., Filly, R. A., Valenti, C., Furbetta, M., and Cao, A. (1977). *Lancet* **1,** 269–271.

Kan, Y. W., Lee, K. Y., Furbetta, M., Angius, A., and Coo, A. (1980). *N. Engl. J. Med.* **302,** 185–188.

Kang, A. H., and Trelstad, R. L. (1973). *J. Clin. Invest.* **521,** 2571–2578.

Kang, E. S., Snodgrass, P. J., and Gerald, P. S. (1972). *Pediatr. Res.* **6,** 875.

Kaufman, S., Holtzman, N. A., Milstein, S., Butler, I. J., and Krumkolz, A. (1975). *N. Engl. J. Med.* **293,** 785–790.

Kawamura, N., Moser, H. W., Kishimoto, Y., Schaumberg, H., Suzuki, K., and Murphy, J. (1978). *Trans. Am. Neurol. Assoc.* **103,** 113–115.

Kelly, T. E., and Taylor, H. A. (1976). *J. Med. Genet.* **13,** 149–151.

Kelly, W. N., and Smith, L. H. (1978). *In* "The Metabolic Basis of Inherited Disease," 4th Edition (J. B. Stanbury, J. B. Wyngaarden, and D. S. Fredrickson, eds.), pp. 1045–1071. McGraw-Hill, New York.

Kelly, W. N., and Wyngaarden, J. B. (1978). *In* "The Metabolic Basis of Inherited Disease," 4th Edition (J. B. Stanbury, J. B. Wyngaarden, and D. S. Fredrickson, eds.), pp. 1011–1036. McGraw-Hill, New York.

Kennedy, J. L., Wertelecki, W., Gates, L., Sperry, B. P., and Caso, V. M. (1976). *Am. J. Dis. Child.* **113**, 16–25.

Kim, Y. J., and Rosenberg, L. E. (1974). *Proc. Natl. Acad. Sci. U.S.A.* **71**, 4821–4825.

Kitagawa, T., Owada, M., Sakiyama, T., Aoki, K., Kamoshita, S., Amenomori, Y., and Kobayashi, T. (1978). *Am. J. Hum. Genet.* **30**, 322–327.

Kleijer, W. J., Wolffers, G. M., Hoogeveen, A., and Niermeijer, M. F. (1976). *Lancet* **2**, 50.

Kleijer, W. J., Hoogeveen, A., Vergeijen, F. W., Niermeijer, M. F., Galjaard, H., O'Brien, J. S., and Warner, T. G. (1979). *Clin. Genet.* **16**, 60–61.

Klein, V., Kresse, H., and von Figura, K. (1978). *Proc. Natl. Acad. Sci. U.S.A.* **75**, 5185–5189.

Klemperer, M. R. (1969). *J. Immunol.* **102**, 168.

Kobayashi, T., Ohta, M., Goto, I., Tanaka, Y., and Kuroiwa, Y. (1979). *J. Neurol.* **221**, 137–149.

Kresse, H. (1973). *Biochem. Biophys. Res. Commun.* **54**, 1111–1118.

Kresse, H., and Neufeld, E. F. (1972). *J. Biol. Chem.* **247**, 2164–2170.

Kresse, H., Paschke, E., von Figura, K., Gilver, W., and Fuchs, W. (1980). *Proc. Natl. Acad. Sci. U.S.A.* **77**, 6822–6826.

Krooth, R. S., and Weinburg, A. N. (1961). *J. Exp. Med.* **113**, 1155–1171.

Krooth, R. S., Howell, R. R., and Hamilton, H. B. (1962). *J. Exp. Med.* **115**, 313–320.

Kurshner, J. B., Basbuto, A. J., and Lee, G. R. (1976). *J. Clin. Invest.* **58**, 1089–1097.

LaBadie, G., Hirschhorn, K., and Beratis, N. G. (1980). *J. Cell Physiol.* **106**, 173–178.

LaBadie, G., Beratis, N. G., and Hirschhorn, K. (1981). *Pediatr. Res.* **15**, 257–261.

La Du, B. N., Howell, R. R., Jacoby, G. A., Seegmiller, J. E., Sober, E. K., Zannoni, V. G., Canby, J. P., and Ziegler, L. K. (1963). *Pediatrics* **32**, 216–227.

Lamberg, S. I., and Dorfman, A. (1973). *J. Clin. Invest.* **52**, 2428–2433.

Latt, S. A., Stetton, G., Jurgens, L. A., Buchanen, G. R., and Gerald, P. S. (1975). *Proc. Natl. Acad. Sci. U.S.A.* **72**, 4066–4071.

Latt, S. A., Schreck, R. R., Loveday, K. S., Dougherty, C. P., and Shuler, C. F. (1980). *In* "Advances in Human Genetics, 10" (H. Harris and K. Hirschhorn, eds.), pp. 267–331. Plenum, New York.

Laurell, C. B., and Erickson, J. (1963). *Scand. J. Clin. Lab. Invest.* **15**, 132–142.

Lawton, A. R., Self, K. S., Royal, S. A., and Cooper, M. D. (1972). *Clin. Immunol. Immunopathol.* **1**, 104–111.

Lawton, A. R., Wu, F. L. Y., and Cooper, M. D. (1975). *In* "Immunodeficiency in Man and Animals, Birth Defects Original Article Series XI" (D. Bergsma, R. A. Good, J. Finstad, and N. Paul, eds.), pp. 28–32. Sinauer Associates, Sunderland, England.

Layzer, R. B., Rowland, L. P., and Rammey, H. M. (1967). *Arch. Neurol.* **17**, 512–523.

Leddy, J. P., Frank, M. M., Guither, T., Baum, J., and Klemperer, M. R. (1974). *J. Clin. Invest.* **53**, 544–553.

Lehmann, A. R., Kirk-Bell, S., and Arlett, C. F. (1977). *In* "Research in Photobiology." Plenum, London.

Leroy, J. G., Ho, M. W., McBrinn, M. C., Zielke, K., Jacob, J., and O'Brien, J. S. (1972). *Pediatr. Res.* **6**, 360–365.

Leroy, J. G., Van Edsen, A. F., Martin, J. J., Dumor, J. E., Hulft, A. E., Okado, S., and Navarro, C. (1973). *N. Engl. J. Med.* **288**, 1365–1369.

Levine, L. S., Zachmann, M., New, M. I., Prader, A., Pollack, M. S., O'Neill, G. J., Yang, S. Y., Oberfield, S. E., and Dupont, B. (1978). *N. Engl. J. Med.* **299**, 911–915.

Levy, H.L., Mudd, S. H., Schulman, J. D., Dreyfuss, P. M., and Abeles, R. H. (1970). *Am. J. Med.* **48**, 390–397.

Lichtenstein, J. R., Kohn, L., Byers, P., Martin, G. R., and McKusick, V. A. (1973a). *Trans. Am. Assoc. Physicians* **86**, 333–339.

Lichtenstein, J. R., Martin, G. R., Kohn, L., Byers, P. H., and McKusick, V. A. (1973b). *Science* **182,** 298–300.

Liebaers, I., Di Natale, P., and Neufeld, E. F. (1977). *J. Pediatr.* **90,** 423–425.

Liebaers, J., and Neufeld, E. F. (1976). *Pediatr. Res.* **10,** 733–736.

Liem, K. O., and Hooghwinkel, G. J. M. (1975). *Clin. Chim. Acta* **60,** 259–262.

Lim, T. W., Leder, I., Bach, G., and Neufeld, E. F. (1974). *Carbohydr. Res.* **37,** 103–109.

Lindblad, B., Lindstedt, S., and Stern, G. (1977). *Proc. Natl. Acad. Sci. U.S.A.* **74,** 4641–4645.

Lipson, M. H., Kraus, J., and Rosenberg, L. E. (1980). *J. Clin. Invest.* **66,** 188–193.

Livni, N., and Legum, C. (1976). *Exp. Cell Biol.* **44,** 1–11.

Lott, I. T., Dulaney, J. T., Milunsky, A., Hoefnagel, P., and Moser, H. W. (1976). *J. Pediatr.* **89,** 438–444.

Lowden, J. A., and O'Brien, J. S. (1979). *Am. J. Hum. Genet.* **31,** 1–18.

Lowden, J. A., Cutz, E., Conen, P. E., Rudd, N., and Doran, T. (1973). *N. Engl. J. Med.* **288,** 225–228.

Lowden, J. A., Callahan, J. W., Norman, M. G., Thain, M., and Prichard, J. S. (1974). *Arch. Neurol.* **31,** 200–203.

Lowden, J. A., Burton, R. M., Desnick, R. J., Goodman, S., Kaback, M. M., Kolodny, E. H., Rattazzi, M. L., and Saifer, A. (1977). *In* "Tay-Sachs Screening: A Manual of Methods." National Tay-Sachs and Allied Disorders Association, New York.

Mahoney, M. J., Rosenberg, L. E., Lindblad, B., Walden-Strom, J., and Zetterstrom, R. (1975). *Acta Paediatr. Scand.* **64,** 44–48.

Manson, J. C., and Brock, D. J. H. (1980). *Lancet* **1,** 330–331.

Mantero, F., Scaronic, C., Pasini, C. V., and Rugiolo, V. (1980). *N. Engl. J. Med.* **303,** 530.

Matalon, R., and Dorfman, A. (1969). *Lancet* **2,** 838–841.

Matalon, R., and Dorfman, A. (1972). *Biochem. Biophys. Res. Commun.* **47,** 959–964.

Matalon, R., Dorfman, A., Nalder, H. L., and Jacobson, C. B. (1970). *Lancet* **1,** 83–84.

Matalon, R., Arbogast, B., Justice, P., Brandt, J. K., and Dorfman, A. (1974a). *Biochem. Biophys. Res. Commun.* **61,** 759–765.

Matalon, R., Arbogast, B., and Dorfman, A. (1974b). *Biochem. Biophys. Res. Commun.* **61,** 1450–1457.

Matalon, R., Arbogast, B., and Dorfman, A. (1974c). *Pediatr. Res.* **8,** 436–441.

Matsuda, I., Arashima, S., Mitsuyama, T., Oka, Y., Ariga, S., Ikeuchi, T., and Ichida, T. (1975). *Clin. Chim. Acta* **63,** 55–60.

Matsuura, F., Nunez, H. A., Grabowski, G. A., and Sweeley, C. C. (1981). *Arch. Biochem.* **207,** 337–352.

McKeon, C., Eanes, R. Z., Fall, R. R., Tasset, D. M., and Wolf, B. (1980). *Clin. Chim. Acta* **101,** 217–223.

McKusick, V. (1972). "Heritable Disorders of Connective Tissue," 4th Edition. Mosby, St. Louis.

McKusick, V. A. (1978). "Mendelian Inheritance in Man," 5th Edition. Johns Hopkins, Baltimore.

McKusick, V., Neufeld, E., and Kelly, T. (1978). *In* "The Metabolic Basis of Inherited Disease," 4th Edition (J. B. Stanbury, J. B. Wyngaarden, and D. S. Fredrickson, eds.), pp. 1282–1307. McGraw-Hill, New York.

McReynolds, J., Mantagos, S., Walser, M., Brusilow, S., and Rosenberg, L. E. (1977). *Pediatr. Res.* **11,** 459.

Menkes, J. H., and Corbo, L. M. (1977). *Neurology* **27,** 928–932.

Merin, S., Livni, N., Berman, E. R., and Yatiu, S. (1975). *Invest. Ophthalmol.* **14,** 437–448.

Meyer, U. A., and Schmid, R. (1978). *In* "The Metabolic Basis of Inherited Disease," 4th Edition (J. B. Stanbury, J. B. Wyngaarden, and D. S. Fredrickson, eds.), pp. 1166–1220. McGraw-Hill, New York.

Migeon, B. R., and Huijing, F. (1974). *Am. J. Hum. Genet.* **26,** 360–368.

Milunsky, A. (1976). *In* "Genetics and the Law" (A. Milunsky and G. J. Annas, eds.), pp. 53–61. Plenum, New York.

Milunsky, A. (1979). "Genetic Disorders and the Fetus." Plenum, New York.

Morrow, G., Schwartz, R. H., Hallock, J. A., and Barness, L. A. (1970). *J. Pediatr.* **77**, 120–123.

Moser, H. W. (1978). *In* "The Metabolic Basis of Inherited Disease," 4th Edition (J. B. Stanbury, J. B. Wyngaarden, and D. S. Fredrickson, eds.), pp. 707–809. McGraw-Hill, New York.

Moser, H. W., Moser, A. H., Van Duyn, M. A., Stowens, D., Barrenger, J. A., and Schulman, J. D. (1981). *Pediatr. Res.* **15**, 637.

Moser, H. W., Moser, A. B., Powers, J. M., Nitowsky, H. M., Schaumberg, H. H., Norum, R. A., and Migeon, B. R. (1982). *Pediatr. Res.* **16**, 172–175.

MRC Working Party on Amniocentesis (1978). *Br. J. Obstet. Gynaecol.* **85**, (Suppl. 2).

Mudd, H. S., and Levy, H. L. (1978). *In* "The Metabolic Basis of Inherited Disease," 4th Edition (J. B. Stanbury, J. B. Wyngaarden, and D. J. Fredrickson, eds.), pp. 458–503. McGraw-Hill, New York.

Mudd, S. H., Levy, H. L., and Abeles, R. H. (1969). *Biochem. Biophys. Res. Commun.* **35**, 121–130.

Mueller, O. T., and Wenger, D. A. (1981). *Clin. Chim. Acta* **109**, 313–324.

Nadler, H. L. (1968). *Pediatrics* **42**, 912–918.

Nadler, H. L., and Walsh, M. M. J. (1980). *Pediatrics* **66**, 690–692.

Nakane, P. K., and Pierce, G. B. (1967). *J. Histochem. Cytochem.* **14**, 929–935.

Navon, R., Pedeh, B., and Adum, A. (1973). *Am. J. Hum. Genet.* **25**, 287–293.

Navon, R., Brand, N., and Sandbank, U. (1980). *Neurology* **30**, 449.

Negishi, H., Morishita, Y., Kodama, S., and Matsuo, T. (1974). *Clin. Chim. Acta* **53**, 175.

Neufeld, E. F., and Cantz, M. (1973). *In* "Lysosomes and Lysosomal Storage Diseases" (H. G. Hers and F. Van Hoof, eds.), pp. 261–275. Academic Press, New York.

New, M. I., Lorenzen, F., Pag, P., Gunczler, B., Dupont, B., and Levine, L. S. (1979). *J. Clin. Endocrinol. Metab.* **48**, 356–359.

Newburger, P. E., Cohen, H. J., Rothchild, S. B., Hobbins, J. C., Malawista, S. E., and Mahoney, M. J. (1979). *N. Engl. J. Med.* **300**, 178.

Ng, W. G., Donnell, G. N., Bergren, W. R., Alfi, O., and Golbus, M. S. (1977). *Clin. Chim. Acta* **74**, 227–235.

NICHD National Registry for Amniocentesis Study Group (1976). *J.A.M.A.* **236**, 1471–1476.

Nitowsky, H. M., Sassa, S., Nakagawa, S., and Jagani, N. (1978). *Pediatr. Res.* **12**, 455.

O'Brien, J. S. (1972). *Proc. Natl. Acad. Sci. U.S.A.* **69**, 1720–1722.

O'Brien, J. S. (1978). *Clin. Genet.* **14**, 55–60.

O'Brien, J. S., Okada, S., Fillerup, D., Veath, M. D., Adornato, B., Brenner, P. H., and Leroy, J. G. (1971). *Science* **172**, 61–63.

O'Brien, J. S., Tennant, L., Veath, M. L., Scott, R. C., and Bucknall, W. E. (1978). *Am. J. Hum. Genet.* **30**, 602–608.

O'Brien, M. L., Buist, N. R. M., and Murphy, W. H. (1978). *J. Pediatr.* **92**, 1006–1012.

Ochs, H. D., Rosenfeld, S. I., Thomas, E. D., Giblett, E. R., Alper, C. A., Dupont, B., Schaller, J. G., Gilliland, B. C., Hansen, J. A., and Widgewood, R. J. (1977). *N. Engl. J. Med.* **296**, 470–475.

Ockerman, P. A., Jelke, H., and Kaijer, K. (1966). *Acta Paediatr. Scand.* **55**, 10–16.

Ogata, M., Mizugaki, J., and Takahara, S. (1974). *Tohoku J. Exp. Med.* **113**, 239–245.

Okada, S., and O'Brien, J. S. (1969). *Science* **165**, 698–700.

Okada, S., Veath, M. L., and O'Brien, J. S. (1970). *J. Pediatr.* **77**, 1063–1065.

Omenn, G. S., and Schrott, H. G. (1973). *Acta Genet. Med. Gemellol.* (*Rome*) **23**, 221–230.

Orkin, S. H., Alter, B. P., Altay, C., Mahoney, M. J., Lazarus, H., Hobbins, J. C., and Nathan, D. G. (1978). *N. Engl. J. Med.* **299**, 166.

Orkin, S. H., Old, J., Weatherall, D. J., and Nathan, D. G. (1979). *Proc. Natl. Acad. Sci. U.S.A.* **76**, 2400.

Painter, R. B., and Young, B. R. (1980). *Proc. Natl. Acad. Sci. U.S.A.* **77**, 7315–7317.

Palo, J., Pollitt, R. J., Pretty, K. M., and Savolainen, H. (1973). *Clin. Chim. Acta* **47**, 69–74.

Paterson, M. C. (1978). *In* "DNA Repair Mechanisms" (P. C. Hanawalt, E. C. Friedberg, and C. F. Fox, eds.), pp. 1–14. Academic Press, New York.

Paterson, M. C., Smith, B. P., and Lohman, P. H. (1976). *Nature* **260**, 444–447.

Patrick, A. D., Wilicox, P., Stephens, R., and Kenyon, V. G. (1970). *J. Med. Genet.* **13**, 49–51.

Patrick, A. D., Young, E., Kleijer, W. J., and Niermeijer, M. F. (1977). *Lancet* **1**, 144–145.

Pattidson, R. M., Moossy, J., Derbes, V. J., and Kloepfer, R. (1963). *Derm. Trop.* **2**, 195–203.

Pearson, C. M., Rimer, D. G., and Mommaerts, W. F. H. M. (1961). *Am. J. Med.* **30**, 502–517.

Peltonen, L., Aarno, P., Toshihiko, H., and Prockop, D. J. (1980a). *Proc. Natl. Acad. Sci. U.S.A.* **77**, 162–167.

Peltonen, L., Palotie, A., and Prockop, D. J. (1980b). *Proc. Natl. Acad. Sci. U.S.A.* **77**, 6179–6183.

Perez-Palacios, G., Ortiz, S., Lopez-Amor, E., Morato, T., Febres, F., Lisker, R., and Saglia, H. (1975). *J. Clin. Endocrinol.* **41**, 946–952.

Perry, T. L., Urguhart, N., Maclean, T., Evans, M. E., and Hausan, S., Davidson, G. F., Applegarth, D. A., MacLeod, P. J., and Lock, J. E. (1975). *N. Engl. J. Med.* **292**, 1269–1273.

Peters, S. P., Glew, R. H., and Lee, R. E. (1977). *In* "Practical Enzymology of the Sphingolipidoses" (R. H. Glew and S. P. Peters, eds.), pp. 71–100. Alan R. Liss, Inc., New York.

Peters, S. P., Aquino, L., Naccarato, W. F., Gilbertson, J. R., Diven, W. F. and Glew, R. H. (1979). *Biochim. Biophys. Acta* **575**, 27–36.

Peterson, B. H., Graham, J. A., and Brooks, G. F. (1976). *J. Clin. Invest.* **57**, 283–290.

Pickering, W. R., and Howell, R. R. (1972). *J. Pediatr.* **81**, 50–55.

Pinnell, S. R., Krane, S. M., Kenzora, J. E., and Glimcher, M. J. (1972). *N. Engl. J. Med.* **286**, 1013–1020.

Poenareo, L., Dreyfus, J. C., Boué, J., Nicolesco, H., Ravise, N., and Bamberer, J. (1976). *Clin. Genet.* **10**, 260–264.

Pollack, M. S., Levine, L. S., Pang, S., Owens, R. P., Nitowski, H., Maurer, P., New, M. I., Duchon, M., Merkatz, I. R., Sachs, G., and Dupont, B. (1979). *Lancet* **1**, 1107–1108.

Pollycove, M. (1978). *In* "The Metabolic Basis of Inherited Disease," 4th Edition (J. B. Stanbury, J. B. Wyngaarden, and D. S. Fredrickson, eds.), pp. 1127–1165. McGraw-Hill, New York.

Pope, R. M., Martin, G. R., Lichtenstein, J. R., Penttinen, R. P., Gerson, B., Rowe, D. W., and McKusick, V. A. (1975). *Proc. Natl. Acad. Sci. U.S.A.* **72**, 1314–1316.

Potter, J. L., Timmons, G. D., Rinehart, L., and Witmer, E. G. (1972). *Clin. Chim. Acta* **39**, 518–523.

Powell, G. F., Rasco, M. A., and Maniscalco, R. M. (1974). *Metabolism* **23**, 505–513.

Powledge, T. M., and Fletcher, J. (1979). *N. Engl. J. Med.* **300**, 168–172.

Prader, A., and Gurtner, H. P. (1955). *Helv. Paediatr. Acta* **10**, 397–403.

Priest, R. E., Moinaddin, J. F., and Priest, F. H. (1973). *Nature* **245**, 264–266.

Quinn, R. S., and Krane, S. M. (1976). *J. Clin. Invest.* **57**, 83–93.

Raiha, N. C. R. (1973). *Pediatr. Res.* **7**, 1–7.

Ramsey, C. A., Coltart, T. M., Blunt, S., Pawsey, S. A., and Gianelli, F. (1974). *Lancet* **2**, 1109–1112.

Rankin, J. K., and Darlington, G. J. (1979). *Somatic Cell Genet.* **5**, 1–10.

Rao, B. G., and Spence, M. W. (1977). *Ann. Neurol.* **1**, 385–392.

Rao, G. J. S., and Nadler, H. L. (1975). *Pediatr. Res.* **9**, 739–743.

Rapin, I., Suzuki, K., Suzuki, K., and Valsamis, M. P. (1976). *Arch. Neurol.* **33**, 120–130.

Rassin, D. K., Fleisher, L. D., Muir, A., Desnick, R. J., and Gaull, G. E. (1979). *Clin. Chim. Acta* **94**, 101–108.

Rattazzi, M. C., and Davidson, R. G. (1972). *In* "Antenatal Diagnosis" (A. Dorfman, ed.), pp. 207–211. Univ. of Chicago Press, Chicago.

Reddy, R. (1977). M.S. Thesis, University of Minnesota, Minneapolis.

Reitman, M. L., Varki, A., and Kornfeld, S. (1981). *J. Clin. Invest.* **67**, 1574–1579.

Renwick, J. H., and Bolling, D. R. (1971). *J. Med. Genet.* **8**, 399.

Revsin, B., and Morrow, G. (1976). *Exp. Cell Res.* **100**, 95–103.

Reynolds, J. W. (1963) *Proc. Soc. Exp. Biol. Med.* **113**, 980–990.

Rhead, W., and Tanaka, K. (1979). *Am. J. Hum. Genet.* **31**, 59A.

Robinson, D., and Thorpe, R. (1974). *Clin. Chim. Acta* **55**, 65–69.

Rodeck, C. H. (1980). *Br. J. Obstet. Gynaecol.* **87**, 449–456.

Rodeck, C. H., and Campbell, S. (1978). *Br. Med. J.* **2**, 728–730.

Rodeck, C. H., and Campbell, S. (1979). *Lancet* **1**, 1244–1245.

Rodeck, C. H., Milbashan, R. S., Peake, I. R., and Bloom, A. L. (1979). *Lancet* **2**, 637–638.

Rodeck, C. H., Eady, R. A. J., and Gosden, C. M. (1980). *Lancet* **1**, 949–952.

Rodeck, C. H., Holman, C. A., and Karnick, J. (1981). *Lancet* **1**, 625–627.

Roerdink, F. H., Gouw, W. L. M., Okken, A., Vander Blij, J. F., Luit-de Haan, G., and Hommes, F. A. (1973). *Pediatr. Res.* **7**, 863–870.

Rogers, L. E., Warford, L. R., Patterson, R. B., and Porter, F. S. (1968). *Pediatrics* **42**, 415–420.

Romeo, G., and Levin, E. Y. (1969). *Proc. Natl. Acad. Sci. U.S.A.* **63**, 856–863.

Romeo, G., Kaback, M. M., and Levin, E. Y. (1970) *Biochem. Genet.* **4**, 659–664.

Ropers, H. H., Zimmerman, J,, and Wienker, T. (1977). *Clin. Genet.* **11**, 114–118.

Rosen, F. S. (1981). *In* "Hematology of Infancy and Childhood" (D. G. Nathan and F. A. Oski, eds.), pp. 457–519. Saunders, Philadelphia.

Rosenberg, L. E. (1978). *In* "The Metabolic Basis of Inherited Diseases," 4th Edition (J. B. Stanbury, J. B. Wyngaarden, and D. S. Fredrickson, eds.), pp. 409–429. McGraw-Hill, New York.

Rosenberg, L. E., and Scriver, C. R. (1980). *In* "Metabolic Control and Disease" (P. K. Bondy and L. E. Rosenberg, eds.), p. 719. Saunders, Philadelphia.

Rosenberg, L. E., Lilljeqvist, A. C., and Hsia, Y. E. (1968). *N. Engl. J. Med.* **278**, 1319.

Rosenberg, L. E., Lilljeqvist, A. C., Hsia, Y. E., and Rosenbloom, F. M. (1969). *Biochem. Biophys. Res. Commun.* **37**, 607–615.

Rosenberg, L. E., Patel, L., and Lillejequist, A. C. (1975). *Proc. Natl. Acad. Sci. U.S.A.* **72**, 4617–4622.

Rosenfeld, S. I., Ruddy, S., and Austen, K. F. (1969). *Clin. Res.* **17**, 358.

Rosenfeld, S. J., Kelly, M. E., Baum, J., and Leddy, J. P. (1976). *J. Clin. Invest.* **57**, 1626.

Rosenmann, A., Schumert, Z., Thesdor, R., Cohen, T., and Brautbar, C. (1980). *Am. J. Med. Genet.* **6**, 295–300.

Roth, S. L., Havemann, K., Gramse, M., Hillig, U., Raukolb, R., and Martini, G. A. (1980). *J. Inher. Metab. Dis.* **3**, 87–88.

Rowe, P. B. (1978). *In* "The Metabolic Basis of Inherited Disease," 4th Edition (J. B. Stanbury, J. B. Wyngaarden, and D. S. Fredrickson, eds.), pp. 430–457. McGraw-Hill, New York.

Ruddy, S., and Austin, K. F. (1978). *In* "The Metabolic Basis of Inherited Disease," 4th Edition (J. B. Stanbury, J. B. Wyngaarden, and D. S. Fredrickson, eds.), pp. 1737–1754. McGraw-Hill, New York.

Salen, G. (1971). *Ann. Intern. Med.* **75**, 843–850.

Sandhoff, K., Andreae, V., and Jatzkewitz, H. (1968). *Life Sci.* **7**, 283–288.

Sandhoff, K., Harzer, K., Wassle, W., and Jatzkewitz, H. (1971). *J. Neurochem.* **18**, 2469–2474.

Sassa, S., Solish, G., Levere, R. D., and Kappas, A. (1975). *J. Exp. Med.* **142**, 722–731.

Saunders, M., Sweetman, L., Robinson, B., Roth, K., Cohn, S., Sherwood, G., and Gravel, R. (1979). *Am. J. Hum. Genet.* **31**, 61A.

Schaumberg, H. H., Powers, J. M., Raine, C. S., Suzuki, K., and Richardson, E. P., Jr. (1975). *Arch. Neurol.* **32**, 577–591.

Schmickel, R. D., Ernest, H., Chu, Y., and Trosko, J. (1975). *Pediatr. Res.* **9**, 317.

Schmid, R., Robbins, R. W., and Trant, R. R. (1959). *Proc. Natl. Acad. Sci. U.S.A.* **45**, 1236–1240.

Schneider, E. L., Ellis, W. G., Brady, R. O., McCulloch, J. R., and Epstein, C. J. (1972). *J. Pediatr.* **81**, 1134–1139.

Schneider, J. A., Verroust, F. M., Kroll, W. A., Garvin, A. J., Horger, E. O., Wong, V. G., Spear, G. S., Jacobson, C., Pellett, O. L., and Becker, F. L. A. (1974). *N. Engl. J. Med.* **290**, 878–882.

Schneider, J. A., Schulman, J. D., and Seegmiller, J. E. (1978). *In* "The Metabolic Basis of Inherited Disease," 4th Edition (J. B. Stanbury, J. B. Wyngaarden, and D. S. Fredrickson, eds.), pp. 1660–1682. McGraw-Hill, New York.

Schulman, J. D., Fujimoto, W. Y., Bradley, K. H., and Seegmiller, J. E. (1970). *J. Pediatr.* **77**, 468–470.

Scriver, C. R. (1967). *In* "Conference on Hereditary Tyrosinemia" (M. Partington, C. R. Scriver, and A. Sass-Korsak, eds.), *Can. Med. Assoc. J.* **95**, 1073–1075.

Scriver, C. R. (1978). *In* "The Metabolic Basis of Inherited Disease," 4th Edition (J. B. Stanbury, J. B. Wyngaarden, and D. S. Fredrickson, eds.), pp. 336–361. McGraw-Hill, New York.

Seegmiller, J. E. (1980). *In* "Metabolic Control and Disease" (P. K. Bondy and L. E. Rosenberg, eds.), p. 873. Saunders, Philadelphia.

Segal, S. (1978). *In* "The Metabolic Basis of Inherited Disease," 4th Edition (J. B. Stanbury, J. B. Wyngaarden, and D. S. Fredrickson, eds.), pp. 160–181. McGraw-Hill, New York.

Seilver, D., Kelleter, R., Kolmel, H. W., and Heene, R. (1973). *Experientia* **29**, 972–973.

Setlow, R. B., Regan, J. D., German, J., and Carrier, W. L. (1969). *Proc. Natl. Acad. Sci. U.S.A.* **64**, 1035–1040.

Setoguchi, T., Salem, G., Tint, G. S., and Mosbach, E. H. (1974). *J. Clin. Invest.* **53**, 1393.

Shafit-Zagardo, B., Devine, E., and Desnick, R. J. (1980). *Biochim. Biophys. Acta* **614**, 459–465.

Shaham, M., Becker, Y., and Cohen, M. M. (1980). *Cytogenet. Cell Genet.* **27**, 155–161.

Shapiro, L. J., Mohandas, T., Weiss, R., and Romeo, G. (1979). *Science* **204**, 1222–1226.

Sharp, H. L., Bridges, R. A., Krivit, W., and Freier, E. (1969). *J. Lab. Clin. Invest.* **73**, 939–940.

Shewan, W. G., Mouat, S. A., and Allen, T. M. (1976). *Br. Med. J.* **1**, 281–282.

Shih, V. E. (1978). *In* "The Metabolic Basis of Inherited Disease," 4th Edition (J. B. Stanbury, J. B. Wyngaarden, and D. S. Fredrickson, eds.), pp. 362–386. McGraw-Hill, New York.

Shih, V. E., Mandell, R., and Tanaka, K. (1973). *Clin. Chim. Acta* **48**, 437–444.

Shiriashi, Y., and Sandberg, A. A. (1978). *Mutat. Res.* **49**, 233–238.

Siegel, R. C. (1977). *J. Biol. Chem.* **252**, 254–259.

Simell, O., Johanson, T., and Aula, P. (1973). *J. Pediatr.* **82**, 54–57.

Simon, M., Pawlotsky, Y., Bourel, M., Fauchet, R., and Genetet, B. (1975). *Nouv. Presse Med.* **4**, 1432–1435.

Simon, M., Bourel, M., Fauchet, R., and Genetet, B. (1976). *Gut* **17**, 332–334.

Simon, M., Alexandre, J. L., Bourel, M., LeMarec, B., and Scordia, C. (1977a). *Clin. Genet.* **11**, 327–341.

Simon, M., Boruel, M., Genetet, B., and Fauchet, R. (1977b). *N. Engl. J. Med.* **297**, 1017–1021.

Simon, M., Alexandre, J. L., Fauchet, B., Genetet, B., and Bourel, M. (1980). *In* "Progress in Medical Genetics, IV" (A. G. Steinberg, A. G. Bearn, A. G. Motulsky, and B. Childs, eds.), pp. 135–168. Saunders, Philadelphia.

Simpson, N. R., Dallaire, L., Miller, J. R., Siminovich, L., Hamerton, J. L., Miller, J., and McKeen, C. (1976). *Can. Med. Assoc. J.* **115**, 739–746.

Sklower, S. L., and Desnick, R. J. (1979). *In* "Birth Defects: Risks and Consequences" (S. Kelly, E. B. Hook, D. T. Jenerich, and I. H. Porter, eds.), pp. 237–252. Academic Press, New York.

Skovby, F., Kraus, J., Redlich, C., and Rosenberg, L. (1980). *Am. J. Hum. Genet.* **32**, 55A.

Sloan, H. R., and Fredrickson, D. S. (1972). *J. Clin. Invest.* **51**, 1923–1930.

Sly, W. S., Quinton, B. A., McAlister, W. H., and Rimoin, D. L. (1973). *J. Pediatr.* **82**, 249–257.

Sperling, O., Liberman, V. A., Frank, M., and De Vries, A. (1971). *Am. J. Clin. Pathol.* **55**, 351–354.

Stanbury, J. B., Wyngaarden, J. B., and Fredrickson, D. S. (1978). "The Metabolic Basis of Inherited Disease," 4th Edition. McGraw-Hill, New York.

States, B., Harris, D., and Segal, S. (1974). *J. Clin. Invest.* **53**, 1003–1013.

Steinberg, D. (1978). *In* "The Metabolic Basis of Inherited Disease," 4th Edition (J. B. Stanbury, J. B. Wyngaarden, and D. S. Frederickson, eds.), pp. 688–706. McGraw-Hill, New York.

Steinherz, R., Raiford, D., Mittal, K. K., and Schulman, J. D. (1981). *Am. J. Hum. Genet.* **33**, 227–233.

Steinitz, K. (1967). *Adv. Clin. Chem.* **9**, 227–265.

Steinmann, B., Tuderman, L., Peltonen, L., Martin, G. R., McKusick, V. A., and Prockop, D. J. (1980). *J. Biol. Chem.* **255**, 8887–8893.

Stevenson, R. E., Taylor, H. A., and Parks, S. E. (1978). *Clin. Genet.* **13**, 305–313.

Stokke, K. T., and Norum, K. R. (1971). *Scand. J. Clin. Lab. Invest.* **27**, 21–31.

Stokke, O., Eldjarn, L., Norum, K. R., Stein-Johnson, J., and Halvorsen, S. (1967). *Scand. J. Clin. Lab. Invest.* **20**, 313.

Stone, N. J., Levy, R. I., Fredrickson, D. S., and Verteo, J. (1974). *Circulation* **49**, 476–488.

Stoop, J. W., Zegers, B. J. M., Hendrickx, T., Siegenbeck Van Heukelom, L. H., Stall, G. E. J., DeBree, P. K., Wadman, S. K., and Ballieux, P. (1977). *N. Engl. J. Med.* **296**, 651–655.

Sunshine, P., Lindenbaum, J. E., Levy, H. L., and Freeman, J. M. (1972). *Pediatrics* **50**, 100.

Suzuki, K. (1977). *In* "Practical Enzymology of the Sphingolipidoses" (R. H. Glew and S. P. Peters, eds.), pp. 101–136. Alan R. Liss, New York.

Suzuki, K., and Suzuki, K. (1970). *Neurology* **20**, 848–851.

Suzuki, K., Schneider, E. L., and Epstein, C. J. (1971). *Biochem. Biophys. Res. Commun.* **45**, 1363–1366.

Sveger, T. (1978). *Pediatrics* **62**, 22–28.

Sweetman, L., Weyler, W., Shafai, T., Young, P. E., and Nyhan, W. L. (1979). *J.A.M.A.* **242**, 1048–1052.

Swift, M. R., and Hirschhorn, K. (1966). *Ann. Intern. Med.* **65**, 496–502.

Tallan, H. H., Pascal, T. A., Schneidman, K., Giliam, B. M., and Gaull, G. E. (1971). *Biochem. Biophys. Res. Commun.* **43**, 303–310.

Tanaka, K., Budd, M. A., and Efron, M. L. (1966). *Proc. Natl. Acad. Sci. U.S.A.* **56**, 236–241.

Tauri, S., Okuno, G., Ikura, Y., Tanaka, T., Suda, M., and Nishikawa, M. (1965). *Biochem. Biophys. Res. Commun.* **19**, 517–523.

Tauri, S., Kono, N., Nasu, T., and Nishikawa, M. (1969). *Biochem. Biophys. Res. Commun.* **34**, 77–83.

Tauro, G. P., Danks, D. M., Rowe, P. B., Vander Weyden, M. B., Schwarz, M. A., Collins, V. L., and Neal, B. W. (1976). *N. Engl. J. Med.* **294**, 466–470.

Tedesco, T. A., and Mellman, W. J. (1975). *Proc. Natl. Acad. Sci. U.S.A.* **57**, 169–174.

Terheggen, H. G., Schwenk, A., Lowenthal, A., Van Sande, M., and Columbo, J. P. (1969). *Lancet* **2**, 748.

Theone, J., Sweetman, L., and Yoshino, M. (1979). *Am. J. Hum. Genet.* **31**, 64A.

Thistlethwaite, D., Darling, J. A. B., Fraser, R., Mason, P. A., Rees, L. H., and Harkness, R. A. (1975). *Arch. Dis. Child.* **50**, 291–297.

Thompson, M. S. (1979). *In* "Genetic Disorders and the Fetus" (A. Milunsky, ed.), pp. 637–651. Plenum, New York.

Thompson, R. A., Haeney, M., Reid, K. B. M., Davies, J. G., White, R. H. R., and Cameron, A. H. (1980). *N Engl. J. Med.* **303,** 22–24.

Tice, R., Windler, G., and Rary, J. B. (1978). *Nature* **273,** 538–540.

Tomlinson, S., and Westall, R. G. (1964). *Clin. Sci.* **26,** 261–270.

Tourian, A. (1976). *Biochem. Biophys. Res. Commun.* **66,** 54–63.

Tourian, A. Y., and Sidbury, J. B. (1978). *In* "The Metabolic Basis of Inherited Disease," 4th Edition (J. B. Stanbury, J. B. Wyngaarden, and D. S. Fredrickson, eds.), pp. 240–255. McGraw-Hill, New York.

Upchurch, K. S., Leyva, A., Arnold, W. J., Holmes, E. W., and Kelly, W. N. (1975). *Proc. Natl. Acad. Sci. U.S.A.* **72,** 4142.

Valenti, C. (1972). *Am. J. Obstet. Gynecol.* **114,** 561–564.

Valle, D. L., Phang, J. M., and Goodman, S. I. (1974). *Science* **185,** 1053–1054.

Valle, D. L., Walser, M., Brusilow, S. W., and Kraiser-Kupfer, M. (1980a). *J. Clin. Invest.* **65,** 371–375.

Valle, D. L., Walser, M., Brusilow, S. W., Faiser-Kupfer, M., and de Monastero, F. (1980b). *Clin. Res.* **28,** 546A.

Van Dyke, D. L., Fluharty, A.L., Schafer, I. A., Shapiro, L. J., Kihara, H., and Weiss, L. (1981). *Am. J. Med. Genet.* **8,** 235–242.

Van Hoof, F., Hue, L., Thi., de Barsy, P., Jacquemin, P., Devos, P., and Hers, H. G. (1972). *Biochimie* **54,** 745–752.

Vidgoff, J., Buist, N. B. M., and O'Brien, J. S. (1973). *Am. J. Hum. Genet.* **25,** 372–381.

Virtanen, I., Ekblom, P., Laurila, P., Nordling, P., Raivio, K. O., and Aula, P. (1980). *Pediatr. Res.* **14,** 1199–1203.

Vogel, A., Holbrook, K. A., Steinmann, B., Gitzelman, R., and Byers, P. H. (1976). *Lab. Invest.* **40,** 201–206.

von Figura, K., and Kresse, H. (1973). *Biochem. Biophys. Res. Commun.* **48,** 262–269.

von Figura, K., van de Kamp, J. J., and Niermeyer, M. F. (1982). *Prenatal Diag.* **2,** 67–70.

Wada, Y., Taka, K., and Minagawa, A. (1963). *Tokohu J. Exp. Med.* **81,** 46–53.

Waldmann, T. A., and McIntire, K. R. (1972). *Lancet* **2,** 1112–1115.

Walters, J. M., Watt, P. W., and Stevens, F. M. (1975). *Br. Med. J.* **4,** 520–522.

Wellner, V. P., Sckura, R., Meister, A., and Larsson, A. (1974). *Proc. Natl. Acad. Sci. U.S.A.* **71,** 2505–2509.

Wendel, U., Rudiger, H. W., Passarge, E., and Mikkelsen, M. (1973). *Humangenetik* **19,** 127.

Wenger, D. A. (1977). *In* "Practical Enzymology of the Sphingolipidoses" (R. H. Glew and S. P. Peters, eds.), pp. 39–70. Alan R. Liss, Inc., New York.

Wenger, D. A., and Olson, G. C. (1981). *In* "Lysosomes and Lysosomal Storage Diseases" (J. W. Callahan and A. J. Lowden, eds.), pp. 157–171. Raven Press, New York.

Wenger, D. A., Clark, C., Sattler, M., and Wharton, C. (1978a). *Clin. Genet.* **13,** 145–153.

Wenger, D. A., Tarby, T. J., and Wharton, C. (1978b). *Biochem. Biophys. Res. Commun.* **82,** 589–595.

Weyler, W., Sweetman, L., Maggio, D. C., and Nyhan, W. L. (1977). *Clin. Chim. Acta* **76,** 321–328.

Willard, H. F., Mahoney, M. J., Mogil, R. J., and Rosenberg, L. E. (1979). *Am. J. Hum. Genet.* **31,** 65A.

Williams, H. E., and Field, J. B. (1963). *Metabolism* **12,** 464–466.

Willner, J. P., Grabowski, G. A., Gordon, R. E., Bender, A. N., and Desnick, R. J. (1981). *Neurology* **31,** 787–798.

Wilson, J. D., and MacDonald, P. C. (1978). *In* "The Metabolic Basis of Inherited Disease," 4th Edition (J. B. Stanbury, J. B. Wyngaarden, and D. S. Fredrickson, eds.), pp. 894–915. McGraw-Hill, New York.

Wolf, B., and Tuck, P. (1979). *Am. J. Hum. Genet.* **31**, 65A.

Wolfe, D. M., and Gatfield, P. D. (1975). *Pediatr. Res.* **9**, 531.

Wong, P. K., Justice, D., Hruby, M., Weiss, E. B., and Diamond, E. (1977). *Pediatrics* **59**, 749–756.

Woo, S. L. C., Gilliam, S. S., and Woolf, L. I. (1974). *Biochem. J.* **139**, 741.

Wood, S., and MacDougall, B. G. (1976). *Am. J. Hum. Genet.* **28**, 489–495.

Woody, N. C., Hutzler, J., and Dancis, J. (1966). *Am. J. Dis. Child.* **112**, 577–585.

Worthy, T. E., Grobner, W., and Kelley, W. N. (1974). *Proc. Natl. Acad. Sci. U.S.A.* **71**, 3031–3035.

Wyngaarden, J. B., and Kelly, W. N. (1978). *In* "The Metabolic Basis of Inherited Disease," 4th Edition (J. B. Stanbury, J. B. Wyngaarten, and D. S. Fredrickson, eds.), pp. 916–1010. McGraw-Hill, New York.

Yaffe, M. G., Kaback, M. M., Goldberg, M., Miles, J., Itabashi, H., McIntyre, H., and Mohandas, T. (1979). *Neurology* **29**, 611.

Young, E. P., and Patrick, A. D. (1970). *Arch. Dis. Child.* **45**, 664–668.

Zannoni, V. G., and La Du, B. N. (1963). *Biochem. J.* **88**, 160–162.

Zoref, E., De Vries, A., and Sperling, O. (1975). *J. Clin. Invest.* **56**, 1093–1099.

Zuchman, M., Vollman, J. A., Hamilton, W., and Prader, A. (1972). *Clin. Endocrinol.* **1**, 369–385.

NOTE ADDED IN PROOF

Since the preparation of this chapter, two additional prenatal diagnoses have been made. First, chronic granulomatous disease has been prenatally diagnosed by the use of the nitroblue tetrazolium (NBT) reduction reaction in neutrophils obtained from fetal blood (Borregaard *et al.*, 1982). It also may be possible that cultured amniotic cells can be used to diagnose this disorder since Fikrig *et al.* (1980) have observed that normal amniotic cells can reduce NBT in response to latex particles. Second, nonketotic hyperglycinemia has been diagnosed prenatally by the determination of amniotic fluid glycine–serine ratios (Garcia-Castro *et al.*, 1982).

Chapter 6

Use of Ultrasound in the Prenatal Diagnosis of Congenital Disorders

STUART CAMPBELL, DAVID GRIFFIN, AND D. LITTLE

Department of Obstetrics and Gynaecology
King's College Hospital Medical School
London, England

LINDSEY ALLAN

Department of Paediatric Cardiology
Guy's Hospital
London, England

I. Introduction

The emphasis in preceding chapters has been on the cellular and biochemical approaches to prenatal diagnosis. This chapter will concentrate on the recogni-

METHODS IN CELL BIOLOGY, VOL. 26

tion of anatomical or functional fetal anomalies before the twenty-sixth week of pregnancy, that is, early enough for selective termination of the severely abnormal fetus to be a possible course of management. An attempt will also be made to present ultrasonic investigation in the context of other diagnostic modalities. Radiology, ultrasound, and fetoscopy all enable direct visualization of the fetus, but only ultrasound and fetoscopy are of value before 26 weeks postmenstrual age. The hazards of ionizing radiation (Polani *et al.*, 1976; Griscon, 1980) are such that they preclude the use of standard radiographic techniques and computerized axial tomography in the second trimester of pregnancy.

Ultrasound and fetoscopy are both valuable techniques in the diagnosis of fetal defects. They should not, however, be regarded as mutually exclusive techniques because, used in a complementary way, they can be most effective. Fetoscopy permits direct visualization of external fetal structures and the identification of fetal vessels on the placental surface suitable for fetal blood sampling. Small fetal parts—such as hands, feet, genitalia, and facial features, the identification of which are sometimes beyond the resolving power of ultrasound—can be clearly seen. The disadvantages, however, are that the position of insertion of the needlescope to examine one part of the fetus (e.g., genitalia) may be totally inappropriate for examination of other parts (e.g., face). Furthermore, the risk of abortion exceeds that of midtrimester amniocentesis (Rodeck, 1980). Diagnostic ultrasound is remarkably free of risk (Lele, 1979; Taylor and Dyson, 1980), and both internal and external structures can be visualized. The fetus is viewed, however, in two-dimensional slices. Skill in interpretation of the echo patterns and the ability to think in three dimensions is essential when making these examinations. Thus ultrasound is the primary method of diagnosing fetal structural abnormalities and indeed could safety be used to screen the whole obstetric population. Fetoscopy is preferred when there may be suspicion of small significant external defects that are beyond the resolution of ultrasound and that cannot be diagnosed by biochemical or cytologic analysis of the amniotic fluid.

II.   Ultrasound Imaging Techniques

Imaging techniques employ pulsed ultrasound of high frequency (2–5 MHz) and low intensity. Short pulses in the region of 1 μsec are transmitted into the maternal abdomen where they are gradually attenuated by absorption, refraction, or reflection from tissue interfaces. The reflected echoes are received by the same transducer during the silent period of about 3 msec between emitted pulses. This long duty cycle also means that the average acoustic power of the system is extremely low and remains well within all recognized safety margins. As the ultrasound pulse crosses a junction (interface) between different tissues it encounters an acoustic mismatch. Part of the sound wave is reflected, the remainder passing on to the next interface. It is the reflected sound waves or echoes that are detected by the transducer, which converts the acoustic signal into the electrical impulses, which are then amplified, processed, and displayed as a visual image on a cathode-ray tube or television screen.

The two basic ultrasound modalities now employed in fetal imaging—and hence in the diagnosis of fetal abnormality—are static B-scanning and real-time scanning.

A.   Static Compound B-Scanning

With static B-scanning the sound wave is passed through the maternal abdomen and uterus via a single transducer mounted on a mechanical gantry. Passage of sound across the interface between the transducer and the skin of the maternal abdomen is facilitated by applying an oil or aqueous jelly to the skin. The transducer is moved in small rotating movements slowly across the abdomen so that the ultrasound beam crosses as many tissue interfaces as possible, because optimal resolution is obtained along the axis of the beam at right angles to each interface. Weak signals from interfaces not at right angles to the beam can also be received by the tranducer because of minor irregularities of surfaces. These backscatter reflections used to be eliminated by signal processing in order to facilitate interpretation of the echogram, but nowadays they can be displayed by gray-scaling techniques and can thus enhance visualization of many soft tissue structures that could not previously be detected. Once the static echogram has been studied, it can be cleared from the screen, ready for a new image to be built up. Static compound B-scanning with gray scale therefore produces high-resolution static images, and by studying multiple, two-dimensional, longitudinal, or cross-sectional "slices" of the fetus, the operator is able to obtain a three-dimensional mental image of its anatomy. This modality therefore produces high-quality images and until recently has been the optimal one for making the diagnosis of fetal abnormality. It is expensive equipment, however; maintenance and running costs are high, and considerable operator expertise is required in its effective use. Furthermore, the scanning process in the exclusion of fetal abnormality takes an average of 20 minutes, too long for screening of an obstetric population to be practical.

B.   Real-Time Scanning

Real-time scanning is a recent development in ultrasonic imaging that is gaining widespread popularity in obstetric diagnosis. There are two main systems at present in common use: linear array and mechanical sector scanners.

1. Linear Array

This modality employs an array of about 60 separate rectangular elements mounted side by side to form a probe of about 15 mm in length, looking vaguely like a harmonica (Fig. 1). An electronic switch selects the first element to produce an ultrasonic pulse, which passes into the patient. The same element receives reflected echoes, which are displayed on the screen. This cycle is then repeated sequentially for each element along the array. The bank of linear echo displays is perceived by the eye as a complete two-dimensional image with correct spatial relationships. The echo-collection process is sufficiently rapid for the entire array to be triggered 40 times per second so that a flicker-free image may be perceived that will allow fetal movements to be observed. The equipment can be small and easily portable to the patient in the clinic or the antenatal ward. However, the general disadvantage of real time was that, until recently, the picture quality (i.e., the resolution of the system) had been inferior to that of the larger

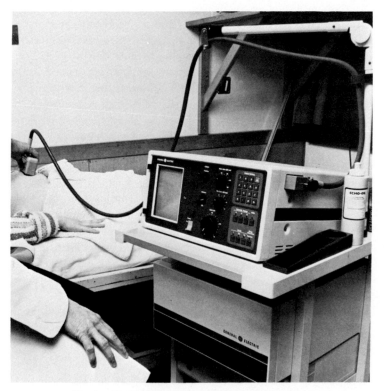

Fig. 1.   Typical high-resolution linear assay scanner.

static scanners. Furthermore, the inability to compound the scan means that many interfaces that can be observed with static scanners cannot be acequately visualized with linear-array machines. New developments in varying the time sequence in which elements are triggered has made it possible to focus the sound beam, resulting in striking improvements in image quality.

2.   MECHANICAL SECTOR SCANNING

In mechanical sector scanning (Fig. 2) three to five transducers are arranged radially around a central rotating spindle. As the transducer rotates past a window in the scanning head it emits an arc (in the region of 90°) of sound pulses. The echoes received during its passage are displayed on the oscilloscope screen as a sector image with its apex corresponding to the center of the rotating spindle. The transducer rotates at such a speed that images produced by each transducer as it passes the window can be displayed in real time in the same way as movie

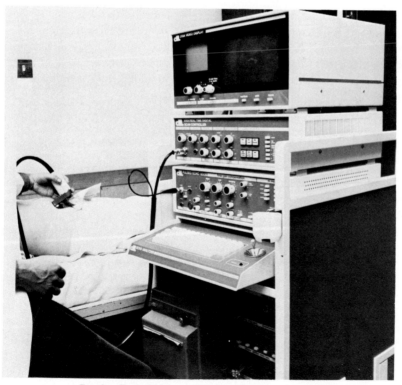

FIG. 2.   Typical high-resolution mechanical sector scanner.

photography. Very high resolution and image quality have been attained by some of these machines, so much so that this modality has become a serious contender with static B-scanning in the prenatal diagnosis of fetal abnormality. An added advantage is that the scanning head can be small and easily manipulated into corners that facilitate visualization of fetal parts inaccessible to linear-array examination.

Already, many fetal abnormalities can be detected by real-time examination. The production of moving images not only enables the study of fetal activity but facilitates the differentiation of fetal organs and the ease and speed with which a three-dimensional mental image of the fetus can be obtained. Because of its ease of use, it is now probable that real-time scanning will be employed for screening the whole antenatal population for certain fetal abnormalities.

III.   Use of Ultrasound in Prenatal Diagnosis

Ultrasound may be used to diagnose fetal defects directly. There are other ways in which ultrasound examination can effectively aid early detection of fetal anomalies, however. It may (1) enhance the safety and efficiency of amniocentesis, (2) diagnose multiple pregnancy, (3) accurately define fetal age, (4) detect disordered fetal growth, (5) show changes in amniotic fluid volume, and (6) enable fetal structural abnormalities to be demonstrated.

A.   Enhancement of the Safety of Amniocentesis

From our experience of over 1000 amniocenteses we believe that the procedure should be performed in the ultrasound department immediately following ultrasonic placental and fetal localization.

The uterus is first scanned to localize and define accurately a pool of amniotic fluid (Fig. 3), and a route to it avoiding fetus and placenta is chosen. The depth of the pool and its distance from the maternal skin can be measured by electronic calipers on the B-mode display to ensure that the needle chosen is long enough or that it is not inserted too deeply. The site chosen is marked with a small indentation (the butt of a needle is an ideal marker) and the skin is cleansed with chlorhexidine in 70% alcohol. Using the ultrasound transducer as a site-line, the needle is immediately inserted into the pool of amniotic fluid. With practice the correct depth can be appreciated by a slight loss of resistance to the needle's passage. A no-touch technique should be employed, and we commonly use an 18- or 21-gauge needle. A local anesthetic may be given, but this only causes delay, increasing the chance that the fetus might move into the path of the needle.

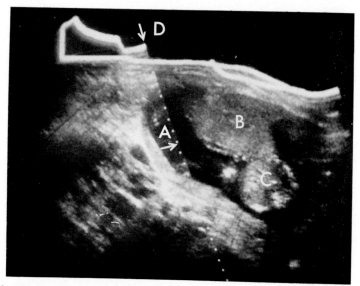

FIG. 3. β-scan echogram of uterus at 17 weeks showing site and direction for amniocentesis. A, Amniotic fluid; B, placenta; C, fetal trunk; D, direction for amniocentesis.

If performed with confidence the procedure usually causes only minor discomfort to the mother and is rapidly completed. Biopsy transducers (Bang and North-eved, 1972) permitting visualization of the tip of the needle are available, but they are cumbersome to use and may increase the risk of infection. Both static and real-time scanning are equally effective in defining the optimal site for amniocentesis. Theoretically, real-time scanning should enable continuous visualization of the needle while in the uterus but, although the needle can be identified, it may be difficult to be certain that the tip of the needle is in view. Thus simultaneous real-time scanning is rarely an advantage. Even if the placenta is anterior, it is usually possible to locate a window lateral to the placental margin, and in the last 7 years we have not found it necessary to penetrate the placenta. If, however, safe access is not afforded to the amniotic fluid at 14 or 16 weeks, it is wise to defer amniocentesis for 2 weeks, when conditions are usually found to be more favorable.

The value of performing amniocentesis under ultrasound control was demonstrated by Harrison et al. (1975), who reported fetal–maternal transfusions of more than 2 ml to occur in 4.5% of patients when amniocentesis was performed under ultrasound control and 9% when it was not. Kerenyi and Walker (1977) showed that the incidence of frankly bloodstained amniotic fluid was 2% when performed under ultrasound control, 12.1% when performed outside the ultrasound department following placenta localization, and 21.4% when performed without prior ultrasonic examination. Nevertheless, none of these studies is without serious flaws in methodology, and there remain some who dispute the value of ultrasound in enhancing the safety of amniocentesis. This may be a consequence of their failing to appreciate the importance of performing amniocentesis coincidentally with ultrasound examination. It should be realized that a pool of liquor accessible at the time of scanning may have moved even 30 minutes later as a result of uterine rotation with fetal movement or changes in maternal bladder distention. Then a safe site marked on the maternal abdomen may be situated over the placenta or fetus some hours later. This fact is highlighted by the recent U.K. report (Medical Research Council Working Party, 1978), which showed that the incidence of bloodstained amniotic fluid was three times more common in those patients in whom amniocentesis was not performed in the ultrasound department compared to those in whom the procedures were performed concurrently.

A further advantage of performing ultrasound concurrently with amniocentesis is the facility to recognize fetal movement and heart activity both immediately before and after the procedure. Although unexplained intrauterine death is rare early in the second trimester, failure to appreciate that it has occurred will result in an unnecessary amniocentesis with an increased risk of intrauterine sepsis. It may also give the mother the false impression that the procedure was responsible for the fetal death. Recognition of activity after amniocentesis is a reassurance to both the patient and physician that the operation has not caused immediate fetal death.

B.   Diagnosis of Multiple Pregnancy

Multiple pregnancy can be easily recognized from 6 weeks postmenstrual age onward. Between the sixth and the twelfth week, multiple pregnancy is diagnosed by counting sacs. A separate fetus should be identified in each sac, for occasionally one embryo may fail to grow and is gradually absorbed. After 12 weeks, the number of fetuses is best determined by counting heads, or bodies if there is an increased risk of anencephaly. This may be performed by making a series of scans across the uterus with a compound B-scanner, although the procedure can be more quickly and reliably performed with real-time apparatus.

Ultrasound contributes to the success of prenatal diagnosis in twin pregnancy by facilitating the removal of clear amniotic fluid from each sac and by directly diagnosing fetal defects, especially if there is discordance for a neural tube defect. Nevin and Armstrong (1975) have shown that alpha-fetoprotein (AFP) can pass across the chorionic membrane, resulting in significantly raised AFP levels in the amniotic fluid surrounding a normal fetus. This is a potential source of diagnostic error and may result in the termination of a normal twin fetus, whose mother has a reduced chance of having a normal child.

Amniocentesis in twin pregnancy should be performed much as described in the previous section. The membrane separating the sacs can usually be seen with compound static B-scanning even between the fourteenth and sixteenth weeks postmenstrual age. Visualization of the membrane is frequently difficult with the linear-array real-time scanner because the interface is usually parallel to the ultrasound beam. With the mechanical sector scanner, however, the beam may be manipulated orthogonal to the membrane, thus readily permitting its identification. Once the membrane has been identified, the needle may be inserted on each side of it. If problems are encountered in distinguishing the separation between sacs, the fetal bodies should be lined up in a single plane and the amniocentesis performed on the side of each fetus furthest from its partner, it being very unusual for the sacs to overlap completely. Some recommend the injection of indigo-carmine into the sac after the first amniocentesis, so that a repeat puncture may be recognized, but our only abortion in twin pregnancy followed this maneuver and it is logical to think that the injection of any foreign material into the gestation sac would carry increased risk of precipitating infection or abortion.

We have reported the direct identification of spina bifida in a twin pregnancy discordant for spina bifida (Campbell and Rodeck, 1979), in which ultrasound correctly identified the fetus, showing a dorsolumbar spina bifida. The pregnancy was allowed to continue. Although the alpha-fetoprotein level was within normal limits in the sac surrounding the unaffected fetus, this was only by virtue of the modest elevation of AFP in the abnormal sac, for there is usually a 2:1 to 3:1 AFP gradient across the chorionic membrane. This gradient is unlikely to occur should only amnion be separating the sacs. At King's College Hospital we have recently been successful in inducing cardiac asystole by air embolism in one malformed fetus under fetoscopic control while allowing the normal fetus to continue uneventfully to term (Rodeck and Campbell, 1981, personal communication). The problems encountered in the diagnosis of neural tube defect in twins have now largely been overcome with the advent of high-resolution mechanical sector real-time scanning, as we are confident of diagnosing even minor sacral lesions with this apparatus.

C. Accurate Determination of Fetal Age

The accurate determination of fetal gestational age is of paramount importance in all patients who are to be subjected to amniocentesis so that (1) amniocentesis may be performed at the correct time and (2) misinterpretation of maternal serum and amniotic fluid alpha-fetoprotein values can be avoided.

The ultrasound dating of pregnancy is based on the principle first propounded by Campbell (1969) that there is little variation in the growth rate between fetuses during the early weeks of pregnancy. Thus the scatter of measurements for a

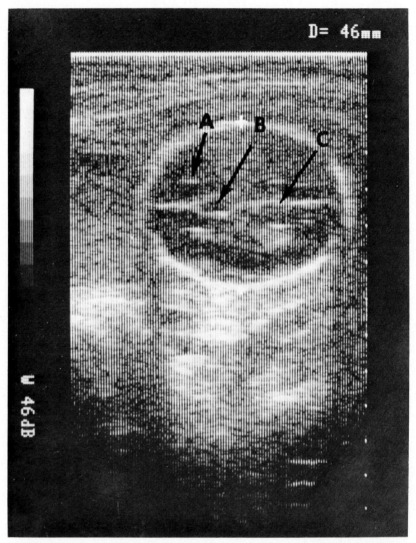

Fig. 4. Echogram showing a typical section of fetal head at 19 weeks. Suitable for head-circumference measurement. The septum pellucidum is one-third of the distance from the synciput and two-thirds from the occiput. The midline echo bisects the head. The lateral border of the anterior horns of the ventricles are easily seen. A, Lateral border of anterior horn; B, septum pellucidum; C, midline echo.

particular week is small and a single measurement of fetal size can give an accurate assessment of postmenstrual age. The earlier the fetus is measured, the more accurate is the assessment, for there is increasing variability in fetal growth (with consequent overlap in ranges from week to week) as pregnancy advances. Fetal age can be accurately determined with a single measurement before 24 weeks postmenstrual age and, even up to 30 weeks, ultrasound measurements provide the most accurate objective prediction of postmenstrual age.

The fetus can be first identified in its sac at 6 weeks postmenstrual age, and the optimal fetal measurement until 12 weeks is that of the crown-rump length (CRL) as described by Robinson (1973). There is a very narrow scatter of measurements during this period, and the 95% confidence limit for fetal age predictions is ± 5 days (Robinson and Fleming, 1975).

Beyond 14 weeks, however, curvature of the spine makes visualization of the full CRL difficult and longitudinal measurement of the fetus increasingly imprecise. Hereafter, cross-sectional images of the fetal head and body will permit measurement of the biparietal diameter (Campbell, 1968), head circumference (Campbell and Thoms, 1977), and abdominal circumference (Campbell and Wilkin, 1975), which are the three major cross-sectional measurements now employed.

The measurement of biparietal diameter (BPD) entails an accurate assessment

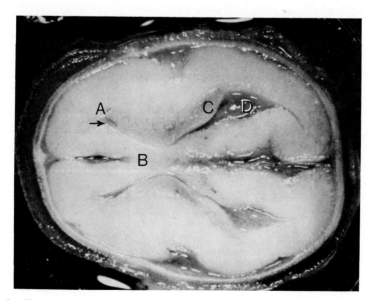

FIG. 5.   Horizontal section of normal fetal brain at upper border of septum pellucidum (18 weeks postmenstrual age). A, Anterior horn of lateral ventricle; B, Septum pellucidum; C, germinal layer of epithelium; D, body of lateral ventricle.

of the extent of lateral angulation (asynclitism) of the fetal head so that the sound directed from one parietal bone to the other produces a strong midline echo, which represents the medial aspect of each cerebral hemisphere. The widest diameter associated with a good midline echo is taken as the biparietal diameter. To measure the head circumference a further estimation of the degree of head extension or flexion is necessary so as to determine the true occipito–frontal diameter. Once the correct section is obtained the head will appear as an ovoid with a central midline echo (Fig. 4) interrupted one-third of the way from the synciput to the occiput by a small rectangular structure previously described as the third ventricle but now recognized from anatomical studies in our laboratory (C. Tsannatos, 1981, personal communication) to be the septum pellucidum (Fig. 5). For measurement of the abdominal circumference, the longitudinal axis of the fetus must first be determined by referring to the fetal spine or, preferably, the fetal aorta. The scanning plane is then aligned orthogonal to these landmarks,

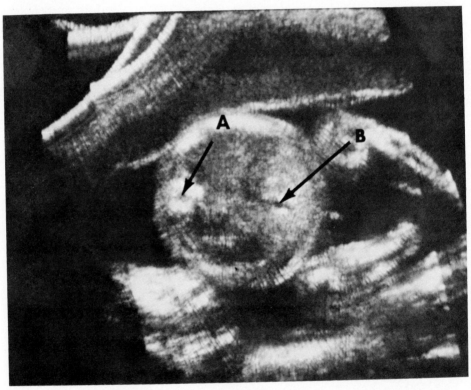

FIG. 6. Echogram of transverse section of fetal abdomen showing the typical circular appearance of an intact neural canal. This section shows the umbilical vein and is suitable for abdomen-circumference measurement. A, Fetal spine; B, umbilical vein.

and a section is measured at the level of the umbilical vein at the midpoint of its passage through the fetal liver (Fig. 6). Frequently, prior to 20 weeks, the fetal umbilical vein cannot be seen, in which case the fetal stomach may be used as a landmark. The head- and abdomen-cicumference measurements, respectively, reflect the size of the fetal brain and liver.

Nomograms of measurements taken during uncomplicated pregnancy are available (Campbell and Newman, 1971), and all predictions are made with reference to these charts. Biparietal diameter measurement is the one most commonly used to estimate fetal age (Campbell, 1975), and the 95% confidence limits for a prediction made before 24 weeks is 5 days. Campbell (1974a) has shown that the measurement of BPD before 24 weeks postmenstrual age (or 65 mm size) more accurately forecasts the date of onset of spontaneous delivery of a mature infant than a prediction based on certain menstrual dates. Consequently, it has been recommended that all pregnancies should be subject to ultrasound dating, and the development of rapid on-screen measuring techniques with real-time scanners makes this a practical course of management, which is followed at King's College Hospital. Certainly for all patients with doubtful menstrual dates, or menstrual irregularity, or bleeding in early pregnancy, or who have been ingesting oral contraceptives within 2 months of the last menstrual period, the early ultrasound estimation of postmenstrual age is an absolute necessity. The importance in relation to the interpretation of maternal serum AFP, amniotic fluid AFP, and the timing of amniocentesis for other disorders has already been

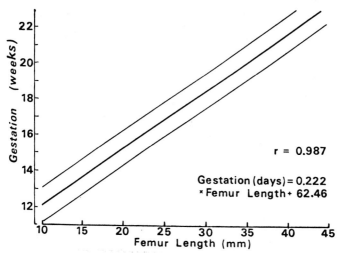

$$r = 0.987$$

$$\text{Gestation (days)} = 0.222 \times \text{Femur Length} + 62.46$$

FIG. 7. Prediction of fetal age from femur-length measurement. Between 12 and 23 weeks, the fetal age can be predicted to within ± 6.7 days (95%)

stressed. In addition, patients at high risk of having a child with a structural abnormality such as microcephaly should have measurements made as early as possible so that subsequent measurements can be appropriately plotted on the growth chart.

Occasionally it may be found that the fetus is in a persistently occipito-posterior position, which renders the BPD inaccessible to measurement. Assessment of femur length before 24 weeks postmenstrual age (Queenan *et al.*, 1980) has been found in our department to be as accurate in predicting fetal post-menstrual age (95% confidence limits ± 6.7 days) as biparietal diameter and may prove a valuable alternative measurement (Fig. 7)

D.   Diagnosis of Fetal Anomaly

Fetal anomalies may be diagnosed by ultrasound either by demonstrating disproportionate growth of a particular fetal part (e.g., the head in microcephaly or the limbs in limb-reduction deformity) or by visualization of a structural defect. Following our report on selective termination of pregnancy after ul-trasound prenatal diagnosis of anencephaly (Campbell *et al.*, 1972), most of the work on early diagnosis has been done in the field of neural tube defects and cranial anomalies. More recently, however, attention has been concentrated on the early detection of other physical defects such as tumors, congenital heart disease, gastrointestinal anomalies, renal and urinary tract disorders, and syn-dromes characterized by shortening of the limbs. More than 700 women at high risk of having an abnormal fetus have now been studied in our department and it is on these that this article is based. Data presented are taken from those studies performed before the twenty-sixth gestational week dated either from certain last menstrual period or from early ultrasound measurement. Among these cases 106 defects were found.

E.   Fetal Growth

Important information on fetal growth and abnormality may be obtained by taking careful fetal measurements. Rapid progress is being made in the develop-ment of accurate on-screen measuring systems with both static and real-time scanners, which has increased both the ease and rapidity with which mea-surements can be performed. Fetal growth can be assessed prenatally by taking serial measurements of the biparietal diameter, head circumference, and abdomi-nal circumference. Measurement of the BPD is the most precise and reproducible but has disadvantages in that occasionally a fetus with a narrow but otherwise normal head (dolichocephaly) will be falsely diagnosed as being growth retarded or microcephalic. Nevertheless, most work on fetal growth has been done by serial

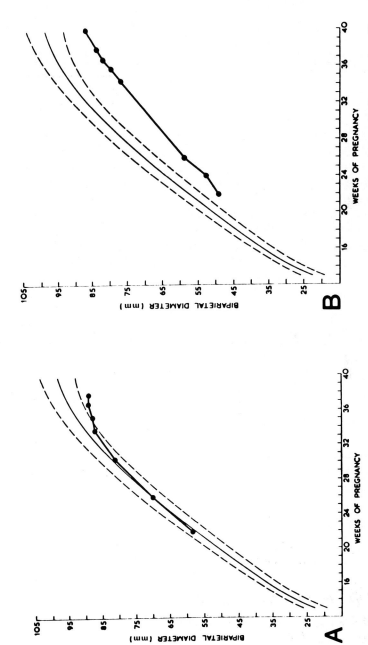

Fig. 8.   Different growth patterns of the fetal biparietal diameter in growth retardation. (A) Late flattening pattern. (B) Low-growth-profile pattern.

measurements of the BPD (Campbell and Dewhurst, 1971). Campbell (1974b), from analysis of cephalometry charts in cases of growth retardation, has described different patterns of intrauterine growth (Fig. 8), which may be important in assessing the short- and long-term risks to the fetus. These patterns generally fall into two main groups. In the first group there is an abrupt slowing and eventual cessation of growth rate after a period of normal growth. This type is called the "late flattening" growth-retardation pattern and is associated with maternal hypertension, intrapartum fetal asphyxia, postnatal hypoglycemia, increased brain:liver ratio, and a typical wasted appearance. These infants usually make up for lost growth in early life (once removed from their hostile intrauterine environment), and if protected from perinatal hypoxia, suffer no neurologic impairment. The "low-profile" growth-retardation pattern demonstrates a persistently low growth rate from early in the second trimester. There is generally no tendency to late cessation of growth and no strong association with toxemia or intrapartum asphyxia. The brain:liver ratio is usually normal. These babies are more stunted than wasted in appearance, and about 20% of small-for-dates babies referred for ultrasonic examination conform to this growth pattern. In many of these cases the fetus is being exposed to a chronic growth-retarding stimulus, such as maternal smoking (Murphy *et al.*, 1980), and in others the babies have a genetic or chromosomal abnormality or may have been victims of intrauterine viral infection, and are examples of reduced growth potential. Measurement of the head-to-abdomen circumference ratio can also help to classify fetuses into the wasted or stunted groups and indeed does so more precisely (Campbell and Thoms, 1977). A wasted fetus with a late flattened BPD growth pattern is generally associated with a high head-to-abdomen circumference ratio, on account of the brain sparing that occurs when growth retardation is caused by impaired intrauterine perfusion. The stunted low-growth-potential fetus with a low-profile growth pattern usually has a normal head-to-abdomen circumference ratio, indicating that both brain and liver are equally affected by the growth-retarding stimulus. Thus the finding of slow BPD growth and a symmetrically small fetus before 24 weeks gestation would be an indication for detailed ultrasound examination, amniocentesis, and chromosomal analysis, in view of the increased risk of genetic defects in this group. Furthermore, the diagnosis of impaired growth potential prenatally is associated with a continued restriction of growth in childhood and perhaps intellectual impairment (Fancourt *et al.*, 1976).

F. Changes in Amniotic Fluid Volume

It is probable that during the early part of the second trimester the amniotic fluid is an extension of the fetal extracellular space, which is why biochemically it resembles an ultrafiltrate of fetal plasma, the skin acting as a semipermeable membrane (Lind and Hytten, 1972). After midpregnancy the fetal skin becomes more stratified and cornified, which prevents diffusion. Thereafter urination and swallowing become the principal processes influencing the change in amniotic fluid volume during the second half of pregnancy. This means that fetal abnormalities that disturb urine production or inhibit swallowing or absorption of amniotic fluid from the intestine will cause large changes in amniotic fluid volume only after the twenty-fourth week of pregnancy. Although gross changes in amniotic fluid volume can be easily assessed, quantification is difficult because the fluid is distributed in small collections around the fetus that obviously shift and change with altered fetal or maternal position. However, the diagnosis of polyhydramnios or oligohydramnios is made when there is excess or virtual absence of echo-free space around the fetus. A more detailed account of the diagnostic and prognostic significance of oligohydramnios will be presented later.

G. Structural Fetal Abnormalities

The ultrasound unit at King's College Hospital has now been in operation for over 4 years and has become a referral center for a large part of the southeastern region of England and further afield. Figures presented should not therefore be taken as representative of a normal population. Many referrals follow the detection of elevated maternal serum or amniotic fluid alpha-fetoprotein (AFP) values, suspicious ultrasound findings such as fetal ascites, oligo- or polyhydramnios, intrafetal cystic structures, and so forth, or are of patients at high risk of repeating an inheritable fetal abnormality. This has resulted in a far higher rate of positive diagnoses than might be expected in the normal population.

Maternal serum AFP (MSAFP) estimation has had a significant effect on the increased detection of central nervous system abnormalities. It is not, however, without its problems. Raised levels may engender considerable maternal anxiety and encourage a large number of unnecessary amniocenteses. The former largely arises from inadequate counseling, and reassurance of the patient with elevated serum AFP concentration that her baby is more likely to be normal than abnormal, particularly when levels are only marginally raised, may save undue distress. At King's College Hospital we believe that an ultrasound backup service experienced in fetal prenatal diagnosis can reduce the necessity for amniocentesis to those with markedly raised AFP levels in whom abnormality cannot be detected by ultrasound or where fetal position repeatedly denies access for adequate examination. It is not difficult with modern ultrasound equipment to detect anencephaly, spina bifida, omphalocele, or hydrocephalus before 23 weeks postmenstrual age. It is more difficult to confirm normality with confidence, although this has been greatly facilitated with high-resolution real-time equipment. Moreover, raised amniotic fluid AFP can be associated with a normal fetus, of which there have been 10 instances in our experience.

1. NEURAL TUBE AND CRANIAL ABNORMALITIES

Following our initial report on the early detection of anencephaly (Campbell *et al.*, 1972), our group of workers at King's College Hospital and Queen Charlotte's Hospital, London have published work on the early diagnosis of spina bifida (Campbell *et al.*, 1975), hydrocephalus (Campbell, 1977), encephalocele (Campbell, 1974c), iniencephaly, holoprosencephaly, and microcephaly (Campbell and Rodeck, 1979). The latest results from the group are presented here and are based on the study of 575 women who were at high risk of having a fetus with craniospinal defect. Indications for referral are shown in Table I. Between 1974 and 1978 most patients were referred because they had had a previous baby with neural tube defect (NTD). In the majority of patients during this time the ultrasound scan was performed without any knowledge of the amniotic fluid AFP (AFAFP) level. Since 1978, however, many patients have been referred from outside because of elevated serum AFP or marginally raised amniotic fluid AFP values (i.e., between 3 and 5 SD above the mean).

a. Anencephaly. Absence of the cranial vault is readily appreciated after the twelfth week of menstrual age, although the decision to terminate on the basis of an ultrasound diagnosis should be deferred to 14 weeks to reduce the chance of error. The diagnosis is facilitated by real-time examination and should not be missed with good equipment and experienced technicians. The fetal head may be deeply located in the pelvis, in which situation visualization may be improved by allowing distention of the mother's bladder. For the past 2 years routine booking

TABLE I

CRANIOSPINAL DEFECTS

Indication for referral[a]	1974–1978	1978–1980 (June)
Previous baby with NTD	249	67
Previous baby with hydrocephalus	21	20
Previous baby with microcephaly	5	17
Family history of NTD	4	19
Patient/husband with NTD	12	4
Raised MSAFP	5	80
Raised AFAFP	15	25
Suspicious ultrasound findings	1	30
	312	262
Total	575	

[a] NTD, Neural tube defects; MSAFP, maternal serum alpha-fetoprotein; AFAFP, amniotic fluid alpha-fetoprotein.

linear-array real-time scanning has been employed at King's College Hospital. In this clinic six anencephalic fetuses have been detected before the twenty-first week, in all of which the diagnosis has been confirmed pathologically following termination of pregnancy. There have been no undiagnosed cases among our patients in that time. In all, 23 cases of anencephaly have been successfully diagnosed (Table II).

b. Spina Bifida. Campbell *et al.* (1975) originally described a method for detecting spina bifida by performing a series of scans along the length of the fetal spine orthogonal to its long axis. The normal spine with an intact neural arch appears as a closed circle (Fig. 6), whereas when closure of the arch is incomplete the spinal canal appears as a saucer or V-shaped complex (Fig. 9)—or in some severe cases as a triple-spiked complex of echoes.

With the static scanner, longitudinal sections of the spine are not reliable in detecting spina bifida because, due to the curvature of the spine, the full length cannot be displayed adequately on a single scan. Recently, with the mechanical sector and focused linear-array scanners, we have been able to manipulate the plane of the scan so that the spine is lying anteriorly; in this position it can be visualized throughout its length in one scan, and the curve of the sacrum may be readily demonstrated (Fig. 10). With this view the integrity of the neural arch and the continuity of overlying skin can be reliably assessed; it is a satisfactory method of eliminating or diagnosing spina bifida. In practice, we employ a combination of longitudinal and transverse sections.

With the static scanner it is rarely possible to see the meninges, and the diagnosis of spina bifida is made on demonstrating the bony defect. However, with the high-resolution mechanical sector scanner we have been able to demon-

TABLE II

STRUCTURAL CRANIOSPINAL ANOMALIES DIAGNOSED BY ULTRASOUND
BEFORE 26 WEEKS GESTATION

Type of anomaly	No. diagnosed
Anencephaly	23
Spina bifida	
Open	32
Closed	2
Encephalocele	8
Iniencephaly	1
Holoprosencephaly	1
Isolated hydrocephalus	6
Microcephaly	4
	77

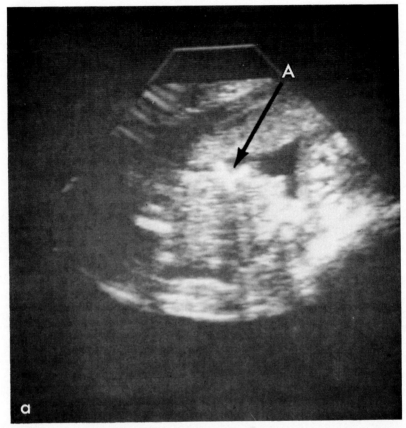

FIG. 9.   Echogram of transverse section of fetal abdomen showing (a) 16-week spine with typical V-shaped defect; (b) 19-week spine showing typical "triple-spike" echo (see opposite page). A, Spina bifida.

strate the bulging meningocele (Fig. 11), and this we believe to have been a major advance in the diagnosis of spina bifida. On two recent occasions identification of sacral lesions has been facilitated by demonstrating the meningocele with the mechanical sector scanners (neither of these lesions was identified with the static B-scanner).

Our success in diagnosing spina bifida is summarized in Table III. Four open spina bifidas were missed, all of which were below the level of the fourth lumbar vertebra (L4), and the pregnancies were terminated because of raised AFAFP levels. Two closed lesions were successfully diagnosed. In one the bony defect was identified, whereas in the other the large skin-covered myelomeningocele was demonstrated. In both of these cases the AFAFP was normal. In this series, amniotic fluid was marginally more successful in the detection of open spina

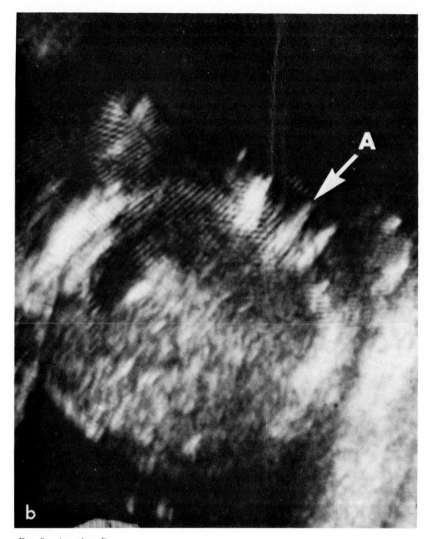

FIG. 9.   (*continued*)

bifida, but both closed lesions were missed and there were 10 false positives including one set of twins. In the first four cases the pregnancies were terminated and the fetuses demonstrated to be normal. Subsequently, the other six pregnancies were allowed to continue on the basis of a normal scan. They all delivered normal babies at term. There have been no false-positive ultrasound diagnoses. In two cases with raised AFAFP levels in which low lesions could not be excluded by ultrasound, we have used fetoscopy (Rodeck and Campbell, 1978)

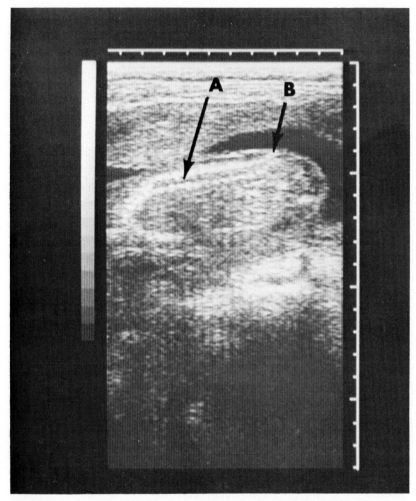

Fig. 10. Echogram of longitudinal section of fetal spine at 18 weeks showing sacral curve. A, Fetal spine; B, sacral curve.

to exclude the diagnosis, but since we have been using mechanical sector scanners in the investigation of these high-risk cases we have had no doubts as to the integrity of the lumbosacral spine.

The majority of fetuses with spina bifida both with and without coexistent hydrocephalus will demonstrate a small biparietal diameter (Fig. 12) and head circumference relative to gestational age, whereas the abdominal circumference will be normal (Roberts and Campbell, 1980). If this anomaly is observed, a diligent search for spina bifida should be made.

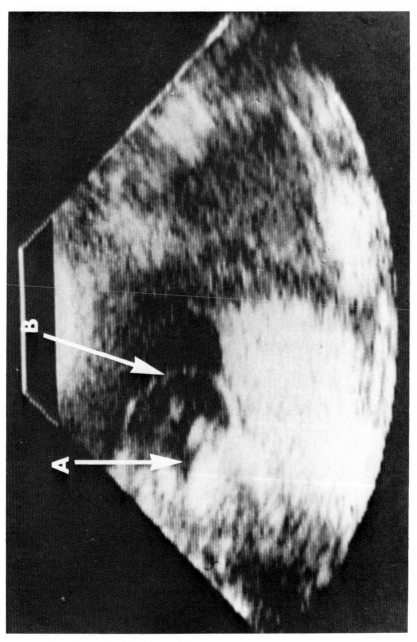

Fig. 11.   Echogram of open spinal defect with myelomeningocele at 18 weeks gestation. A, Spina bifida; B, myelomeningocele.

TABLE III

ULTRASOUND AND ALPHA-FETOPROTEIN IN THE EARLY DETECTION OF CRANIOSPINAL DEFECTS

	Total	Ultrasound			Amniotic fluid alpha-fetoprotein		
		Detected	Not detected	False positive	Detected	Not detected	False positive
Anencephaly	23	23	0	0	23	0	0
Spina bifida							
Open	36	32[a]	4[b]	0	35	1	10
Closed	2	2	0	0	0	2	0
Encephalocele	9	8	1	0	7	2	0
Iniencephaly	1	1	0	0	1	0	0
Isolated hydrocephaly	6	6	0	0	1[c]	4	0
Holoprosencephaly	1	1	0	0	—	—	—
Microcephaly	4	4	0	0	—	—	—
Totals	82	77	5	0	67	9	10

[a] Two confirmed by fetoscopy.
[b] All below L4.
[c] Omphalocele present.

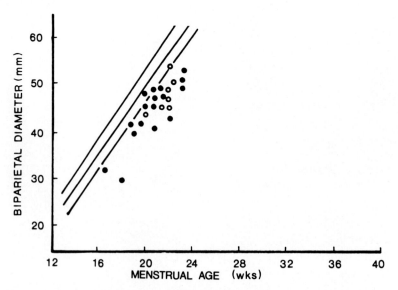

FIG. 12.   Biparietal diameter values in fetuses with spina bifida compared with normal range (mean, fifth, and ninety-fifth percentile limits). Fetuses born with enlarged ventricles were found to have smaller BPD values and head-circumference measurements. ○, No hydrocephaly; ●, hydrocephaly.

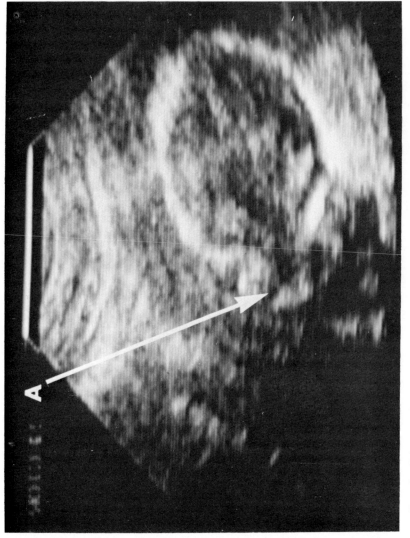

FIG. 13. Echogram of transverse section of fetal head at 20 weeks showing encephalocele. A, Encephalocele.

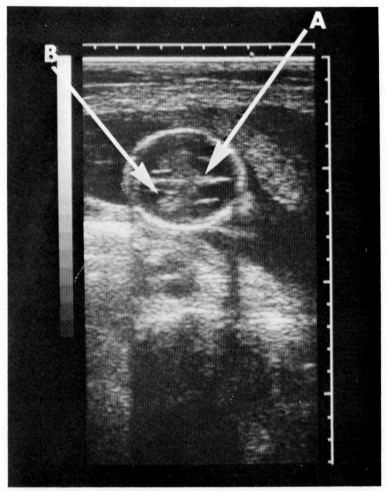

FIG. 14.   Echogram of transverse section of fetal head at 16 weeks showing anterior and posterior horns of the cerebral ventricles. The posterior horn is seen to contain the choroid plexus. The VHR is normal. A, Anterior horn; B, posterior horn.

    c. Encephalocele.   Encephalocele is recognized as a bulge in the occiput or a defect in the normal rounded outline of the fetal head (Fig. 13). Defects may range from a simple bulging occipital meningocele containing minimal neural tissue to major vault defects with more than half of the fetal brain contained within the sac (exencephaly). We have diagnosed eight of the nine cases of encephalocele in our series before 26 weeks, and our one failure was a lesion measuring 1 cm in the occipital region. The baby was found to have no

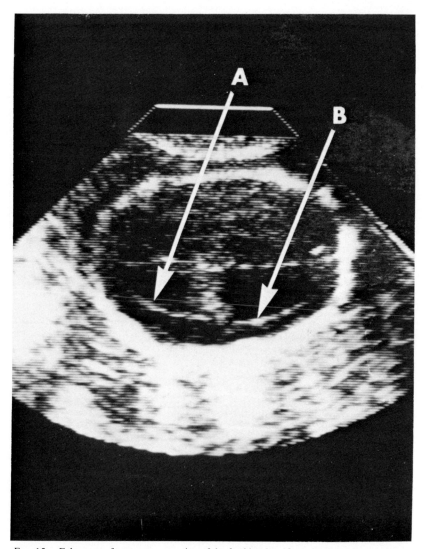

FIG. 15.   Echogram of a transverse section of the fetal head at 18 weeks showing enlargement of the anterior and posterior horns of the cerebral ventricles with a high VHR. Head zone artifact obscures ventricular echoes from the proximal cerebral hemisphere. A, Lateral border anterior horn; B, lateral border posterior horn.

neurologic defects at birth. Among patients with a history of having delivered a fetus with an encephalocele or unspecified neural tube defect it is particularly important to identify those with Meckel's syndrome. Half of our cases with this syndrome have been referred simply as cases of "previous neural tube defect."

This obscures the much higher recurrence rate for Meckel's syndrome of one in four. Multicystic kidneys, polydactyly, and encephalocele characterize the syndrome, but microcephaly and hydrocephaly rather than encephalocele can be present.

    d. Hydrocephaly. Lorber (1961) observed that nearly all neonates with spina bifida had pathologically dilated ventricles, and it appears from our experience that the majority (about 80%) of fetuses with spina bifida are similarly affected. The presence of pathologically dilated ventricles is readily diagnosed in early pregnancy, and we have largely concentrated on the study of anterior horns of the lateral ventricles. Scans of the head should be made as for head-circumference measurements, so that the ultrasound beam will cross the parietal eminences in the transcoronal plane and the occipito–frontal diameter in the sagittal plane (Campbell and Thoms, 1977). When scans are made at the cranial extremity of the septum pellucidum it is always possible to detect a line in each hemisphere running parallel to the midline echo between it and the lateral walls of the skull (Fig. 14). These lines represent the lateral margin of the anterior horn of each lateral ventricle, and the measurement of their distance from the midline is essential to the detection of hydrocephaly (Fig. 15). The ventricle to hemisphere ratio (VHR) is obtained by measuring the distance from the lateral margin of the anterior horn to the midline (V) and dividing it by the maximum width of the cerebral hemisphere (H) at the same level. Campbell (1980) measured the

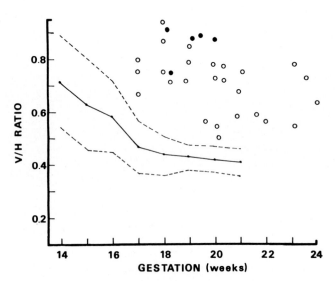

    Fɪɢ. 16.   Ventricle to hemisphere ratios of fetuses who were found to have hydrocephalus associated with spina bifida (○) or isolated hydrocephalus (●) compared with normal range (mean, fifth, and ninety-fifth percentile limits).

VHR of 102 normal fetuses examined between 12 and 24 weeks postmenstrual age and plotted the mean ($\pm$ 2 SD) against postmenstrual age (Fig. 16). The VHR in 26 cases of hydrocephalus associated with spina bifida and 4 cases of isolated hydrocephalus lie well above the normal range, indicating good discrimination between normal and abnormal. In practice a VHR above 0.5 at 18 weeks gestation is a sufficient criterion for diagnosis of pathologic ventricular dilatation. It is important to realize that the biparietal diameter and head circumference are always within normal limits for gestational age and that in cases associated with spina bifida often fall below the normal limits. In two cases of fetuses with isolated hydrocephalus, aqueduct stenosis was demonstrated, and our highest VHR was found in a fetus at 16 weeks with aqueduct stenosis.

It is occasionally possible to find that the posterior horns of the lateral ventri-

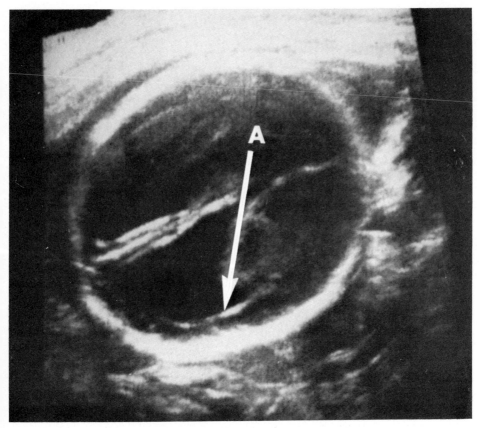

FIG. 17.   Echogram of transverse section of fetal head at 24 weeks showing dilated posterior horn. A, Lateral border of posterior horn.

cles are dilated without significant distention of the anterior horns (Fig. 17), but this is a rare occurrence and there are no good data on the size of the posterior horns in normal pregnancy. With better resolution real-time equipment, considerable detail of cerebral structures is visible, although the anatomical significance of many of these has yet to be elucidated.

e. Microcephaly. Slow fetal head growth can be due to growth retardation, and it is essential to relate the growth of the fetal head to that of the abdominal girth in order to make the diagnosis of microcephaly. Unfortunately, ventricle size is of no value in making the diagnosis, because in our series the VHR has always been normal. Head- and abdomen-circumference measurements may remain within normal limits until the second half of the middle trimester, when progressive retardation of head growth relative to normal abdominal growth causes the head to abdomen ratio to fall below the normal range. Reduced abdominal growth may complicate the diagnosis, however, and we were unable to diagnose confidently one microcephalic fetus until 26 weeks gestation. Representative measurement of the abdominal circumference for comparision may be complicated by the distortion of the abdominal outline consequent upon gross fetal hyperflexion. For this reason we also recommend measurement of the femur length as an indicator of somatic growth. Table IV summarizes our experience with this condition. We have successfully made the diagnosis on four occasions and followed this up with termination of pregnancy. Pathologic confirmation of microcephaly was made in each case, and we have had no false-negative or false-positive diagnoses from the 18 high-risk referrals. Although these results are encouraging it would be optimistic to expect the success rate to continue because it seems likely that in some instances slowing of the fetal head growth may not become apparent until after 26 weeks gestation when termination of pregnancy is ethically impossible.

f. Other Cranial Abnormalities. We have diagnosed other cranial abnormalities such as iniencephaly, holoprosencephaly, and hydranencephaly. Iniencephaly is characterized by gross hyperextension of the fetal head, the occiput fusing with the cervical vertebrae. A case of holoprosencephaly demonstrated a

TABLE IV

EXPERIENCE OF KING'S COLLEGE HOSPITAL WITH ULTRASOUND DIAGNOSIS OF MICROCEPHALY
(18 REFERRALS)

17 Previously affected fetus or infant
1 Routine ultrasound (diabetic clinic)

4 Positive
No false negative
No false positive

single ventricle in association with phocomelia in a diabetic mother (Fig. 18). Hydranencephaly was characterized by the absence of any normal ventricular pattern, the normal shaped head being echo-free apart from a symmetrical central echo thought to represent the mid-brain. This fetus was found to have trisomy 13-15 and cyclopea, which could be recognized on retrospective examination of real-time recordings.

2.   Fetal Tumors

In all four referrals because of ultrasound findings suspicious of fetal tumor the lesions have been found in the neck. Table V summarizes our findings. Teratoma is a rare condition, but pterygium coli is found in association with Turner's syndrome and is therefore a much more common lesion. The cystic swellings are typically lateral and dorsal to the fetal neck and are distinguished from en-

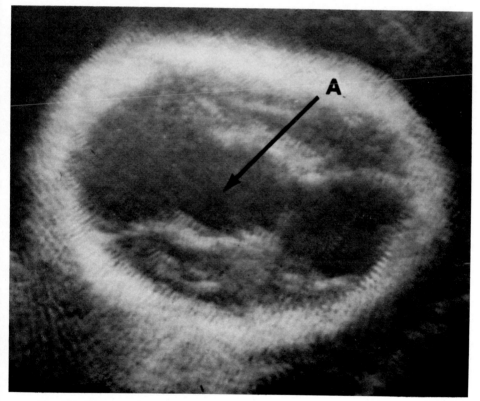

Fig. 18.   Echogram of transverse section of the fetal head at 17 weeks showing holoprosencephaly. A, Holoprosencephaly.

TABLE V

EXPERIENCE OF KING'S COLLEGE HOSPITAL WITH ULTRASOUND DIAGNOSIS OF FETAL TUMORS
(FOUR REFERRALS)

4 Positive
2 Pterygium colli (1 Turner's syndrome)
1 Lymphangiectasia
1 Teratoma of the neck

2 Misclassified
No false negative
No false positive

cephalocele by demonstrating that their maximum width is at the level of the cervical spine (Fig. 19). A similar appearance may be seen in fetuses with gross edema in the absence of an XO genotype.

3. GASTROINTESTINAL ANOMALIES (TABLE VI)

a. Bowel Obstruction. High bowel obstruction is usually associated with polyhydramnios. In duodenal atresia the fluid-filled stomach and duodenum gave a typical appearance of twin cystic spaces (the double bubble) in the upper abdomen (Fig. 20), whereas with jejunal atresia three or four dilated bowel segments may be identified. Esophageal atresia may be diagnosed if there is failure to identify the stomach bubble on repeated scanning. We have successfully diagnosed two cases of duodenal atresia and one jejunal atresia, but we have failed to recognize one omphalocele and have made one false-positive diagnosis of duodenal atresia: this fetus appeared to have a double bubble, but this disappeared on subsequent examination.

b. Omphalocele. This lesion is being recognized with increasing frequency as it is associated with elevated MSAFP levels. The fetal abdomen and the insertion of the umbilical cord can be readily identified between 16 and 24 weeks postmenstrual age. Omphalocele can be recognized as a bulge in the anterior abdominal wall. We have successfully detected seven such cases before 24 weeks, all patients having been referred with raised AFAFP levels and a suspected diagnosis of neural tube defect. In those cases where the lesion was extensive, termination of pregnancy was recommended. However, minor lesions may be suitable for surgical repair, and it is therefore important to identify structures within the omphalocele. The liver is usually present within the sac and can be identified by visualizing the umbilical vein within its substance. If large amounts of bowel and bladder are contained within the sac then it is clearly inoperable. It is important to try to distinguish between omphalocele and gastroschisis, in which extruded abdominal contents are not contained within a

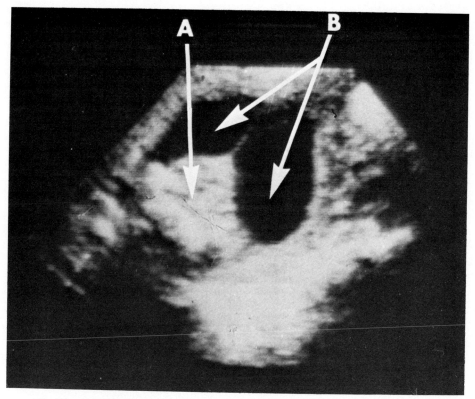

FIG. 19.   Echogram of transverse section of the fetal neck at 22 weeks demonstrating a pterygium colli. A, Cervical spine; B, pterygium colli.

TABLE VI

EXPERIENCE OF KING'S COLLEGE HOSPITAL WITH ULTRASOUND DIAGNOSIS OF GASTROINTESTINAL ANOMALIES, 1978–JUNE 1980 (55 REFERRALS)

40 Raised MSAFP or AFAFP
15 Suspicious ultrasound findings ("cysts in abdomen," polyhydramnios)

10 Positive
7 Omphalocele
2 Duodenal atresia
1 Jejunal atresia

1 False negative (omphalocele)
1 False positive (duodenal atresia)

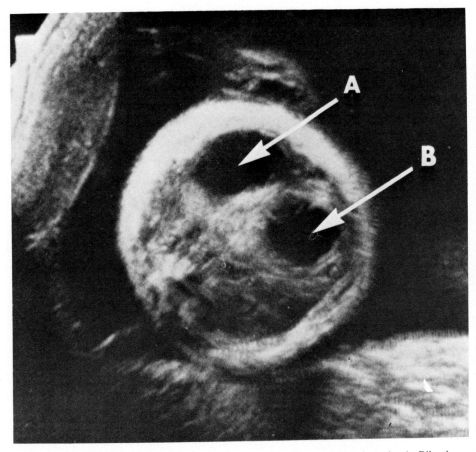

F$_{IG}$. 20.   Echogram showing typical "double bubble" effect of duodenal atresia. A, Dilated stomach; B, dilated duodenum.

peritoneal sac. Gastroschisis is usually an isolated phenomenon, whereas 50% of cases of omphalocele are associated with other chromosomal or cardiac abnormalities that should always be investigated if the decision to continue with the pregnancy is considered.

4.   RENAL TRACT ANOMALIES

Normal renal outlines may be identified from 14 weeks postmenstrual age and reliably from 18 weeks (Fig. 21). They are best visualized on real-time scanning and are located below the level of the umbilical vein on either side of and anterior

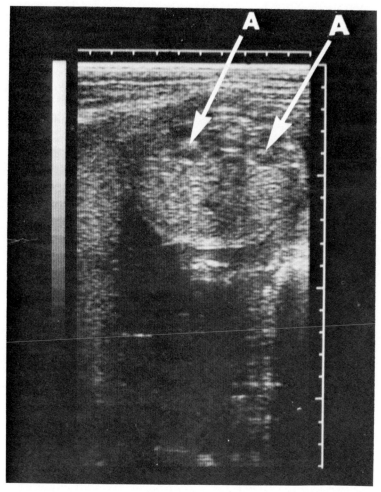

Fɪɢ. 21. Fetogram at 22 weeks showing typical renal outlines with central echo from renal pelvis. A, Renal pelvis.

to the spine. Visualization is often facilitated by fetal trunk or particularly breathing movements, which help to distinguish the kidneys from surrounding tissue masses. Relative to the surrounding tissue the kidney is normally less echogenic and contains a small central echo-free circle representing the renal pelvis. Later in the second trimester lobulation becomes apparent. Grannum et al. (1980) have published data on fetal kidney size in relation to abdominal-circumference measurements and have found that the fetal kidney circumference is approximately

30% of the abdominal circumference at any stage of gestation. Evidence of renal function can be obtained by identification of the fetal bladder, which is usually recognizable from 16 weeks gestation.

  a. Renal Agenesis. The diagnosis of renal agenesis is based on the absence of normal kidney echoes and bladder filling in the presence of severe oligohydramnios. The diagnosis is often made difficult by gross fetal flexion resulting from oligohydramnios and an absence of fetal breathing or motor activity.

  b. Multicystic Dysplasia. Multicystic kidneys are typically enlarged, especially when found in association with encephalocele in Meckel's syndrome. The variable size of the cysts is reflected in the ultrasonic appearance of the kidney. If the cysts are very small, a uniform increase in echogenicity is apparent, lending a speckled appearance (Fig. 22). Larger cysts may be seen arranged in a symmetrical rosette around the renal pelvis (Fig. 23) or may be randomly distributed throughout the renal parenchyma, which often shows increased echogenicity. In the case of infantile polycystic disease the condition is always bilateral, and further evidence of cystic dysplasia should be sought in other organs such as liver and lungs. Normal renal function is usually absent in these cases, hence bladder filling will not be apparent even following the administration of a diuretic to the mother, and there is commonly coexistent oligohydramnios.

  c. Isolated Renal Cysts. Isolated renal cysts can be identified as large cystic spaces attached to the kidneys. Differentiation from other intraabdominal cysts may be facilitated by observing synchronous movement of the cyst and renal tissue with fetal motor or respiratory activity. Dilatation of the renal pelvis may be seen if the cyst is large enough to cause obstruction of the ureters. As these isolated cysts may coexist with normally functioning renal tissue and are frequently unilateral, normal bladder filling may be observed.

  d. Obstructive Uropathy. There is a wide spectrum of pathologic, clinical, and ultrasonic features associated with this group of conditions characterized by dilatation of all or part of the urinary outflow tract. The gestational age at which outflow-tract dilatation becomes obvious seems to be closely related to the degree of renal impairment, and if significant dilatation is found before the twenty-fourth week of gestation, then the prognosis for the fetus is extremely poor and termination of pregnancy is advised. If either the urethra is stenosed or there are posterior urethral valves, the fetal bladder is continuously distended and enlarged ureters and renal pelvis are apparent. If the obstruction is ureteric, then there is absence of bladder filling and, again, dilatation of the renal pelvis. Renal aplasia or multicystic dysplasia frequently coexist with and may indeed be consequent upon ureteric or pelvic agenesis (Bernstein, 1980). In some cases of urethral obstruction, enlargement of the ureters and renal pelvis is so great that they may be difficult to distinguish from the distended bladder. Gross dilatation may be seen in conjunction with absent abdominal wall musculature of the "prune belly" syndrome.

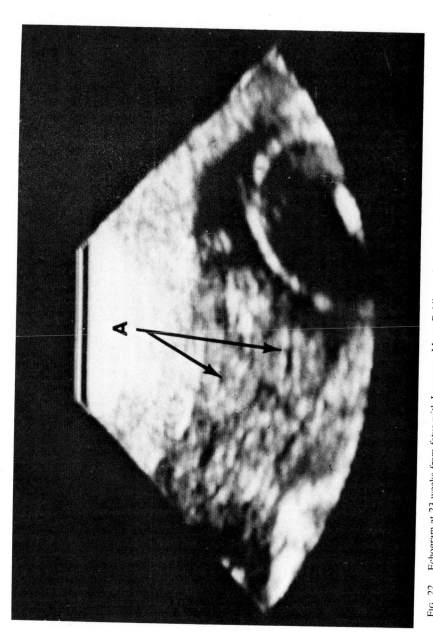

Fig. 22. Echogram at 23 weeks from fetus with Lawrence–Moon–Beidle syndrome showing the echogenic renal parenchyma in polycystic kidney disease. The fetal kidneys were not enlarged. A, Fetal kidney.

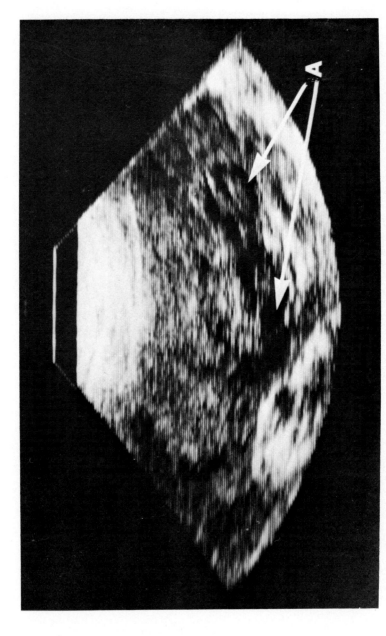

FIG. 23.   Echogram of fetus at 23 weeks showing the large cystic spaces in multicystic renal dysplasia. There is gross oligohydramnios indicating fetal renal failure. A, Multicystic kidneys.

In some cases evidence of obstruction may not develop until a later stage in gestation, and one such fetus was identified at 28 weeks with a grossly dilated bladder that failed to empty. Over the succeeding 4 weeks the ureters and later the renal pelvis gradually dilated; delivery was effected at the thirty-fifth week postmenstrual age to prevent renal parenchymal damage, and the child has progressed well following surgery. In this case, ultrasound played a useful part in management of the case where timely therapeutic intervention was able to prevent irreparable renal damage.

Most instances of obstructive uropathy and multicystic dysplasia or aplasia are sporadic and the risk of recurrence in future pregnancy is slight, except when found in association with recognized syndromes such as Meckel's syndrome. Infantile polycystic disease, however, is inherited as an autosomal recessive with a one in four chance of recurrence. Expert histologic and possibly histochemical study of affected fetal kidneys may enable distinction of etiologic types and facilitate counseling of the parents of an affected fetus.

Table VII summarizes our experience to June 1980 in the diagnosis of renal tract disorders. Of the 39 referrals, 19 mothers had experienced previous pregnancies with an affected fetus. In previous ultrasound examinations suspicious findings had been noted in 20 patients, including cystic spaces in the abdomen, oligohydramnios, fetal ascites, or encephalocele. In 10 of these 39 referrals positive diagnoses of urinary tract or renal disorders were made. Three diagnoses were missed. One was referred at 20 weeks gestation because of elevated MSAFP and severe oligohydramnios. On static B-scan examination it was thought that the renal outlines and fetal bladder could be identified, and amniotic fluid obtained by amniocentesis had a normal AFP concentration. Labor was induced at 28 weeks and a grossly abnormal fetus was delivered with renal cystic

TABLE VII

EXPERIENCE OF KING'S COLLEGE HOSPITAL WITH ULTRASOUND DIAGNOSIS OF RENAL ANOMALIES, 1978–JUNE 1980 (39 REFERRALS)

19 Previously affected fetus or infant
20 Suspicious ultrasound findings ("cysts in abdomen," oligohydramnios, fetal ascites, encephalocele)

10 Positive
5 Obstructive uropathy
1 Renal cysts
2 Infantile polycystic kidneys
2 Polycystic kidneys (Meckel's syndrome)

3 False negative (2 renal cystic dysplasia; 1 renal agenesis)
No false positive

dysplasia that died at 3 days from renal failure. It is our belief that this abnormality would have been diagnosed were we in possession of a high-resolution real-time scanner at that time. The remaining two cases were both referred late in pregnancy. In one, gross intrauterine growth retardation was suspected; in the other, we were able to detect gross hydrocephalus and spina bifida but further examination was hampered by severe oligohydramnios. All three infants suffered neonatal death. There were no false-positive diagnoses.

5. OLIGOHYDRAMNIOS

It is pertinent at this point to comment on oligohydramnios, which is commonly but not invariably associated with renal and urinary tract disorders. Table VIII summarizes the serious prognostic consequences of severe oligohydramnios diagnosed before the twenty-sixth week. Of the five fetuses with obstructive uropathy, three pregnancies were terminated (TOP) and two continued to premature delivery and neonatal death (NND). An attempt to release back pressure on the kidneys and preserve renal function was attempted in one case by catheterizing the fetal bladder, but no subsequent bladder filling was observed. The baby died from renal failure in the neonatal period. Large cystic swellings lateral and posterior to the fetal neck, diagnosed as pterygium coli, were observed in another fetus, which subsequently died *in utero*. Although cell culture was unsuccessful, Turner's syndrome was suspected from this ultrasound finding. A further fetus in which the kidneys appeared normal had severe congenital heart disease. Another

TABLE VIII

PROGNOSTIC CONSEQUENCES OF OLIGOHYDRAMNIOS <26 WEEKS
(1978–JUNE 1980)

Type of consequence	No. of fetuses affected
Obstructive uropathy (3 TOP, 2 NND)[a]	5
Renal agenesis (NND)	1
Bilateral renal cystic dysplasia (NND)	1
Pterygium colli (abortion)	1
Congenital heart defect (NND)	1
Termination of pregnancy	1
Spontaneous abortion	1
Preterm labor (NND)	2
Normal term baby (alive and well)	1
	14

[a] TOP, Termination of pregnancy; NND, neonatal death.

pregnancy was electively terminated following elevated MSAFP, although ultrasound examination showed no abnormality: pathology in this case was normal.
Only 1 pregnancy of the 14 showing severe oligohydramnios resulted in a normal
infant born at term and continuing in good health. Fetal abnormality should
therefore be diligently sought when severe oligohydramnios is found in the
second trimester, and the pregnancy closely supervised should no abnormality be
found.

6.   FETAL ASCITES

Fetal ascites can of course be associated with rhesus isoimmunization and the
hydropic fetus. Detection of fetal ascites before 26 weeks gestation is of grave
prognostic significance. There have now been reported a number of cases of

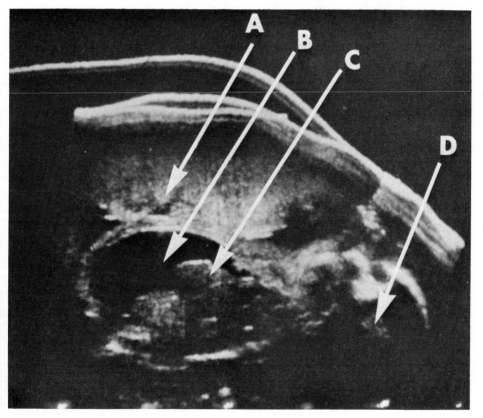

FIG. 24.   Echogram of longitudinal section of fetus showing gross fetal ascites. A, Placenta; B,
ascites; C, liver; D, head.

unexplained fetal ascites, some of which have been present for several weeks and have thereafter spontaneously resolved. Possible etiologic factors are transient fetal cardiac failure, viral infection, and nephrotic syndrome. Figure 24 shows a case of fetal ascites. The fetal cardiac outline was considered to be abnormal on static scanning, and retrospective examination of the real-time videotape revealed an abnormality with dilatation of the left atrium and a thick-walled left ventricle. Postnatally the fetus was found to have aortic stenosis. A more detailed account of examination of the fetal heart will be presented later in this article.

7. Limb-Reduction Deformities

The advent of high-resolution real-time scanning, particularly the mechanical sector scanner, has greatly facilitated the measurement of fetal limb length.

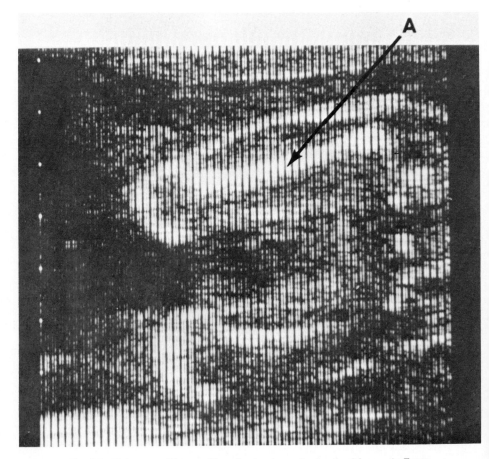

Fig. 25.   Echogram of fetus at 22 weeks showing entire length of femur. A, Femur.

When performing limb measurements it is important to recognize that the soft tissue extremities of the limb should be visible beyond the bone being measured so that full bone visualization is assured (Fig. 25). Nomograms for the femur (Fig. 26), tibia and fibula, humerus and radius and ulna have now been constructed from the eleventh to twenty-fourth gestational week (Queenan *et al.*, 1980). Although gross limb-reduction deformities such as diastrophic dwarfism and severe phocomelia may be easily diagnosed, achondroplasia may not show significant reduction in limb growth until 24 to 26 weeks gestation. Serial measurements to this gestational age should be performed before distinguishing the normal from abnormal fetus. In Table IX our experience in the diagnosis of limb reduction is shown. Limb deformities or reductions may coexist as part of recognized syndromes, with more serious underlying pathology less amenable to an-

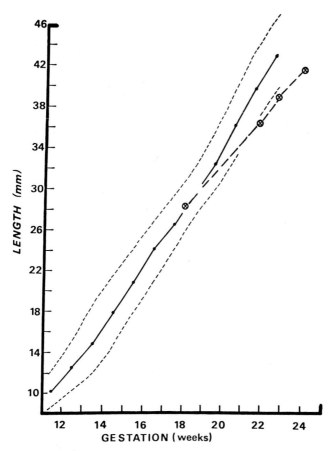

FIG. 26.   Growth of femur in a fetus with achondroplasia compared with normal range (Mean ± 2S.D.)

TABLE IX

EXPERIENCE OF KING'S COLLEGE HOSPITAL WITH ULTRASOUND DIAGNOSIS OF LIMB-REDUCTION
DEFORMITIES (29 REFERRALS)

27 Previously affected fetus or infant
2 Drugs in early pregnancy

3 Positive
1 Phocomelia
1 Diastrophic dwarf
1 Achondroplasia

No false negative
No false positive

tenatal diagnosis. Examples of these are the absence of the radius in the thrombocytopenia absent-radius (TAR) syndrome or radio–ulna synostosis associated with congenital heart disease in the Holt–Oram syndrome. It may be possible also to detect reduced calcification, shortening, or intrauterine fractures in cases of osteogenesis imperfecta.

8. CARDIAC ANOMALIES

It is possible to study the fetal heart, using two-dimensional ultrasound, from around 16 weeks gestation. At this stage some normal anatomy can be defined, namely four cardiac chambers, two atrioventricular valves, and the aortic root. By 20 weeks gestation a more detailed examination can be performed and most normal features of the heart identified. A simultaneous M-mode echocardiogram, as is possible with the Advanced Technical Laboratories Mark III sector scanner used in our department, will add to the diagnostic accuracy. The cardiac examination becomes more difficult toward term as the fetus becomes more fixed in position, often with the fetal back anterior. In our study of 500 pregnancies a normal fetal heart was accurately predicted in 486. Eight abnormalities have been accurately detected. These are listed in Table X. There were three errors during the study: one prediction of ventricular septal defect was made when none existed; there were two false negatives, namely an ostium primum atrial-septal defect at 19/52 and in one patient, in whom an adequate study was impossible at 15/52 gestation, autopsy showed a univentricular heart of left-ventricular type. Right atrial and ventricular dilatation were found in five hearts. This is thought to be a nonspecific sign of intrauterine cardiac failure. All were associated with fetal ascites, two due to rhesus isoimmunization; three had nonimmune hydrops fetalis.

All the abnormalities we have detected have occurred in what we consider to be "high-risk" groups. The high-risk groups include those pregnancies where

TABLE X

CARDIAC ANOMALIES DETECTED BY ULTRASOUND IN A STUDY OF 500 PREGNANCIES

	Gestational age at detection	Confirmation
Primum atrial-septal defect	16	Anatomy
Hypoplastic aortic arch	18	Anatomy
Left ventricular hypertrophy	26	Anatomy
Tetralogy of Fallot assent pulmonary valve	32	Anatomy
Aortic stenosis	34	Anatomy
Right ventricular hypertrophy	35	Anatomy
Tetralogy of Fallot A-V canal	37	Anatomy
Double outlet right ventricle A-V canal	38	Cardiac catheterization

there is a family history of congenital heart disease, maternal diabetes, fetal arrhythmia, fetal ascites, and fetal anomaly. The last group, that of fetal anomaly, is particularly important as up to one-third of congenital heart disease is associated with other anomalies, and conversely six of our cardiac abnormalities occurred in association with extracardiac lesions, although this was a selected population. The abnormalities detected in each group are listed in Table XI.

Detection of a severe cardiac abnormality early in pregnancy may in the future allow termination of pregnancy, but at the present time the application of cardiac scanning is to optimize the neonatal condition by obviating delay in diagnosis, and planning the route and place of delivery, with knowledge of the abnormality. The combination of more than one congenital lesion should perhaps indicate that a chromosomal defect or a specific syndrome should be sought. In the future it should be possible during a routine obstetric scan to identify the cardiac sections

TABLE XI

HIGH-RISK GROUPS FOR FETAL CARDIAC ABNORMALITIES

	No. scanned	Abnormality detected
Family history of CHD	38	1
Maternal diabetes	48	—
Fetal ascites	14	3
Fetal arrhythmia	5	1
Fetal anomaly	22	6

[a] Three abnormalities fell into more than one high-risk group.

TABLE XII

Routine Ultrasound 1978–June 1980)

Antenatal clinic	Pregnancy diabetic clinic
4 Anencephaly	1 Anencephaly
1 Encephalocele	2 Hydrocephalus
1 Spina bifida	1 Microcephaly
1 Omphalocele	1 Holoprosencephly
1 Obstructive uropathy	
3 Fetal tumors	
——	——
11	5

that contribute most information to the diagnosis of normality, but the elucidation of abnormality is difficult and likely to remain a specialist subject.

IV.   The Place of Early Routine Ultrasound Scanning in the Diagnosis of Fetal Anomalies

Although specialized scanning is highly successful in diagnosing the anomalies described here, the pickup rate of severe anomalies may be considerably lower when scanning is performed on routine basis for simple fetal measurements and placental localization. Consistently successful diagnosis of many of these conditions will only be possible if specific attention is paid to individual organs. However, during ultrasound examinations performed by our group between 1978 and June 1980 (Table XII), 11 anomalies were picked up in the antenatal clinic as a result of routine scanning. More detailed attention is paid to scanning patients in the pregnancy diabetic clinic, and five further anomalies were detected in this group. Recently in routine booking scans performed at 16 weeks postmenstrual age, more specific attention is being paid to the diagnosis of fetal anomalies and of neural tube defects in particular.

References

Bang, J., and Northeved, A. (1972). *Am. J. Obstet. Gynecol.* **114,** 599.

Bernstein, J. (1980). *In* "Pediatric Kidney Disease" (C. Edelmann, ed.), Vol. II, p. 551. Little, Brown, Boston.

Campbell, S. (1968). *J. Obstet. Gynaecol. Br. Commonw.* **75,** 568.

Campbell, S. (1969). *J. Obstet. Gynaecol. Br. Commonw.* **76,** 603.

Campbell, S. (1974a). *In* "Clinics in Perinatology" (A. Milunsky, ed.), Vol. 1, No. 2, p. 507. Saunders, Philadelphia.

Campbell, S. (1974b). *Clin. Obstet. Gynecol.* **1,** 41.

Campbell, S. (1974c). *In* "Birth Defects" (A. G. Molnsky and E. Leftz, eds.), p. 240. Excerpta Medica, Amsterdam.

Campbell, S. (1975). *In* "Fetal Physiology and Medicine" (R. W. Beard and P. W. Nathanielz, eds.), pp. 271–301. Saunders, London.

Campbell, S. (1977). *Clin. Obstet. Gynecol.* **20,** 351.

Campbell, S. (1980). *In* "Genetic Disorders and the Fetus" (A. Milunsky, ed.), pp. 431–467. Plenum, New York.

Campbell, S., and Dewhurst, C. H. (1971). *Lancet* **2,** 1002.

Campbell, S., and Newman, G. B. (1971). *J. Obstet. Gynaecol. Br. Commonw.* **78,** 513.

Campbell, S., and Rodeck, C. H. (1979). Presented at October 4 symposium on the diagnosis and management of neural tube defects, Royal College of Obstetricians and Gynecologists, London, England.

Campbell, S., and Thoms, A. (1977). *Br. J. Obstet. Gynaecol.* **84,** 165.

Campbell, S., and Wilkin, D. (1975). *Br. J. Obstet. Gynaecol.* **82,** 689.

Campbell, S., Johnston, F. D., Holt, E. M., and May, P. (1972). *Lancet* **2,** 1226.

Campbell, S., Pryse-Davies, J., Coltart, T. M., Seller, M. J., and Singer, J. D. (1975). *Lancet* **1,** 1065.

Fancourt, R., Campbell, S., Harvey, D., and Norman, A. P. (1976). *Br. Med. J.* **1,** 1435.

Grannum, P., Bracken, M., Silvermann, R., and Hobbins, J. C. (1980). *Am. J. Obstet. Gynecol.* **136,** 249.

Griscon, N. T. (1980). *In* "Genetic Disorders and the Fetus" (A. Milunsky, ed.), pp. 469–494, Plenum, New York.

Harrison, R., Campbell, S., and Kraft, I. (1975). *J. Obstet. Gynecol.* **46,** 389.

Kerenyi, T. D., and Walker, B. (1977). *J. Obstet. Gynecol.* **50,** 61.

Lele, P. P. (1979). *Ultrasound Med. Biol.* **5,** 307–320.

Lind, T., and Hytten, F. E. (1972). *In* "International Symposium on Physiological Biochemistry of the Fetus" (A. Hodari and F. Mariona, eds.), p. 54. Thomas, Springfield, Ill.

Lorber, J. (1961). *Arch. Dis. Child.* **36,** 381–389.

Medical Research Council Working Party (1978). *Br. J. Obstet. Gynaecol.* **85,** 826.

Murphy, J. F., Drumm, J. E., Mulcahy, R., and Daly, L. (1980). *Br. J. Obstet. Gynaecol.* **87,** 462–460.

Nevin, N. C., and Armstrong, M. J. (1975). *Br. J. Obstet. Gynaecol.* **82,** 826.

Polani, P. E., Alberman, E., Berry, A. C., Blunt, S., and Singer, J. D. (1976). *Lancet* **2,** 516.

Queenan, J., O'Brien, G. D., and Campbell, S. (1980). *Am. J. Obstet. Gynecol.* **138,** 297.

Roberts, A. B., and Campbell, S. (1980). *Br. J. Obstet. Gynaecol.* **87,** 927–928.

Robinson, H. P. (1973). *Br. Med. J.* **4,** 28.

Robinson, H. P., and Fleming, J. E. (1975). *Br. J. Obstet. Gynaecol.* **82,** 702–710.

Rodeck, C. H. (1980). *Br. J. Obstet. Gynaecol.* **87,** 449.

Rodeck, C. H., and Campbell, S. (1978). *Lancet* **1,** 1128.

Taylor, J. W. T., and Dyson, M. (1980). *In* "Principles and Practice of Ultrasonography in Obstetrics and Gynecology" (R. C. Sanders and A. E. James, eds.), 2nd Edition, pp. 15–24. Appleton-Century-Crofts, New York.

Chapter 7

Fetoscopy and Fetal Biopsy

MAURICE J. MAHONEY

Departments of Human Genetics, Pediatrics, and Obstetrics and Gynecology
Yale University School of Medicine
New Haven, Connecticut

Fetoscopy, literally a "viewing of the fetus," refers to endoscopic visualization of the fetus and placenta *in utero*. The procedure is used in the fourth and fifth months of pregnancy to obtain a limited view of fetal anatomy, to aspirate fetal blood samples, and to obtain biopsy specimens of fetal skin or fetal liver (Mahoney and Hobbins, 1979; Rodeck, 1980). Because the operation carries considerably more risk than do midtrimester amniocentesis and ultrasonography, diagnostic fetoscopy has been restricted to a small number of referral centers that number fewer than 50 throughout the world.

I. Rationale for Fetoscopy

The advent of genetic amniocentesis in the late 1960s spawned intense activity toward early (i.e., second-trimester) diagnosis in fetal medicine. Amniocytes

METHODS IN CELL BIOLOGY, VOL. 26

could reveal the karyotype and many biochemical phenotypes of the fetus but failed to disclose many other biochemical and physiological attributes, especially parameters of specialized cells and organs. In general, enzymes and other proteins found in cultured skin fibroblasts are present in cultured amniocytes, but proteins specific to liver, blood cells, brain, and other specialized tissues are not. Yet many serious diseases are expressed primarily in one of those specialized tissues. Hollenbert *et al.* (1971) and Kan *et al.* (1972) recognized the potential for diagnosis of hemoglobinopathies if a small volume of fetal blood could be obtained. Diagnosis would be possible because adult hemoglobins are synthesized in reticulocytes from the midtrimester fetus. Thus central to the development of fetoscopy was the goal of a safe method of fetal blood sampling.

Another spur to the development of fetoscopy in the 1970s was the desire for a better anatomic definition of the fetus than could be obtained using ultrasonography or radiography. Early reports of fetoscopy (summarized in Mahoney and Hobbins, 1979) emphasized views of the fetus and behaviors of the fetus such as swallowing and limb movements.

It was recognized from the beginning that fetoscopy carried higher risks of pregnancy loss or other fetal damage than genetic amniocentesis or ultrasonography. At this stage of development, experienced fetoscopists are reporting a 2–4% risk of miscarriage and a probable increase, though less than 1.5-fold, in prematurity (International Fetoscopy Group, 1981). The risk of miscarriage as a consequence of amniocentesis is one in several hundred at experienced centers, and at present there are no recognized risks of ultrasonography for the unborn baby.

In prenatal diagnosis fetoscopy is used only when seeking serious disorders whose diagnosis will influence pregnancy-management decisions, and only when a safer technique is unavailable. When studies of amniotic fluid and amniocytes or anatomic definition of the fetus by ultrasonography can establish a diagnosis, these methods are preferred. With the rapid evolution of prenatal diagnosis via amniocentesis and ultrasound examination, as detailed in other articles of this volume, we have seen changing indications and a changing role for fetoscopy.

Diagnoses that have been accomplished or excluded using fetoscopy are summarized in Table I. Some of these would be sought by other means today. For example, the requirement for fetal blood to diagnose hemoglobinopathies has been halved since the advent of prenatal diagnosis by DNA analysis using the methods of molecular genetics (Kan and Dozy, 1978). Similarly, the sophistication of fetal imaging with ultrasound has made it the preferred modality for all but small details of fetal anatomy such as digits, nails, and ears.

As advancing technology decreases the use of fetoscopy in some spheres, it increases it in others. Experience with fetal skin biopsy and fetal liver biopsy is now being accumulated and attempts are under way to find a means of fetal muscle biopsy. In addition, ideas for intrauterine fetal therapy, which would

TABLE I

DIAGNOSES ESTABLISHED OR EXCLUDED BY FETOSCOPY

I. By visualization of fetal anatomy
    Multiple malformation syndromes characterized by:
    Limb or digit abnormalities, external ear deformities, facial or palatal clefts, multiple pterygia
        (Benzie, 1977; Mahoney and Hobbins, 1977)
    Amniotic bands
    Neural tube defects (Rodeck and Campbell, 1978)
    Anatomy of external genitalia
    Exstrophy of cloaca
    Gastroschisis
    Omphalocele
II. By fetal blood
    Hemoglobinopathies, several (Alter *et al.*, 1976)
    Coagulopathies: classic hemophilia, hemophilia B, homozygous von Willebrand disease
        (Firschein *et al.*, 1979; Mibashan *et al.*, 1979)
    Chronic granulomatous disease (Newburger *et al.*, 1979)
    $Alpha_1$-antitrypsin deficiency
    Congenital hereditary neutropenia
    Congenital dyserythropoietic anemia, Type II
    Rapid karyotype (aneuploidies, mosaicism)
    Red-cell blood type (rhesus) (Philip *et al.*, 1978)
III. By skin biopsy
    Bullous ichthyosiform erythroderma (Golbus *et al.*, 1980)
    Congenital ichthyoses: harlequin-type (Elias *et al.*, 1980), lamellar type, Sjögren–Larssen
        syndrome
    Epidermolysis bullosa dystrophica
    Epidermolysis bullosa letalis (Rodeck *et al.*, 1980)
IV. By liver biopsy
    Ornithine transcarbamylase deficiency

[a] Diagnoses without specific references were reported at Second Annual Meeting of International Fetoscopy Group (1981).

make use of fetoscopic access to the fetal bloodstream at the umbilical cord, are undergoing initial trials (C. H. Rodeck, unpublished experience).

II. Method of Fetoscopy

Successful fetoscopy combines careful ultrasound examination with skillful endoscopic technique. Initial scanning is performed with either a B-mode contact scanner (3.5–5 MHz) or a real-time scanner and identifies the fetal lie, placental site, umbilical cord attachments at the placenta, and any peculiarities of uterine

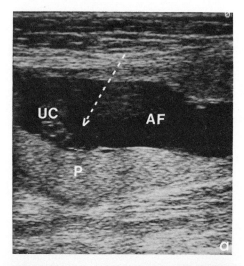

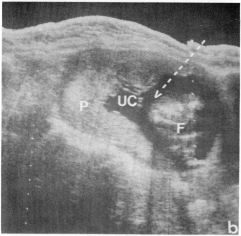

FIG. 1. (a) Sonogram of an 18-week pregnancy showing a large pocket of amniotic fluid (AF), posterior placenta (P), and loops of unbilical cord (UC). Entry into the amniotic cavity would be made along the path of the arrow, through the maternal abdomen and anterior uterine wall, and would provide a ready view of the chorionic plate of the posterior placenta and the umbilical cord at its placental attachment site. (b) Sonogram of a 19-week pregnancy showing an anterior–fundal placenta (P) with umbilical cord attachment site (UC). The arrow shows the path of entry for the fetoscope; this path would go through an edge of the anterior part of the placenta. Parts of the fetus (F) are also present in this view.

or intrauterine anatomy. A site that will avoid the fetus and also avoid the placenta, if possible, is chosen on the maternal abdomen for safe entry of the endoscope into the amniotic cavity. Figure 1 illustrates an appropriate path of entry. Traversing an edge of the placenta is sometimes necessary when the placenta is large and anterior. Improvement of the fetal lie often can be accomplished by external pressure or by having the pregnant woman get off the examining table, walk about for a short period, or do other simple exercises.

The object of the fetoscopy must be kept clearly in mind and accomplished in as short a time as practical. If a portion of fetal anatomy is to be visualized, that area of the fetus should be initially identified by ultrasound and then approached promptly by the endoscope. If blood or another tissue is to be obtained for biopsy, the sample should be obtained without efforts at visualizing other parts of the fetus.

Fetal visualization is most successful at 15–18 postmenstrual weeks of gestation. The area that can be examined through the endoscope, 2–4 cm², is small, and recognizable landmarks are difficult to find if the fetus is of large size. Fetal blood sampling is most often performed from 18 to 22 weeks gestation when the fetal blood volume is large enough that significant depletion does not occur. Moderate sedation (10 mg diazepam and 25 mg meperidine, intravenously) is useful to stop fetal movements temporarily for the period of fetoscopy.

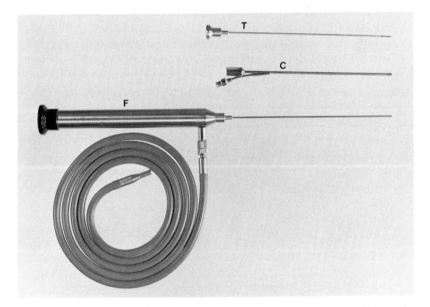

FIG. 2. Instruments used in fetoscopy. The fetoscope (F) (Needlescope, Dyonics) contains a narrow cylindrical lens, 15 cm long, surrounded by fibers to transmit light into the amniotic cavity. An introducing trocar (T) and a cannula (C) with a Y-side arm are used to enter the cavity. The figure is 25% actual size.

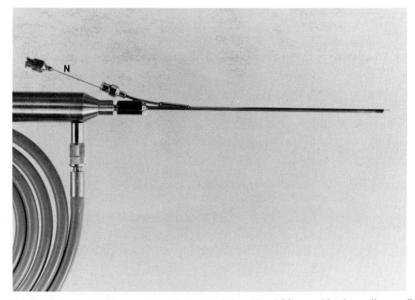

FIG. 3.   Cannula with fetoscope through its central channel and 26-gauge blood-sampling needle
(N) through the Y-side arm. The tip of the needle is seen beyond the end of the cannula.

An endoscope (fetoscope) used in fetoscopy and fetal tissue sampling is pic-
tured in Fig. 2. The cannula with sharp pointed trocar within is inserted through
the locally anesthesized skin and on into the amniotic cavity. The trocar is
removed and replaced by the endoscope. Most scopes in use today use a self-
focusing lens, which is a solid rod surrounded by fibers that transmit light into
the amniotic cavity; its diameter is usually 1.7–2.3 mm. A Y-cannula is used for
blood sampling to carry the aspirating needle alongside the lens (Fig. 3). The
cannula will measure 2–3.5 mm. The needle can be seen as it exits the cannula,
so blood sampling is performed under direct vision.

III.   Methods of Blood Sampling

A.   Fetoscopy

Fetoscopy affords the opportunity of controlled direct-vision blood sampling
either from the umbilical cord or from vessels on the chorionic plate of the
placenta. When pure blood is required for diagnostic studies the umbilical cord is
the favored site for vessel puncture, either at or close to its attachment to the
placenta. Figure 4 depicts the umbilical cord insertion site which is so important

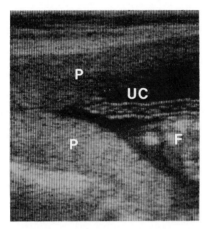

FIG. 4. Umbilical cord (UC) inserting onto the anterior aspect of a fundal placental (P). Fetal parts (F) are seen posterior to the umbilical cord.

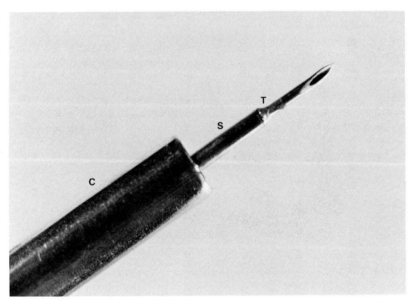

FIG. 5. Magnified view of a blood-sampling needle with a 3-mm long 27-gauge tip (T) fused to a 21-gauge shaft (S). The needle extends beyond the end of the cannula (C) and is useful for sampling from umbilical cord vessels. Magnification, 7×.

to identify ultrasonically before starting the procedure. The umbilical cord is also relatively fixed at the fetal abdomen and can be punctured at that site as an alternative.

If amniotic fluid admixture can be tolerated in the blood sample, vessels on the placental surface can be punctured and blood aspirated as it spurts from the puncture site. This method usually results in mixtures of 1 part blood plus 1 to 10 parts amniotic fluid. Occasionally maternal blood is also sampled in this manner. Maternal blood contamination is tolerable for some diagnoses but not for most and should be avoided whenever possible. Blood specimens are always checked for maternal contamination immediately after removal from the womb. This is accomplished with an electronic cell sizer (Channelyser, Coulter Electronics) that easily differentiates the larger fetal red cells [average mean volume, 140 femtoliters (fl)] from the smaller adult cells (average mean volume, 85 fl).

A 25- or 26-gauge needle, or a 21-gauge needle with a 27-gauge tip (Fig. 5), is used for fetal blood sampling during fetoscopy. Between 50 and 800 μl of fetal blood is aspirated into a 1-ml or 3-ml syringe. The syringe may contain a measured volume of anticoagulant or 50 μl heparin or sodium citrate; or the blood may be expelled into a small vial containing the anticoagulant. The puncture wound in the fetal vessel made by the small-gauge sampling needle stops bleeding in a few seconds.

B.   Placentacentesis

An alternative method for obtaining fetal blood to the use of fetoscopy is placentacentesis. After the placenta is localized by ultrasound a 19- or 20-gauge spinal needle is pushed through an anesthetized site on the maternal abdomen to the chorionic plate of the placenta. A sample of blood is then aspirated and checked to see whether it contains adequate numbers of fetal cells. If the sample is unsatisfactory, the needle is reoriented and another sample taken. Pure fetal blood is rarely obtained by this method and, in most persons' hands, the risks are higher than those associated with fetoscopy.

IV.   Method of Tissue Sampling

In addition to blood, two solid tissues of the fetus have been biopsied: skin and liver. Skin can be obtained conveniently with a small pinch forceps such as the one shown in Fig. 6. The forceps usually replaces the fetoscope in the cannula after a biopsy site has been identified. An instrument that will pass down the Y-arm of the cannula and permit direct-vision biopsy has been tried but has been unreliable thus far.

One-millimeter skin of scalp fragments are readily obtained and can be pro-

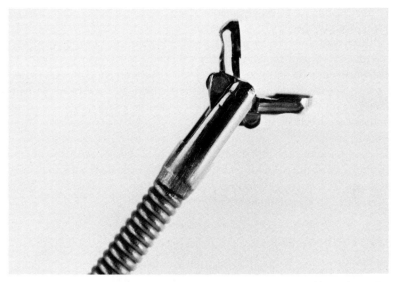

FIG. 6. Biopsy forceps that will pass through a cannula and obtain 1-mm skin specimens from the fetus. Magnification, 6×.

cessed for various studies. If histology is desired, the biopsy specimens are placed in appropriate fixatives for either light or electron microscopy. Alternatively the specimen can be placed in tissue culture for later karyotyping or biochemical assay, or can undergo direct chemical analysis after homogenization or other treatment. Healing after skin biopsy is usually complete because biopsy sites have not been identifiable at full-term birth.

Liver biopsy is accomplished using an aspiration needle-biopsy instrument that will pass alongside the fetoscope within the Y-cannula. The site for biopsy is chosen midway between the right nipple and the umbilicus. This technique was developed by Charles Rodeck in London. Very limited experience exists to assess its risks, but no significant bleeding has been noted thus far. The pieces of liver tissue can be readily processed for microenzyme assays or for histochemical staining.

V. Analysis of Fetal Blood

A. Routine Assays (Blood Counts, Karyotypes)

The small fetal samples aspirated from within the womb may be examined as whole blood or separated into plasma and cellular components. If the latter is desired the sample is placed in plastic microcentrifuge tubes and spun at an appropriate speed, usually 1500–2000 rpm.

T-cell karyotypes are easily obtained with the standard methods used to process peripheral blood lymphocytes in a cytogenetics laboratory. Volumes are reduced depending on the size of the fetal blood sample, but otherwise the sequence of phytohemagglutinin stimulation, colchicine arrest, and hypotonic swelling–fixation is identical. Either whole blood or a buffy coat can be used, and mitoses are available in 48 hours.

Common parameters of peripheral blood such as red-cell, white-cell, and platelet counts, white-cell differential counts, hematocrit, and hemoglobin determinations are measured with microadjustments to standard hemotologic laboratory methods. Similarly, Ficoll–Hypaque can be used to concentrate lymphocytes for standard immunologic tests.

B.   Hemoglobinopathies

The most frequent prenatal diagnosis of a biochemical disorder has been β-thalassemia. Nearly 2000 diagnoses have been reported using fetal blood samples. The methods used for diagnosis have been applicable to other thalassemias and to sickle cell disorders as well. Only general aspects of these methods will be cited here plus references to more detailed descriptions.

The most widely used method has been determination of globin-chain synthesis by fetal red blood cells. Cells, as few as 50 million, are incubated with [^{3}H] leucine, and the newly synthesized globin chains, radioactivity labeled, are separated by carboxymethyl cellulose column chromatography (Alter et al., 1976). A β/γ-globin chain ratio is crucial to diagnosis of the β-thalassemias, and the presence or absence of β^s-globin to the sickle cell disorders. Column separation of hemoglobins rather than globins is an alternative (Hollenberg et al., 1971).

Electrophoretic separations have also been developed. With isoelectric focusing and densitometry, Dubart et al. (1980) demonstrated satisfactory results with as little as 0.1 mg of unlabeled hemoglobin. Alter et al. (1981) separated radiolabeled globin chains in Triton–polyacrylamide slab gels and used fluorography for quantitation.

The various methods of hemoglobinopathy diagnosis are useful, even when maternal blood contaminates the fetal blood sample, if the fetal cells can be sufficiently concentrated. Two ways of accomplishing this have been successful. One utilizes an antibody to the fetal red cell antigen, i, and effects a concentration by one or more precipitations of the fetal cells. The other leads to selective hemolysis of adult cells (which have higher carbonic anhydrase activity) in NH_4Cl–NH_4 HCO_3 solution, the Ørskov reaction (Dubart et al., 1980). This latter method can concentrate fetal cells when their original proportion is only 2–3%.

C. Coagulopathies

Next to the hemoglobinopathies, the X-linked hemophilias have been the most frequently attempted prenatal diagnoses using fetal blood. Again, only general comments will be made about the specialized hematologic assays.

Bioassays of clotting activities of Factor VIII and Factor IX in blood from midtrimester fetuses indicate average activities for this stage of development of about 50 U/100 ml and 25 U/100 ml, respectively. Activity assays can be successfully used to diagnose severe deficiency of either factor, provided a pure blood sample can be obtained in which no clotting has occurred. Adequate samples can be taken from the umbilical cord vessels but usually not from placental vessels. Amniotic fluid causes some degree of clotting when it is mixed with blood.

In addition to bioassays of clotting activity, immunologic assays for the clotting-factor antigens can be used for prenatal diagnosis. A sensitive radioimmunoassay for VIII-related antigen and VIII-coagulant antigen permits diagnosis of most cases of severe Factor VIII deficiency despite contamination of the fetal blood sample with amniotic fluid (Firschein *et al.*, 1979). Most individuals with severe Factor VIII deficiency (classic hemophilia) have very little or no VIII-coagulant antigen and normal concentrations of VIII-related antigen. Amniotic fluid does not significantly change the relative antigen concentrations. A few families with classic hemophilia have circulating, but inactive, VIII-coagulant antigen; pure blood for a clotting assay is needed in these families. The majority of severe Factor IX-deficiency individuals have inactive Factor IX antigen, and fetal diagnoses in their families likewise require a pure blood sample.

References

Alter, B. P., Modell, C. B., Fairweather, D., Hobbins, J. C., Mahoney, M. J., Frigoletto, F. D., Sherman, A. S., and Nathan, D. G. (1976). *N. Engl. J. Med.* **295,** 1473.

Alter, B. P., Coupal, E., and Forget, B. G. (1981). *Hemoglobin* **5,** 357.

Benzie, R. J. (1977). *Birth Defects* (Orig. Articles Series) **13**(3D), 181.

Dubart, A., Goosens, M., Beuzard, Y., Monplaisir, N., Testa, U., Basset, P., and Rosa, J. (1980). *Blood* **56,** 1092.

Elias, S., Mazur, M., Sabbagha, R., Esterly, N. B., and Simpson, J. L. (1980). *Clin. Genet.* **17,** 275.

Firschein, S. I., Hoyer, L. W., Lazarchick, J., Forget, B. F., Hobbins, J. C., Clyne, L. P., Pitlick, F. A., Muir, W. A., Merkatz, I. R., and Mahoney, M. J. (1979). *N. Engl. J. Med.* **300,** 937.

Golbus, M. S., Sagebiel, R. W., Filly, R. A., Gindhart, T. D., and Hall, J. G. (1980). *N. Engl. J. Med.* **302,** 93.

Hollenberg, M. D., Kaback, M. M., and Kazazian, H. H., Jr. (1971). *Science* **174,** 698.

International Fetoscopy Group (1981). Data reported at the Second Annual Meeting, Athens, Greece.

Kan, Y. W., and Dozy, A. M. (1978). *Lancet* **2,** 910.

Kan, Y. W., Dozy, A. M., Alter, B. P., Frigoletto, F. D., and Nathan, D. G. (1972). *N. Engl. J. Med.* **287,** 1.

Mahoney, M. J., and Hobbins, J. C. (1977). *N. Engl. J. Med.* **297,** 258.

Mahoney, M. J., and Hobbins, J. C. (1979). *In* "Genetics Disorders and the Fetus" (A. Milunsky, ed.), pp. 501–526. Plenum, New York.

Mibashan, R. S., Thumpston, J. K., Singer, J. D., Rodeck, C. H., Edwards, R. J., White, J. M., and Campbell, S. (1979). *Lancet* **1,** 1309.

Newburger, P. E., Cohen, H. J., Rothchild, S. B., Hobbins, J. C., Malawista, S. E., and Mahoney, M. J. (1979). *N. Engl. J. Med.* **300,** 178.

Philip, J., Brandt, N. J., Fernandes, A., Freiesleben, E., and Trolle, D. (1978). *Clin. Genet.* **14,** 324.

Rodeck, C. H. (1980). *Br. J. Obstet. Gynaecol.* **87,** 449.

Rodeck, C. H., and Campbell, S. (1978). *Lancet* **1,** 1128.

Rodeck, C. H., Eady, R. A. J., and Gosden, C. M. (1980). *Lancet* **1,** 949.

Chapter 8

Miniaturization of Biochemical Analysis of Cultured (Amniotic Fluid) Cells

HANS GALJAARD

Department of Cell Biology and Genetics
Erasmus University Rotterdam
Rotterdam, The Netherlands

I. Introduction

Since the first prenatal diagnoses of genetic metabolic diseases in the late 1960s (Fujimoto *et al.*, 1968; Nadler, 1968, 1969; Fratantoni *et al.*, 1969; de Mars *et al.*, 1969; Nadler and Messina, 1969), the scope has become much wider and the methodology has improved. At present about 50 different inborn errors of metabolism have been diagnosed *in utero*, at least 20 others can also be detected by amniotic fluid (cell) analysis, and most recently fetal blood has successfully been used to diagnose metabolic defects that are not expressed in cultured cells

METHODS IN CELL BIOLOGY, VOL. 26

(for reviews see Galjaard, 1980; Kleijer *et al.*, 1980; Milunsky, 1980; Rodeck, 1980).

From published data on collective series it can be deduced that at least 2000 pregnancies at risk for a metabolic disease have been monitored (Epstein and Golbus, 1977; Galjaard, 1976, 1980; Milunsky, 1976, 1980) The number of requests for biochemical analysis of amniotic fluid cells is about 5% of the total number of prenatal diagnoses. The preventive value, however, is about 10 times higher than in the case of chromosomal aberrations and neural tube defects, where 2–3% of the fetuses are found to be affected, compared with 25% in the case of prenatal monitoring for genetic metabolic disease (see Table I).

The categories for which prenatal monitoring is most often requested are the lipidoses and mucopolysaccharidoses, and as far as individual diseases are concerned, the largest series of prenatal analyses have been performed for G_{M2}-gangliosidosis (Tay-Sachs type), mucopolysaccharidoses IH (Hurler's disease) and II (Hunter syndrome), glycogenosis II (Pompe's disease), and galactosyl-ceramide lipidosis (Krabbe's disease) (Galjaard, 1979, 1980).

There are several reasons for a centralization of the activities involved in the prenatal diagnosis of metabolic diseases.

1. The number of requests for each disease is small, even in countries with a relatively large population; centralization is therefore the only way to enable a few groups to acquire and to maintain sufficient expertise with the analysis of rare metabolic defects.

2. It becomes more and more clear that there may be considerable clinical, biochemical, and genetic heterogeneity within each of the metabolic diseases

TABLE I

PRENATAL DIAGNOSES OF GENETIC METABOLIC DISEASES

	Total no. monitored	% Affected
United States and Canada, reported by Epstein and Golbus (1977)	522	24
Western Europe and Israel, reported by Galjaard (1979)	632	23
Abnormalities in carbo- hydrate metabolism	60	
Mucopolysaccharidoses	120	
Mucolipidoses	23	
Lipidoses	327	
Aminoacidopathies	60	
Other genetic diseases	42	

(see McKusick, 1978; Stanbury, *et al.*, 1978; Galjaard, 1980). A correct interpretation of the analytical data therefore requires the availability of proper comparative cell material and sufficient knowledge about the metabolic pathways investigated. Because there are very few groups with expertise both in the study of specific metabolic pathways and in the cultivation and molecular analysis of cultivated human cells, skin fibroblasts and amniotic fluid samples can best be referred to these few expert centers.

When conventional biochemical methods are used for the analysis of an enzyme deficiency or the intracellular storage of certain metabolites, relatively large amounts of cell material are required. The biochemist will consider 1–10 mg of cellular protein as a minute quantity, but for the cell biologist it implies the necessity to cultivate 3×10^6–3×10^7 cells. In the case of amniotic fluid, which contains only a few viable fetal cells (see chapter by Hoehn and Salk) such large numbers of cells can only be obtained after prolonged cultivation of fibroblast-like cells. Depending on the assay method and the enzyme activity to be measured, time intervals between amniocentesis and biochemical diagnosis of 3 to 6 weeks have been reported; in some instances of metabolite analysis even longer periods were needed (for reviews see Nadler, 1972; Milunsky, 1973, 1975, 1980; Galjaard, 1976, 1979, 1980). Such long waiting periods are of course a psychological burden for the parents at risk.

In a few instances genetic metabolic defects, such as the hypoxanthine-guanine-phosphoribosyl transferase (HGPRT) deficiency in Lesch–Nyhan syndrome (Fujimoto *et al.*, 1968; Boyle *et al.*, 1970; Halley and Heukels-Dully, 1977) and the DNA-repair defect in xeroderma pigmentosum (Ramsey *et al.*, 1974; Halley *et al.*, 1979), have successfully been demonstrated by autoradiography after incubation of living cultured cells with radioactive precursors. This approach in principle enables metabolic defects to be detected at the level of individual cells, and hence rapid prenatal diagnoses can be made. A disadvantage is the qualitative nature of this technique. This may particularly cause problems in cases where a partial metabolic defect in an affected fetus has to be distinguished from decreased values in a normal heterozygote.

In histochemistry a variety of preparative and analytical techniques have been developed for the quantitative analysis of enzymes and metabolites in microscopic structures and single cells that are isolated from tissue sections (for reviews, see Glick, 1963, 1971, 1977a,b; Dubach and Schmidt, 1971; Lowry and Passonneau, 1972; Neuhoff, 1973; Ciba Foundation 1980). Some of these techniques and principles of microscopic spectrofluorometry have been successfully adapted for the microchemical analysis of small numbers of cultured cells (Galjaard *et al.*, 1972, 1973, 1974a,b, 1977; Jongkind *et al.*, 1974). The application of these microtechniques has allowed prenatal diagnoses of different lysosomal storage diseases to be made within 7–20 days after amniocentesis (Galjaard *et al.*, 1973, 1974c; Niermeijer *et al.*, 1975, 1976; Kleijer *et al.*, 1976a,b, 1979a,b). Also, several radiometric assays have been miniaturized (Jacoby *et al.*, 1972; Wendel *et al.*, 1973a,b; Willcox and Patrick, 1974; Willers *et al.*, 1975; de Bruyne *et al.*, 1976; Hösli, 1977). The use of these methods made it possible to establish prenatal diagnoses for several inborn errors of amino acid metabolism and nucleic acid metabolism within a period of 2 weeks (Wendel *et al.*, 1973a; Willcox and Patrick, 1974; Niermeijer *et al.*, 1975; Aitken *et al.*, 1980).

At present, microtechniques are available for the rapid prenatal diagnosis of at least 20 different genetic metabolic diseases (for reviews, see Galjaard *et al.*, 1977; Patrick, 1978; Kleijer *et al.*, 1979a; Galjaard, 1980). In the future further methodological improvements are to be expected. More sensitive radiometric methods are being developed for the assay of enzymes with natural substrates (Håkansson, 1979; Svennerholm, 1979; Svennerholm *et al.*, 1979). The synthesis of chromogenic and fluorogenic derivatives of natural substrates (Gal *et al.*, 1975, 1977; Gatt *et al.*, 1978, 1980) will lead to higher sensitivity and greater simplicity of certain enzyme assays. Finally there are several other micromethods that in principle can also be adapted for the analysis of cultured (amniotic fluid) cells (Lowry and Passonneau, 1972; Neuhoff, 1973; Glick, 1977a,b; Kronberg *et al.*, 1980; Poehling and Neuhoff, 1980; Ciba Foundation, 1980).

In this chapter the present possibilities of miniaturization of biochemical analysis of small numbers of cultured cells will be discussed and examples of application in prenatal diagnosis presented. In addition a few examples will be given where qualitative enzyme assays of single cultured human cells have contributed to the characterization of different amniotic fluid cell types, the study of genetic heterogeneity using somatic cell hybridization, and the investigation of exchange of enzymes between normal and mutant human fibroblasts.

II.   Isolation and Handling of Small Numbers or Single Cultured Cells

A.   Cell Homogenates

In most instances biochemical analyses are performed on cell homogenates. This limits the possibility of miniaturization of the assay, because harvesting of cultured cells by trypsinization or by scraping and subsequent homogenization by sonication or repeated freezing and thawing requires between 10,000 and 100,000 cells. Crystalline preparations of trypsin (2.5 mg/ml salt solution) must be used, and after subsequent repeated rinsing with culture medium and isotonic saline, the cultured cells can be suspended in a volume of 100 μl of saline or of the appropriate buffer. To prevent enzyme denaturation the protein concentration must be higher than 0.2 mg/ml. Bovine serum albumin must be added in case the concentration of cellular protein is too low. Interferometric determinations have shown that the dry weight of individual human fibroblasts and amniotic fluid cells varies from 1×10^{-10} to 10×10^{-10} g, with an average value of 3×10^{-10} g (Galjaard *et al.*, 1974a). This implies that a minimum of 60,000 cells have to be suspended in 100 μl. If biochemical analyses are not performed directly, cultured cells must not be suspended but should instead be stored as a pellet at $-70°C$. In the analysis of certain cell constituents—such as glycosaminoglycans, cystine, or neuraminidase activity—special precautions must be taken during preparation of the cell sample (Neufeld and Cantz, 1973; Schneider, 1974; Fortuin and Kleijer, 1978; Wenger *et al.*, 1978; Hoogeveen *et al.*, 1980).

When cell homogenates are used the results of the biochemical analysis are usually expressed per unit weight of cellular protein. When little cell material is available it is of course advantageous to use one of the more sensitive protein-assay methods (Udenfriend *et al.*, 1972; Böhlen *et al.*, 1974; Bradford, 1976; Butcher and Lowry, 1976; Kinoshita *et al.*, 1977; Neuhoff *et al.*, 1979). Each of these has certain advantages and limitations, but they all have a sensitivity in the order of 10^{-8} g, which corresponds to a few hundred cultured fibroblasts. We found the fluorescamine method without hydrolysis the most suitable method for the study of cultured cell homogenates (Jongkind and Verkerk, personal communication).

B.   Isolation of Small Numbers or Single Cultured Cells

The activity of several enzymes in cultured fibroblasts or amniotic fluid cells is high enough to allow for microchemical analysis on a few hundred, a few dozen, or even single cells (see Table II and for review, see Galjaard, 1980). For the isolation of such small numbers of cells we have used a method originally described for the dissection of microscopic structures from tissue sections (Lowry, 1953). As is illustrated in Fig. 1, cells are grown on 5-cm dishes with a bottom of thin plastic film, which we used to make ourselves but which are now commercially available in sterilized packages (Heraeus, Hanau, Federal Republic of Germany). In the case of amniotic fluid cell cultures, clones of a few hundred cells are usually present at 7–9 days after amniocentesis in the sixteenth week of pregnancy. After removal of the medium with diluted saline, the whole dish is quickly frozen in liquid nitrogen or Freon, and subsequently the cells are freeze-dried overnight *in vacuo* at $-20°C$ to $-45°C$. For research studies on single cells of a specific type in a mixed culture it may be important to preserve optimal morphology. In that case the medium should be rinsed with 0.15 *M* ammonium acetate (pH 6.8) to prevent deposition of salt crystals during subsequent freezing. Also the temperature of freeze-drying is more critical and

TABLE II

GENETIC METABOLIC DISEASES THAT CAN BE DIAGNOSED *in Utero* WITH ULTRAMICROCHEMICAL ASSAYS OF CULTURED AMNIOTIC FLUID CELLS[a]

Disease	Enzyme/metabolite tested	Activity in normal amniotic fluid cells ($\times 10^{-14}$ moles/hour/cell)	Minimum cell nos. that can be assayed
	Fluorometric		
Glycogenosis II	α-1,4-glucosidase	0.2–2.7	1–100
Mucopolysaccharidosis I H/S	α,L-iduronidase	0.2–3	1–100
Mucopolysaccharidosis VII	β-glucuronidase	1–3	1–100
Mucolipidosis I	*N*-acetylneuraminidase	0.5–1.1	10–100
Mucolipidoses II/III	Multiple lysosomal enzyme deficiency	See other enzymes	10–100
Mannosidosis	α-mannosidase	1–5	1–100
Fucosidosis	α-fucosidase	2–10	1–10
Gaucher disease	β-glucosidase	3–13	1–10
Mucosulfatidosis	arylsulfatases, A, B+C	0.2–0.8	100–1000
Fabry's disease	α-galactosidase	0.2–2	1–100
G_{M1}-Gangliosidosis	β-galactosidase	5–50	1–10
G_{M2}-Gangliosidosis 1	β-*N*-acetylhexosaminidase A+B	70–400	1–10
G_{M2}-Gangliosidosis 2	β-*N*-acetylhexosaminidase A	40–240	300–1000
	Spectrophotometric		
Mucopolysaccharidosis I H/S	α-L-iduronidase	0.5–1.3	10^4
Mucopolysaccharidosis III B	α-*N*-acetylglucosaminidase	0.07–0.17	10^4
Mucopolysaccharidosis VI	arylsulfatase B	6–18	10^3–10^4
Metachromatic leukodystrophy	arylsulfatase A	3–16	10^3–10^4
Wolman's disease	acid lipase	60–200	10^3
	Radiometric		
Maple-syrup urine disease	[^{14}C]ketoacid or [^{14}C]leucine	—	10^4
Cystinosis	L-[^{35}S]cystine	—	10^4
Lesch–Nyhan syndrome	[^{3}H] or [^{14}C]hypoxanthine	—	1–100
Combined immunodeficiency	[^{14}C]adenine	—	10–10^3
Xeroderma pigmentosum	UV radiation, [^{3}H]thymidine	—	1–100

[a] Data derived from Galjaard, H. (1980). "Genetic Metabolic Diseases." Elsevier-North Holland Biomedical Press, Amsterdam, New York, with kind permission.

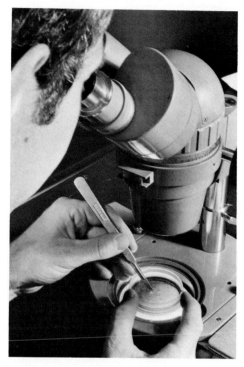

FIG. 1.   Freehand microdissection of small groups or single cells from a freeze-dried culture dish.

should be kept around −43°C (for review, see Pearse, 1968, 1973). For enzyme assays in (prenatal) diagnosis, the exact conditions of quenching and lyophilization are not so important.

After freeze-drying the culture dish can be brought to room temperature, and by freehand dissection, pieces of the plastic bottom containing a counted number of lyophilized cells can be cut under a stereomicroscope (Figs. 1 and 2). Isolation of 10 pieces, each with a few dozen or a few hundred cells, does not take more than 30–60 minutes. The isolation of single cells for research purposes requires more time, especially when specific cell types have to be selected (Fig. 2). An experienced worker isolates a hundred individual cells in 3–5 hours; to prevent rehydration during the isolation procedure the humidity must be kept around 40%.

The pieces of plastic foil containing a known number of lyophilized cells can be transferred into the appropriate substrate for biochemical analysis without prior homogenization. Model studies have shown that soluble enzymes as well as membrane-bound proteins are liberated into the substrate as soon as freeze-dried cells are immersed in aqueous solutions (see Bonting and Rosenthal, 1960; Galjaard *et al.*, 1974a). When the isolated cells are not used for immediate

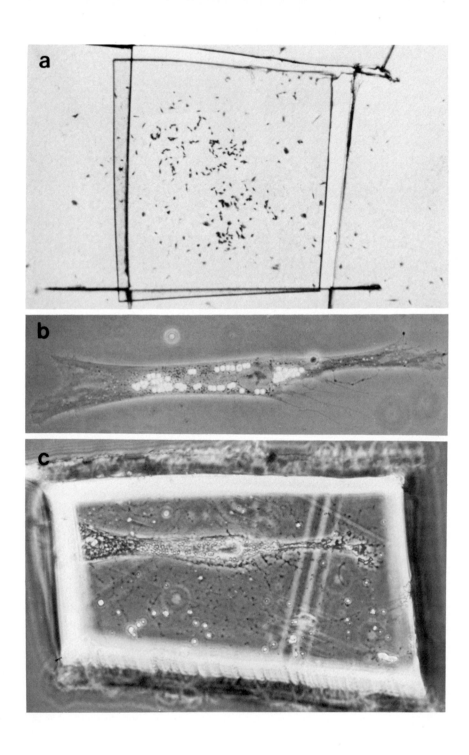

microchemical analysis, the pieces of plastic foil containing the freeze-dried cells can be stored *in vacuo* at −70°C for a long period without biochemical or morphological alterations.

C. Incubation of Small Numbers or Single Cultured Cells

A prerequisite for sensitive microchemical analysis is the incubation of the available cell material in the smallest possible volume. In the case of homogenates prepared from trypsinized cell cultures, the highest possible concentration is in the order of 10^4 cells in 100 μl. After homogenization by sonication or repeated freezing and thawing, aliquots of this volume can be used for the necessary biochemical assays and the protein determination. Commercially available disposable plastic capped microtubes and micropipets (ranging from 1 to 50 μl) can be used, and in case of small incubation volumes (around 1–10 μl) the incubation mixture should be covered with paraffin oil:hexadecane (60:40 v/v) to prevent evaporation.

When small numbers or single cultured cells are being analyzed, incubation must be carried out in smaller volumes. Originally, we have used the "oil-well" technique described by Lowry's group (Matschinsky *et al.*, 1968; Lowry and Passonneau, 1972; Galjaard *et al.*, 1974a). Teflon racks with holes drilled nearly to the bottom part are filled with a paraffin oil:hexadecane mixture, and dissected pieces of plastic foil containing a counted number of freeze-dried cells are transferred to each of the wells. Microscopic observation is possible by transmitted light through the thin bottom of the Teflon rack under the wells (Fig. 3). Often it is easier to transfer the pieces of plastic with the lyophilized cell(s) first and then add the oil. With special quartz constriction micropipets, submicroliter volumes of the appropriate substrate are added to the various wells. Direct microscopic visualization shows when the cell(s) are dissolved in the microdroplet of substrate (Fig. 3). The minimum incubation volume for groups of 20–50 cells is 0.3–0.5 μl, and for enzyme assays of single cultured cells we use 0.08–0.10 μl. These volumes can reliably be pipetted (error less than 1%) when self-made constriction pipets are used; these are calibrated colorimetrically with 5% *p*-nitrophenol in 0.4 *M* KOH, and volumes as small as 0.001 μl can be handled. The Teflon racks can be placed in an incubator to achieve the right temperature for incubation. Incubation volumes above 1 μl require a minimum

FIG. 2. Isolated cultured human cells. (a) Clone of a few dozen cultured amniotic fluid cells, isolated for prenatal diagnosis of a genetic metabolic disease; (b) living cybrid under phase-contrast microscopy (fusion of enucleated cell from one type of patient—cytoplasm labeled with latex particles—with whole cells from another patient—still containing the nucleus; (c) the same cybrid after isolation from a freeze-dried culture (prepared by Dr. A. d'Azzo and A. Hoogeveen, Dept. of Cell Biology and Genetics, Erasmus University, Rotterdam).

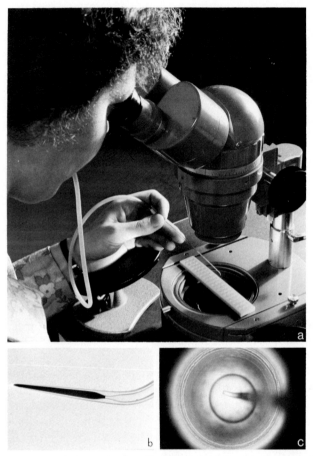

Fig. 3.   Ultramicrochemical analysis of small numbers or single cells using Lowry's "oil-well" technique. (a) Introduction of submicroliter volumes of substrate to isolated cells in each well of a Teflon rack; (b) photograph of a self-made constriction micropipet filled with colored reagent; (c) view through the microscope when a microdroplet of substrate is introduced on top of isolated cells covered with paraffin oil to prevent evaporation.

protein concentration of 0.2 mg/ml and below 1 μl bovine albumin must be added to a concentration of 1 mg/ml. Afterward the reaction mixture can be sucked into a microcapillary (Drummond 1-mm microcaps), and both microspectrophotometric and microfluorometric measurements can be made (see Section III).

In the case of microfluorometric analyses an alternative, more direct, and easier procedure can be followed (Jongkind *et al.*, 1974). Pieces of plastic containing one or more freeze-dried cells are placed on a holder with thin transparent nonfluorescent foil (50-μm foil from Habia, Sweden, or a variety of holders made by Tecnomara, Zürich, Switzerland, can be used). Each individual cell or group of cells is covered with a microdroplet of substrate, which is then covered with oil to prevent evaporation (Fig. 7). After incubation the fluorescence can be measured directly; neither the presence of paraffin oil nor the size of the droplet interferes with the measurements if an inverted microscope fluorometer is used (see Section III).

When microspectrophotometric assays have to be performed in (sub)microliter volumes, the "parafilm method" described by Hösli (1977) is an attractive alternative for the "oil-well" procedure. Here the freeze-dried cells are placed in small holes drilled with a special device into a parafilm sheet. After transfer of the microdroplet of substrate, the holes are closed airtight with another sheet of parafilm, thus avoiding evaporation. After incubation the reaction mixture is pipetted into microcuvets, and extinction measurements can be carried out without any interference of oil.

Bladon and Milunsky (1978, 1980) have used another approach to the microchemical analysis of cultured (amniotic fluid) cells, which is based on previous work by Rotman (1961) and Wudl and Paigen (1974). A cell suspension is dispersed in uniformly spaced and sized droplets of 0.001 to 1 μl, which are deposited under oil in the chambers of glass microslides (Lab Tek No. 4802). After freezing and thawing to disrupt the trypsinized cells, contact with a fluorogenic substrate is established by diffusion. This procedure is quite complicated, but its main limitation is that the cultured (amniotic fluid) cells are harvested in the conventional way by trypsinization, which implies that a minimum number of 10^4–10^5 cultured cells must be available.

A number of investigators have used different types of microtiter plates to grow and analyze cell numbers in the order of 2000 to 10,000. Richardson and Cox (1973) grew 200-μl samples of amniotic fluid in wells of a microtest II tissue-culture plate (Falcon plastics) and studied the incorporation of ^{3}H- and ^{14}C-labeled hypoxanthine in colonies of several thousands of cells. They also harvested relatively small numbers of cells from the wells by freezing and thawing in a 5-μl volume of 2.5 M merthiolate, 7.4 mM β-mercaptoethanol, 0.025% Triton X-100, and 2.7 mM NADP, and analyzed the hexosaminidase isoenzyme pattern. No practical applications of this method are, however, known to the author. A similar approach has been followed by Wendel et al. (1973a), who cultivated cells in wells of a microtiter plate, and after incubation with ^{14}C-labeled ketoacids, measured the radioactivity of liberated ^{14}CO$_2$ trapped in a glass-fiber platelet soaked with 3.5 N NaOH. This method, with minor modifications, has successfully been used in the prenatal diagnosis of maple-syrup urine disease (Wendel et al., 1973b; Niermeijer et al., 1975). Cultivation of amniotic fluid cells in wells of microtiter plates and incorporation with $^{64}CuCl_2$ has proved to be a useful method for the (prenatal) diagnosis of Menkes disease (Horn, 1976).

III. Microspectrophotometry and Microfluorometry

A. Microspectrophotometry

According to Lambert–Beer's law for colorimetric measurements, the extinction is proportional to the concentration, the optical path, and the extinction coefficient of the substance to be measured. The simplest way to improve the sensitivity of a colorimetric assay, therefore, is to incubate the available cell material in a small volume and to measure the extinction in the smallest possible volume using cuvets with the longest possible optical path.

Several commercially available spectrophotometers have adaptations for microcuvets with a volume of 20–100 μl and a 10-mm optical path. In most instances the smaller cuvets are difficult to fill and to clean, and also the optics of normal colorimeters are not suitable for a precise adjustment of the smallest microcuvets (see Glick, 1963, 1971; Galjaard et al., 1974a; de Josselin de Jong et al., 1980). The optics and precision of adjustment of microscope spectrophotometers are much more suitable for extinction measurements in microliter volumes.

We have successfully used microcapillaries of 1 mm diameter for extinction measurements in a 1-μl volume using a microscope spectrophotometer and low magnification (Galjaard et al., 1974a, 1977). As is shown in Fig. 4, a holder with several capillaries can be used; these are filled in a simple way by introducing them in the microdroplet of reaction mixture in an "oil-well" (see Fig. 3). The colored final product of the biochemical reaction will be enclosed by oil, preventing evaporation during the measurements.

The possibility of colorimetric assays in a final volume of 1 μl implies that 3000 times less cell material is needed to obtain the same extinction volume, as compared with the conventional 3-ml cuvets in a normal spectrophotometer. The loss of sensitivity because of the short optical path in case of a 1-mm capillary cuvet was found to be compensated by the possibility of reliable measurements of very low extinction values in case of a microscope spectrophotometer.

Recently an instrument has been designed that combines the advantages of the good optics and accurate adjustment system of a microscope-spectrophotometer with the rapid and easy handling of a conventional colorimeter (de Josselin de Jong et al., 1980). With this instrument, absorption measurements can be carried out in cuvets with a 10-mm optical path and volumes varying from 3 ml down to 10 μl (Figs. 5 and 6). Model experiments showed that absolute amounts of 10^{-10}

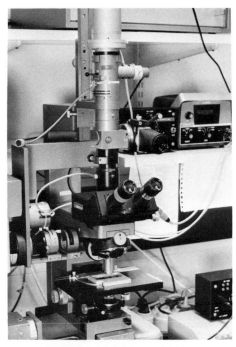

FIG. 4. Microspectrophotometer with holder containing microcapillaries used for extinction measurements of 1-μl volumes, according to Galjaard *et al.* (1974a), with permission.

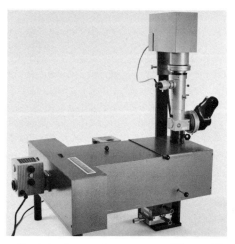

FIG. 5. New design of a (micro)spectrophotometer permitting rapid and reliable extinction measurements in volumes varying from 3 ml down to 10 μl, according to de Josselin de Jong *et al.* (1980), with permission.

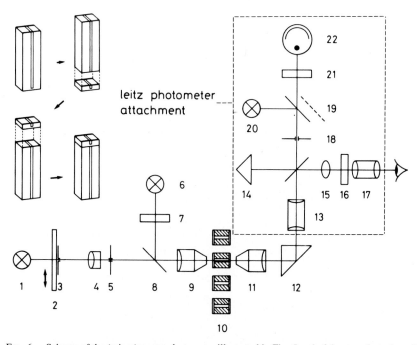

FIG. 6.   Scheme of the (micro)spectrophotometer illustrated in Fig. 5 and of the manufacturing of 10-μl cuvets from conventional cuvets. 1, Measuring lamp; 2, graded interference filter; 3, slit; 4, achromat; 5, measuring spot; 6, adjustment lamp; 7, shutter; 8, glass coverslip; 9, condenser; 10, stage with curets; 11, objective; 12, prism; 13, projective; 14, triple mirror; 15, adaption lens; 16, shutter; 17, observation tube; 18, measuring diaphragm; 19, movable mirror; 20, tungsten lamp; 21, shutter; 22, photomultiplier.

to 10^{-11} moles of p-nitrocatechol could be measured with an error of 5%. This is more than a hundred times less than in normal colorimetry, hence less than 1% of the amount of cell material is needed for a (prenatal) diagnosis. From the minimum amount of final product that can be measured and the mean activity of various enzymes in cultured amniotic fluid cells (see Table II), it can be deduced how many cells are required for (micro)colorimetric analyses. At present, spectrophotometric assays are most often used for the prenatal diagnosis of certain mucopolysaccharidoses, metachromatic leukodystrophy, and Wolman's disease (Table II). The synthesis of natural substrates with a chromogenic terminal group (Gal *et al.*, 1975; Goldberg *et al.*, 1978) may further widen the scope.

B.   Microfluorometry

The synthesis of a variety of methylumbelliferyl derivatives for the assay of lysosomal hydrolases has further increased the interest for fluorometry in the diagnosis of genetic metabolic disease (Leaback, 1976; Koch-Light Lab., list of substrates). The minimum amount of 4-methylumbelliferone that can be measured in a 500-μl volume using a conventional fluorometer is in the order of 10^{-11}–10^{-12} moles. By comparing this value with the activity per cell of enzymes that can be assayed with methylumbelliferyl substrates, it can be calculated how many cells are needed. In this calculation it must be taken into account that a diagnostic assay should be based on triplicate assays, that the protein content must be determined in case of cell homogenates, and that low values in heterozygotes or high residual activities in affected patients should give measurable values. This implies that about 10 times more cells are needed than the

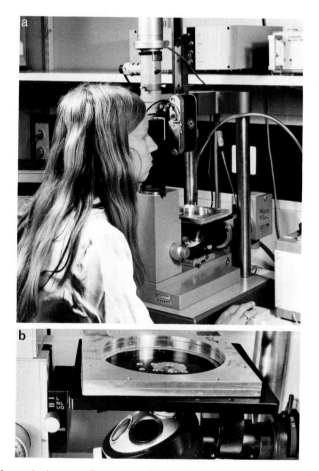

FIG. 7. Inverted microscope fluorometer with epi-illumination (a) enabling direct fluorescence measurements in submicroliter volumes of reagent covered by paraffin oil (b), according to Jongkind *et al.* (1974).

minimum for a single assay on the basis of enzyme activities in normal (amniotic fluid) cells (Table II).

The sensitivity of a fluorometric assay can be increased by lowering the blank value, by increasing the concentration of the fluorescent product, and by increasing the intensity of the exciting light. As far as the latter is concerned, it is important to excite as many molecules as possible, and to avoid quenching and decomposition of the fluorescent end product.

A low blank value requires first of all the highest possible quality of the substrate, water, and other chemicals used. Furthermore, it is advantageous to use a small amount of substrate during incubation, and by subsequent dilution the concentration of interfering substances can be reduced. In model experiments with methylumbelliferyl derivatives the sensitivity of lysosomal enzyme assays could be increased 10-fold by reduction of the incubation volume to 3 μl and subsequent fluorescence measurements in a 500-μl final volume (Galjaard et al., 1974a). If the dilution factor becomes too large, the number of molecules that are excited in a conventional fluorometer becomes too low. This problem can be solved by increasing the concentration of the fluorescent end product and by intensifying the exciting light beam.

Fluorescence measurements in (sub)microliter volumes can easily be performed with a microscope fluorometer. The optics and precise adjustment system permit reliable measurements in volumes as small as 0.001 μl (Rotman, 1961; Wudl and Paigen, 1974; Jongkind et al., 1974). In model experiments we have found that a minimum amount of 10^{-14} moles methylumbelliferone could be measured both in 1-μl droplets in microcapillaries using transmitted light (Fig. 4) and in 0.02- to 0.1-μl droplets under oil using an inverted microfluorometer with epi-illumination (Fig. 7).

The possibility of measuring such small amounts of fluorescent end product made it possible to perform quantitative assays in individual cultured cells (see Table II and Section V on practical applications).

IV.   Radiometric (Micro)Analysis and Other Methods

Although radiometric methods are generally considered to be very sensitive, scintillation counting of carrier-free ^{14}C in 2 hours with an error of about 3% still requires more than 10^{-14} moles, which is in the same order as the sensitivity of microfluorometry. The wide scope of radiometric methods makes them, however, very useful in the early diagnosis and prenatal analysis of genetic metabolic diseases. The metabolic defects of more than half of the diseases that can be diagnosed in utero are analyzed with radiometric methods (Galjaard, 1980). The sensitivity of the instruments for the actual measurement of radioactivity can hardly be improved, but the conditions of incubation, chromatography, electrophoresis, and recovery of radioactive end products can be adapted to smaller amounts of cell material. A high specific radioactivity of the chemicals used and a low blank value are of course of great importance.

A good example of the contribution of improved methodology is the prenatal monitoring for cystinosis. The first case was reported by Schulman et al., (1970), where 7-8 weeks were needed to obtain sufficient cultured cells for the analysis of [^{35}S]cystine incorporation. Schneider et al. (1974), using ion-exchange chromatography after [^{35}S]cystine incorporation, reported a prenatal diagnosis after 5 weeks of cultivation, and they also showed a radioautogram after thin-layer chromatography according to a method by States and Segal (1969). Willcox and Patrick (1974) reported a simple method based on the latter procedure and were able to demonstrate cystine accumulation after 2-3 weeks of amniotic fluid cell cultivation. They incubate early cultures with L-[^{35}S]cystine, harvest the cells, remove the protein, and apply aliquots of the supernatant to 1-cm streaks of cellulose plate; after drying, the strips are exposed for 1-3 days to Kodirex X-ray film, and densitometric scanning clearly shows cystine accumulation (Fig. 8). States et al. (1975) have also described a sensitive method based on paper electrophoresis followed by scintillation counting of cut sections. Another example where miniaturization of the incubation volume with radioactive-labeled substrate and of the chromatographic separation has led to a faster prenatal diagnosis is the method for adenosine deaminase (ADA) described by Aitken et al. (1980). When incubation is carried out in a few microliters with 8-[^{14}C]adenosine of high specific radioactivity, the ADA activity can be measured on groups of 10-50 cells; this implies that a prenatal diagnosis of combined immune deficiency can now be made within 7-9 days after amniocentesis. Similar methods are available for the analysis of HGPRT activity (deficient in Lesch-Nyhan syndrome) (Willers et al., 1975; de Bruyne et al., 1976; Hösli, 1977) and other inborn errors of nucleic acid metabolism.

The procedure of cultivation of cells in wells of microtiter plates, incubation with radioactive-labeled precursors, and recovery of liberated $^{14}CO_2$ as described by Wendel et al. (1973a,b), not only permit rapid prenatal diagnosis of maple-syrup urine disease, but can also be used for the sensitive analysis of other aminoacidopathies (see Galjaard, 1980).

A number of genetic diseases are associated with a deficiency of one isoenzyme only, such as in Tay-Sachs disease (hexosaminidase A) or metachromatic leukodystrophy (arylsulfatase A) or mucopolysaccharidosis IV (arylsulfatase B). Electrophoretic separation often gives a correct diagnosis, but in cases of a high residual isoenzyme activity this qualitative approach has its limitations. Column chromatography followed by quantitative analysis is a reliable alternative, and examples of miniaturization have been reported (Ellis et al., 1975). For hexosaminidase isoenzyme analyses a simple batchwise fractionation with DEAE-cellulose (d'Azzo et al., 1978) permitted prenatal diagnoses of Tay-Sachs disease within 7-10 days after amniocentesis. Christamanou and Sandhoff

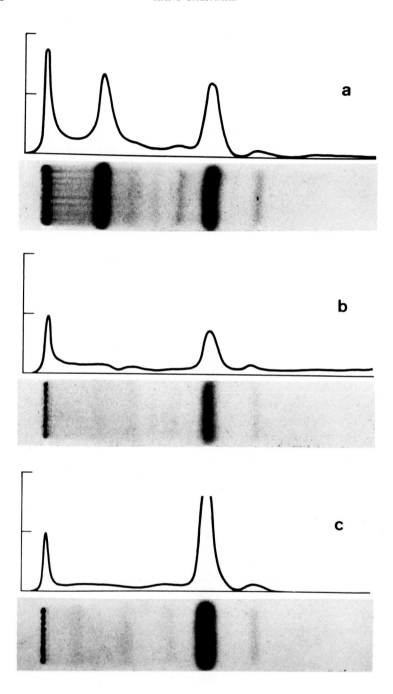

(1977) reported on a very sensitive assay for arylsulfatase isoenzymes using methylumbelliferyl substrate and inhibition of arylsulfatase A by $AgNO_3$. A slight modification of this method combined with microscope fluorometry made it possible to establish a prenatal diagnosis of metachromatic leukodystrophy within 10 days after amniocentesis (van der Veer *et al.*, to be published).

In the field of quantitative histochemistry and cytochemistry there are several other micromethods that could be adapted for the study of small numbers or single cultured cells. Polyacrylamide gel electrophoresis can be carried with minute quantities of cell material using microcapillaries and special equipment (for reviews, see Neuhoff, 1973). Also chromatography for amino acids has been miniaturized (Neuhoff *et al.*, 1974; Quentin *et al.*, 1974), as well as two-dimensional electrophoresis (Poehling and Neuhoff, 1980). In certain instances the principles of NAD (P) (H) cycling described by Lowry's group (Lowry, 1963; Matschinksy, 1971; Lowry and Passonneau, 1972) or that of biolumines-cence (Seitz and Neary, 1976; Glick, 1977a,b) might be used for the early detection of genetic defects. In the future it is likely that more attention will be paid to the quantitative analysis of cultured cells *in situ*, in order to avoid the need of harvesting, homogenization, or isolation of small numbers of cells. In those instances where the (prenatal) diagnosis of genetic metabolic defects re-quires the use of natural substrates, it will be of great help if more substrates become available with a high purity and a high specific radioactivity (Håkansson, 1979; Svennerholm *et al.*, 1979; Vanier *et al.*, 1979).

V.   Examples of Application

A.   Prenatal Diagnosis

The first applications of microfluorometric assays on isolated groups of a few hundred freeze-dried amniotic fluid cells were in the monitoring of pregnancies at risk for glycogenosis II (Galjaard *et al.*, 1972, 1973; Niermeijer *et al.*, 1975) and Fabry's disease (Galjaard *et al.*, 1974c). The activity of lysosomal α-1,4-glucosidase and α-galactosidase, respectively, could be measured within 9–14 days after amniocentesis using microliter volumes of methylumbelliferyl substrate. Since then similar procedures have been developed for other lysosomal

---

FIG. 8.   Microradiometric assay of cystine accumulation in small numbers of cultured human cells. (a) Densitometry after autoradiography, thin-layer chromatography and [^{35}S]cystine incorpora-tion by cultured cells from a patient with cystinosis (middle peak clearly shows incorporation into cystine); (b) cells from a heterozygous individual; (c) cells from a normal control showing radioactiv-ity at the origin (left peak) and at the area of glutathione-*N*-ethylmaleinide (right peak). Photographs were kindly provided by Dr. A. D. Patrick, Institute of Child Health, University of London; derived from work by Willcox and Patrick (1974), with permission.

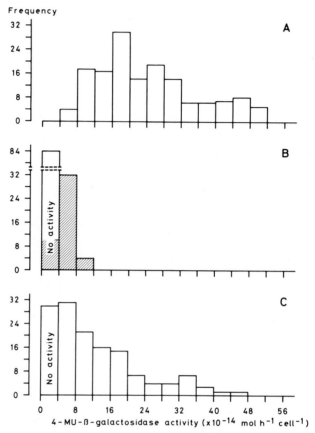

Fᴉɢ. 9.   The use of ultramicrochemical analysis of single (hybrid) cells in genetic complementation studies. (A) Distribution of β-galactosidase activity in single normal human fibroblasts. (B)
β-Galactosidase activity in two cell strains from patients with different types of enzyme deficiency.
(C) Restoration of β-galactosidase activity in binucleated heterokaryons after hybridization of the two
enzyme-deficient cell strains. (D) Binuclear cell in phase contrast after fusion of two human cell
strains. (E) The same cell after isolation by micro-dissection from a freeze-dried culture dish. From
work by Galjaard *et al.* (1974a, 1975), with permission.

enzymes (Table II), which have been successfully used in rapid prenatal diagnosis (Kleijer *et al.*, 1976a,b, 1979a,b; for review, see Galjaard, 1980).

When microchemical assays are performed on isolated groups of dozens or a
few hundred cells there is quite some variation in the activity per cell, even
between cell groups within the same culture dish. This variation also exists when
activities of individual cells are compared (Fig. 9), irrespective of the subcellular
localization of these enzymes (Galjaard *et al.*, 1974d, 1975; Reuser *et al.*,
1976a,b). The differences among single cells are probably due to differences in
their total dry weight and to the fact that they may be in different stages of the cell

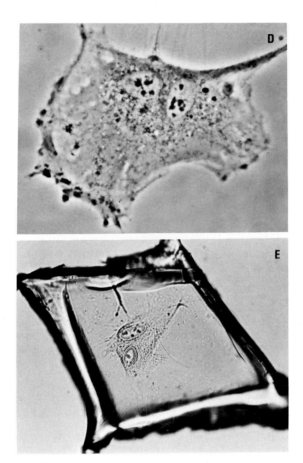

Fig. 9. (*continued*)

cycle. Variation among different cell groups in amniotic fluid cell cultures may also be caused by the presence of various cell types (see article by Hoehn and Salk). We have studied several lysosomal hydrolases in different types of amniotic fluid cells and compared their activity per cell (Table III). Various types of epitheloid cells and fibroblast-like cells did not differ, but the activity of large multinucleated cells was found to be 5 to 10 times higher. By combined interferometric determination of the dry weight of single cells and microchemical analysis, van der Veer *et al.* (1978) were able to express the lysosomal enzyme activity of individual cells per unit dry weight. Their results showed that no differences exist among the various cell types (Table III).

Kleijer *et al.* (1976a) performed β-galactosidase assays in isolated groups of 10–30 freeze-dried cells of different types of amniotic fluid cells in three pregnancies at risk for G_{M1}-gangliosidosis. results were obtained at 9–12 days after

TABLE III

LYSOSOMAL ENZYME ACTIVITIES IN DIFFERENT TYPES OF AMNIOTIC FLUID CELLS[a,b]

	α-1,4-Glucosidase (activity per cell)	β-Galactosidase (activity per cell)	N-Acetyl-β-hexosaminidase		
			Activity per cell	Cellular dry weight[c]	Activity per unit dry weight
Epithelioid I	0.15	11.2	—	—	—
Epithelioid II	0.19	11.0	99	38	2.6
Fibroblast-like	0.25	7.9	94	37	2.4
Large multinuclear	2.67	58.2	197	91	2.2

[a] Data derived from van der Veer et al. (1978) with kind permission.

[b] Microbiochemical enzyme assays were performed on different cell types within the same culture and activities are expressed $\times 10^{-14}$ moles/hour/cell; values are the mean of assays on 6–50 groups containing 1–200 cells.

[c] The dry weight of individual cells was determined by interference microscopy and the data are expressed $\times 10^{-11}$ grams; values are the mean of measurements of 7–22 individual cells.

amniocentesis, and a good correlation was observed between the data from microchemical assays on few freeze-dried cells and those obtained by conventional biochemical analysis of cell homogenates. The same authors also successfully employed microfluorometric assays in the rapid prenatal diagnosis of disorders with multiple lysosomal enzyme deficiencies such as mucolipidosis II ("I-cell" disease) and combined β-galactosidase/neuraminidase deficiency (Kleijer et al., 1979b).

The application of microspectrophotometric analyses in prenatal diagnosis has remained more limited. Reduction of the incubation volume followed by extinction measurements in microcuvets has accelerated the prenatal diagnosis of metachromatic leukodystrophy (Niermeijer et al., 1974) and that of mucopolysaccharidosis I H/S (Kleijer, personal communication). The same approach could also be used to improve the prenatal diagnosis of other mucopolysaccharidoses, Wolman's disease, and lipidoses for which natural substrates with a chromogenic terminal group are available (see Section III).

Sensitive radiometric assays have not yet been widely used in the (prenatal) diagnosis of genetic disease. As has already been mentioned in Section IV, relatively small numbers of cultured cells (about 10^4) can be incubated in wells of a microtiter plate with radioactive-labeled ketoacids or amino acids to allow for rapid prenatal diagnosis of maple-syrup urine disease (Wendel et al., 1973b; Niermeijer et al., 1975). The same approach could also be followed for some other aminoacidopathies (see Galjaard, 1980). Incubation in small volumes, thin-layer chromatography on small strips of paper or polyethyleneimine cellulose, followed by autoradiography and scanning or by scintillation counting, have yielded prenatal diagnoses within 10–20 days for cystinosis (Willcox and Patrick, 1974) and combined immune deficiency (Aitken et al., 1980).

During the last few years the technique of fetal blood sampling seems to improve further and further. An article by Rodeck (1980) reports nearly a 100% success rate in obtaining pure fetal blood by ultrasound-guided fetoscopy, and only 3% fetal loss occurred in his series. Most other obstetricians, however, still have problems in obtaining fetal blood without admixture with maternal blood. It may be possible to separate maternal blood cells and fetal cells by using immunological techniques and fluorescence-activated cell sorting, as has been used by Herzenberg et al. (1979) to recover fetal lymphocytes from the maternal circulation. In most instances relatively few fetal white blood cells will be available, hence microchemical techniques will be helpful in the detection of metabolic defects. We have investigated the feasibility of using fetal white blood cells in the monitoring of pregnancies at risk for glycogenosis II, G_{M1}-gangliosidosis, mucopolysaccharidosis 1 H, and sialidosis (see Galjaard, 1980). In all instances a clear enzyme deficiency was found compared with control fetal white blood cells, and thus prenatal diagnosis of these and many other metabolic diseases will be possible within 1–2 days after fetoscopy in the sixteenth to eighteenth week of pregnancy as soon as this technique is considered safe enough.

B.   Single-Cell Analysis in Research

In those instances where enzyme activities or metabolite concentrations can be determined in single cultured cells, a variety of applications in basic research arise. In the previous section studies were already mentioned where enzyme assays had been performed on different cell types within one culture (van der Veer et al., 1978). It is also possible to analyze biochemical characteristics of cells that possess the same morphology but that differ genetically. Measurements of the activity of glucose-6-phosphate dehydrogenase (G-6-PD) in single fibroblasts using Lowry's method of NADP (H) cycling made it possible to detect the proportion of G-6-PD$^+$ and G-6-PD$^-$ cells in a culture of a female heterozygote for G-6-PD deficiency (Galjaard et al., 1974b,d). Once micromethods would be available for the determination of other X-linked metabolic defects in single cells, female carriers could be detected much faster than with the present techniques of cloning of skin fibroblasts.

In mixed cultures of normal cells and mutant cells, microchemical analysis in single cells has contributed to the study of intercellular exchange. No transfer of α-glucosidase and β-galactosidase activity was observed in mixed cultures of normal fibroblasts and those from patients with glycogenosis II or G_{M1}-gangliosidosis, whereas a clear transfer of hexosaminidase activity from normal to Sandhoff fibroblasts occurred (Galjaard et al., 1974b,d; Reuser et al., 1976a,b). These observations formed the basis for further analyses of the fate of exogenous enzyme that had been ingested by mutant cells. Similar techniques could be used to study the in vitro interaction between cells from different species.

Another area where quantitative enzyme assays in single cells have contributed is that of somatic cell hybridization (for review, see Bootsma and Galjaard, 1979). The genetic background of clinical and biochemical heterogeneity within a particular metabolic disease can be investigated by fusing fibroblasts from two patients with a different expression of "the same" disease, followed by complementation analysis of the cell-fusion products. If restoration of the metabolic defect occurs in hybrid cells or in heterokaryons, this implies that two different gene mutations are involved in the different variants. Unfortunately, there is no selection system for human × human hybrids or heterokaryons, and complementation analyses must therefore be performed by biochemical analysis of a cell homogenate of a mixed cell population or by assays at the single-cell level. In complementation studies of DNA-repair defects in different variants of xeroderma pigmentosum, Bootsma's group was able to use an autoradiographic method that enabled DNA repair to be studied in single heterokaryons (de Weerd-Kastelein *et al.*, 1972). For most other metabolic defects this is not possible, and therefore most subsequent complementation analyses have been carried out on homogenates of mixed unfused and fused cells.

In case of a high cell-fusion efficiency it will not cause any difficulty to show restoration of enzyme activity in a mixed cell population, but the results cannot be quantitated. Also in experiments with a low fusion index, as in some interspecies cell hybridizations, the effect of restoration of enzyme activity in a few cells might be diluted by too many of the enzyme-deficient parental cells. In such instances microchemical assays of individual heterokaryons is advantageous. An example of the latter approach has been reported by Galjaard *et al.* (1975), who demonstrated restoration of β-galactosidase activity in single heterokaryons 2 days after fusion of β-gal⁻ fibroblasts derived from two different types of patients. It could also be shown that in a proportion of the cells with the genome from both patients the enzyme activity was restored to control values (see Fig. 9).

A similar technique could be used in hybridization studies of cells from different species or from the same species but with different morphological or biochemical characteristics (see chapter by Darlington in this volume). In investigations of cell differentiation and gene transfer (see Ringertz and Savage, 1976), as well as in studies on the restoration of genetic metabolic defects (de Wit-Verbeek *et al.*, 1978; d'Azzo *et al.*, 1980), the use of "cybrids" may be an important tool. When no selection system is available, the interaction between enucleated cytoplasm of one cell type and the nucleus of another cell type can also be studied by microchemical assays of single "cybrids." Fluorescence cell sorting after cytochalasin B treatment yields a nearly pure population of cytoplasts (Schaap *et al.*, 1979; Jongkind *et al.*, 1980), and labeling of a specific cell type with latex particles allows the identification of cybrids (d'Azzo *et al.*, 1980), which can then be isolated by dissection from freeze-dried cultures as described earlier (see Figs. 1 and 2b,c).

In conclusion, during the last decade a variety of micromethods has permitted the biochemical analysis of small numbers and in some instances even of single cultured cells. The application of these microtechniques has been valuable in rapid prenatal diagnosis of genetic metabolic diseases, and in the future they are likely to contribute in the analysis of fetal blood (cells) and in the detection of female carriers for X-linked disease. In basic research, enzyme assays of single cultured cells has been helpful in studies on *in vitro* cell differentiation, metabolic interaction, and somatic cell hybridization.

ACKNOWLEDGMENTS

I want to thank all my colleagues who either have provided their data on prenatal diagnosis or who have kindly provided illustrations of their experimental work. In particular I acknowledge the contributions of A. d'Azzo, A. Hoogeveen, P. Hartwijk, J. F. Jongkind, J. E. de Josselin de Jong, W. J. Kleijer, and E. van der Veer, all of the Department of Cell Biology and Genetics, Rotterdam. The illustrations have been made by W. Visser, T. van Os, and J. Fengler, and Ms. M. van Woensel typed the manuscript.

REFERENCES

Aitken, D., Hoogeveen, A., Kleijer, W. J., and Galjaard, H. (1980). *Clin. Genet.* **17**, 291–298.
Bladon, M., and Milunsky, A. (1978). *Clin. Genet.* **14**, 359–366.
Bladon, M. T., and Milunsky, A. (1980). *Clin. Chim. Acta* **105**, 325–334.
Böhlen, P., Stein, S., Imal, K., and Udenfriend, S. (1974). *Anal. Biochem.* **58**, 559–562.
Bonting, S. L., and Rosenthal, J. M. (1960). *Nature* **185**, 686–687.
Bootsma, D., and Galjaard, H. (1979). *In* "Models for the Study of Inborn Errors of Metabolism" (F. A. Hommes, ed.), pp. 241–255. Elsevier-North Holland, Amsterdam.
Boyle, J. A., Raivo, K. A., Schulman, J. D., Seegmiller, J. E., Graf, M. L., and Jacobson, C. E. (1970). *Science* **169**, 688.
Bradford, M. M. (1976). *Anal. Biochem.* **72**, 248–254.
Butcher, E. C., and Lowry, O. H. (1976). *Anal. Chem.* **76**, 502–503.
Christamanou, H., and Sandhoff, K. (1977). *Clin. Chim. Acta* **79**, 527–531.
Ciba Foundation (1980). Symposium on Trends in Enzyme Histochemistry and Cytochemistry, No. 73 (new series). Excerpta Medica, Amsterdam and Oxford.
d'Azzo, A., Hoogeveen, A., and deWit-Verbeek, H. A. (1978). *Clin. Chim. Acta* **88**, 1–7.
d'Azzo, A., Konings, A., Verkerk, A., Jongkind, J. F., and Galjaard, H. (1980). *Exp. Cell Res.* **127**, 484–488.
de Bruyne, C. H. H. M., Oei, T. L., and Hösli, P. *Biochem. Biophys. Res. Commun.* **68**, 483–488.
de Josselin de Jong, J. E., Hartwijk, P. J. M., Van de Giessen, H. P., and Galjaard, H. (1980). *Anal. Biochem.* **106**, 397–401.
de Mars, R., Santo, G., and Felix, J. S. (1969). *Science* **164**, 1309.
de Weerd-Kastelein, E. A., Keijzer, W., and Bootsma, D. (1972). *Nature* **238**, 80–83.
deWit-Verbeek, H. A., Hoogeveen- A., and Galjaard, H. (1978). *Exp. Cell Res.* **113**, 215–218.
Dubach, U. C., and Schmidt, U., eds. (1971). "Advances in Quantitative Histo- and Cytochemistry." Huber, Bern.
Ellis, R. B., Ikonne, J. U.. and Manson, P. K. (1975). *Anal. Biochem.* **63**, 5–11.
Epstein, C. J., and Golbus, M. S. (1977). *Am. Sci.* **65**, 703–711.
Fortuin, J. J. H., and Kleijer, W. J. (1978). *Clin. Chim. Acta* **82**, 79–83.
Fratantoni, J. C., Neufeld, E. F., Uhlendorf, B. W., and Jacobson, C. B. (1969). *N. Engl. J. Med.* **280**, 686–688.

Fujimoto, W. Y., Seegmiller, J. E., Uhlendorf, B. W., and Jacobson, C. B. (1968). *Lancet* **2**, 511–512.

Gal, A., Brady, R. O., Hibbert, S. R., and Pentchev, P. G. (1975). *N. Engl. J. Med.* **293**, 632–636.

Gal, A., Brady, R. O., Pentchev, P. G., Scott, F., Suzuki, K., Tanaka, H., and Schneider, E. L. (1977). *Clin. Chim. Acta* **77**, 53–59.

Galjaard, H. (1976). *Cytogenet. Cell Genet.* **16**, 453–467.

Galjaard, H. (1979). *In* "Proceedings of Third European Conference on Prenatal Diagnosis" (J. D. Murken, S. Stengel-Rutkowski, and E. Schwinger, eds.), pp. 73–84. Enke, Stuttgart.

Galjaard, H. (1980). "Genetic Metabolic Diseases: Early Diagnosis and Prenatal Analysis." Elsevier-North Holland, Amsterdam.

Galjaard, H., Fernandes, J., Jahodova, M., Koster, J. F., and Niermeijer, M. F. (1972). *Bull. Eur. Soc. Hum. Genet.* **6**, 79–91.

Galjaard, H., Mekes, M., de Josselin de Jong, J. E., and Niermeijer, M. F. (1973). *Clin. Chim. Acta* **49**, 361–375.

Galjaard, H., van Hoogstraten, J. J., de Josselin de Jong, J. E., and Mulder, M. P. (1974a). *Histochem. J.* **6**, 409–429.

Galjaard, H., Hoogeveen, A., Keijzer, W., deWit-Verbeek, H. A., and Vlek-Noot, C. (1974b). *Histochem. J.* **6**, 491–509.

Galjaard, H., Niermeijer, M. F., Hahnemann, M., Mohr, J., and Sørensen, S. A. (1974c). *Clin. Genet.* **5**, 368–477.

Galjaard, H., Reuser, A. J. J., Heukels-Dully, J. J., Hoogeveen, A., Keijzer, W., deWit-Verbeek, H. A., and Niermeijer, M. F. (1974d). *In* "Enzyme Therapy in Lysosomal Storage Diseases" (J. M. Tager, G. J. M. Hooghwinkel, and W. Th. Daems, eds.). North Holland Publ. Co., Amsterdam.

Galjaard, H., Hoogeveen, A., Keijzer, W., deWit-Verbeek, H. A., Reuser, A. J. J., Mae Wan Ho, and Robinson, D. (1975). *Nature* **257**, 60–62.

Galjaard, H., Hoogeveen, A., van der Veer, E., and Kleijer, W. J. (1977). *In* "Proceedings of 5th Int. Congress on Human Genetics" (S. Armendares and R. Lisker, eds.), pp. 194–206. Excerpta Medica, Amsterdam.

Gatt, S., Dinur, T., and Barenholz, U. (1978). *Biochim. Biophys. Acta* **530**, 503–507.

Gatt, S., Dinur, T., and Barenholz, Y. (1980). *Clin. Chem.* **26**, 93–96.

Glick, D. (1963). "Quantitative Chemical Techniques of Histo- and Cytochemistry," Vols. I and II. Interscience, New York.

Glick, D. (1971). *In* "Recent Advances in Quantitative Histo- and Cytochemistry" (U. C. Dubach and U. Schmidt, eds.), pp. 35–53. Huber, Bern.

Glick, D. (1977a). *J. Histochem. Cytochem.* **25**, 1087–1101.

Glick, D. (1977b). *Clin. Chem.* **23**, 1465–1471.

Goldberg, R., Barenholz, Y., and Gatt, S. (1978). *Biochim. Biophys. Acta* **531**, 237–241.

Håkansson, G. (1979). "Biochemical Studies of the Norrbottnian Type of Gaucher Disease," Thesis, Dept. of Neurochemistry, Univ. of Göteborg, Sweden.

Halley, D., and Keukels-Dully, M. J. (1977). *J. Med. Genet.* **14**, 100–102.

Halley, D. J. J., Keijzer, W., Jaspers, N. G. J., Niermeijer, M. F., Kleijer, W. J., Boué, J., Boué, A., and Bootsma, D. (1979). *Clin. Genet.* **16**, 137–146.

Herzenberg, L. A., Bianchi, D. W., Schröder, J., Cann, H. M., and Iverson, G. M. (1979). *Proc. Natl. Acad. Sci. U.S.A.* **76**, 1453–1455.

Hoogeveen, A. T., Verheijen, F. W., d'Azzo, A., and Galjaard, H. (1980). *Nature* **285**, 500–502.

Horn, N. (1976). *Lancet* **1**, 1156–1157.

Hösli, P. (1977). *Clin. Chem.* **23**, 1476–1484.

Jacoby, L. B., Littlefield, J. W., Milunsky, A., Shih, V. E., and Wilroy, R. S. (1972). *Am. J. Hum. Genet.* **24**, 321–324.

Jongkind, J. F., Ploem, J. S., Reuser, A. J. J., and Galjaard, H. (1974). *Histochem.* **40**, 221–229.

Jongkind, J. F., Verkerk, A., Schaap, G. H., and Galjaard, H. (1980). *Exp. Cell Res.* **130,** 481-484.

Kinoshita, T., Inuma, F., Atsumi, K., and Tsuji, A. (1977). *Anal. Biochem.* **77,** 471-477.

Kleijer, W. J., van der Veer, E., and Niermeijer, M. F. (1976a). *Hum. Genet.* **33,** 299-305.

Kleijer, W. J., Wolffers, G. M., Hoogeveen, A., and Niermeijer, M. F. (1976b). *Lancet* **2,** 50.

Kleijer, W. J., Niermeijer, M. F., Boué, A., and Galjaard, H. (1979a). In "Proceedings of Third European Conference on Prenatal Diagnosis" (J. D. Murken, S. Stengel-Rutkowski, and E. Schwinger, eds.), p. 85. Enke, Stuttgart.

Kleijer, W. J., Hoogeveen, A., Verheijen, F. W., Niermeijer, M. F., Galjaard, H., O'Brien, J. S., and Warner, T. G. (1979b). *Clin. Genet.* **16,** 60-61.

Kleijer, W. J., Patrick, A. D., Aula, P., Berg, K., Goldman, H., Mannutti, M. M., and Potier, M. (1980). *Prenatal Diagnosis,* special issue, December, pp. 39-42.

Kronberg, H., Zimmer, H. G., and Neuhoff, V. (1980). *Electrophoresis* **1,** 27-32.

Leaback, D. H. (1976). *FEBS Lett.* **66,** 1-3.

Lowry, O. H. (1953). *J. Histochem. Cytochem.* **1,** 420-428.

Lowry, O. H. (1963). *Harvey Lect.* **58,** 1.

Lowry, O. H., and Passonneau, J. V. (1972). "A Flexible System of Enzymatic Analysis. Academic Press, New York.

Matschinsky, F. M. (1971). In "Recent Advances in Quantitative Histo- and Cytochemistry" (U. C. Dubach and U. Schmidt, eds.), pp. 142-182. Huber, Bern.

Matschinsky, F. M., Passonneau, J. V., and Lowry, O. H. (1968). *J. Histochem. Cytochem.* **16,** 29-39.

McKusick, V. A. (1978). "Mendelian Inheritance in Man," 5th Edition. Johns Hopkins Univ. Press, Baltimore.

Milunsky, A. (1973). "The Prenatal Diagnosis of Hereditary Disorders." Thomas, Springfield, Ill.

Milunsky, A., ed. (1975). "The Prevention of Genetic Disease and Mental Retardation. Saunders, Philadelphia.

Milunsky, A. (1976). *N. Engl. J. Med.* **295,** 377-380.

Milunsky, A., ed. (1980). "Genetic Disorders and the Fetus." Plenum, New York.

Nadler, H. J. (1968). *Pediatrics* **42,** 912.

Nadler, H. L. (1969). *J. Pediatr.* **74,** 132-143.

Nadler, H. L. (1972). *Biochimie* **54,** 677-681.

Nadler, H. L., and Messina, A. M. (1969). *Lancet* **2,** 1277.

Neufeld, E. F., and Cantz, M. (1973). In "Lysosomes and Storage Diseases" (H. G. Hers and F. van Hoof, eds.). Academic Press, New York.

Neuhoff, V. (1973). "Micromethods in Molecular Biology." Springer Verlag, Heidelberg.

Neuhoff, V., Behbehani, A. W., Quentin, C. D., and Prinz, A. (1974). *Hoppe Seylers Z. Physiol. Chem.* **355,** 891-894.

Neuhoff, V., Philipp, K., Zimmer, H. G., and Mesecke, S. (1979). *Hoppe Seylers Z. Physiol. Chem.* **360,** 1657-1670.

Niermeijer, M. F., Fortuin, J. J. H., Koster, J. F., Jahoda, M., and Galjaard, H. (1974). In "Enzyme Therapy in Lysosomal Storage Diseases" (J. M. Tager, G. J. M. Hooghwinkel, and W. Th. Daems, eds.), pp. 25-35. North Holland-American Elsevier, Amsterdam and New York.

Niermeijer, M. F., Koster, J. F., Jahodova, M., Fernandes, J., Heukels-Dully, M. J., and Galjaard, H. (1975). *Pediatr. Res.* **9,** 498-503.

Niermeijer, M. F., Sachs, E. S., Jahodova, M., Tichelaar-Klepper, C., Kleijer, W. J., and Galjaard, H. (1976). *J. Med. Genet.* **13,** 182-194.

Patrick, A. D. (1978). In "Towards the Prevention of Fetal Malformation" (J. B. Scrimgeour, ed.), pp. 165-176. Edinburgh Univ. Press, Edinburgh.

Pearse, A. G. E. (1968). "Histochemistry: Theoretical and Applied," Vol. I. Churchill & Livingstone, London.

Pearse, A. G. E. (1973). "Histochemistry: Theoretical and Applied," Vol. II. Churchill & Livingstone, London.

Poehling, H. M., and Neuhoff, V. (1980). *Electrophoresis* **1**, 90-102.

Quentin, C. D., Behbehani, A. W., Schulte, F. J., and Neuhoff, V. (1974). *Neuropaediatrie* **5**, 138-145; 238-278.

Ramsey, C. A., Coltart, T. M., Blunt, S., Pawsey, S. A., and Gianelli, F. (1974). *Lancet* **2**, 1109-1112.

Reuser, A. J. J., Jongkind, J. F., and Galjaard, H. (1976a). *J. Histochem. Cytochem.* **24**, 578-586.

Reuser, A. J. J., Halley, D., deWit-Verbeek, H. A., Hoogeveen, A., van der Kamp, M., Mulder, M. P., and Galjaard, H. (1976b). *Biochem. Biophys. Res. Commun.* **69**, 311-318.

Richardson, B. J., and Cox, D. M. (1973). *Clin. Genet.* **4**, 376-380.

Ringertz, N. R., and Savage, R. E. (1976). "Cell Hybrids." Academic Press, New York.

Rodeck, C. H. (1980). *Br. J. Obstet. Gynaecol.* **87**, 429-436.

Rotman, B. (1961). *Proc. Natl. Acad. Sci. U.S.A.* **47**, 1981-1991.

Schaap, G. H., van der Kamp, A. W. M., Öry, F. G., and Jongkind, J. F. (1979). *Exp. Cell Res.* **122**, 422-426.

Schneider, J. A. (1974). *In* "Heritable Disorders of Amino Acid Metabolism" (W. L. Nyhan, ed.), pp. 618-637. Wiley, New York.

Schneider, J. A., Verroust, F. M., Kroll, W. A., Garvin, A. J., Horger, E. D., Wong, V. G., Spear, S. S., Jacobson, C., Pellett, O. L., and Becker, P. L. A. (1974). *N. Engl. J. Med.* **290**, 878-882.

Schulman, J. D., Fujimoto, W. Y., Bradley, K. H., and Seegmiller, J. E. (1970). *J. Pediatr.* **77**, 468-470.

Seitz, W. R., and Neary, M. P. (1976). *In* "Methods of Biochemical Analysis" (D. Glick, ed.), Vol. 23, pp. 161-188. Wiley Interscience, New York.

Stanbury, J. B., Wyngaarden, J. B., and Frederickson, D. S. (1978). "The Metabolic Basis of Inherited Disease," 4th Edition. McGraw-Hill, New York.

States, B., and Segal, S. (1969). *Anal. Biochem.* **27**, 323-329.

States, B., Blazer, B., Harris, D. and Segal, S. (1975). *J. Pediatr.* 558-562.

Svennerholm, L. (1979). *In* "Proceedings of Third European Conference on Prenatal Diagnosis" (J. D. Murken, S. Stengel-Rutkowski, and E. Schwinger, eds.), pp. 276-283. Enke, Stuttgart.

Svennerholm, L., Håkansson, G., Mansson, J. E., and Vanier, M. T. (1979). *Clin. Chim. Acta* **92**, 53-64.

Udenfriend, S., Stein, S., Böhlen, P., Dairman, W., Leimgruber, W., and Weigele, M. (1972). *Science* **178**, 871-872.

van der Veer, E., Kleijer, W. J., de Josselin de Jong, J. E., and Galjaard, H. (1978). *Hum. Genet.* **40**, 285-292.

Vanier, M. T., Revol, A., and Boué, A. (1979). *In* "Proceedings of Third European Conference on Prenatal Diagnosis" (J. D. Murken, S. Stengel-Rutkowski, and E. Schwinger, eds.), pp. 292-298. Enke, Stuttgart.

Wendel, U., Rudiger, H. W., and Passarge, E. (1973a). *Humangenetik* **19**, 127-128.

Wendel, U., Wöhler, W., Goedde, H. W., Langenbeck, U., Passarge, E., and Rüdiger, H. W. (1973b). *Clin. Chim. Acta* **45**, 433-440.

Wenger, D. A., Farby, T. J., and Wharton, C. (1978). *Biochem. Biophys. Res. Commun.* **82**, 589-595.

Willcox, P., and Patrick, A. D. (1974). *Arch. Dis. Child.* **49**, 209-212.

Willers, J., Agarwal, D. P., Singh, S., Schloot, W., and Goedde, H. W. (1975). *Humangenetik* **27**, 323-328.

Wudl, L., and Paigen, K. (1974). *Science* **184**, 992-994.

Chapter 9

The Use of Growth Factors to Stimulate the Proliferation of Amniotic Fluid Cells[1]

CHARLES J. EPSTEIN[2]

Departments of Pediatrics and of Biochemistry and Biophysics
University of California, San Francisco
San Francisco, California

I. Requirements for More Rapid Growth of Amniotic Fluid Cells

Unlike other types of culture systems in which rapidity of cell proliferation, though desirable, is not essential, the use of amniotic fluid cells for the prenatal diagnosis of genetic disorders operates under significant time constraints. These constraints derive from two sources. The first is the natural desire of the parents of the fetus to obtain an answer as rapidly as possible; the second are the medical and legal restrictions, which define the earliest time at which amniotic fluid can be safely obtained and the stage of pregnancy beyond which therapeutic abortion is no longer feasible or allowable. These problems are further compounded by

[1]This work was supported in part by grants from the March of Dimes Birth Defects Foundation, the Maternal and Child Health Service (MCT-00445), and a contract from the California State Department of Health Services.

[2]Formerly an investigator of the Howard Hughes Medical Institute.

269

the occasional need to repeat an amniocentesis because of a failure to obtain fluid or of the cells to grow, whether for intrinsic or technical reasons, or to grow large numbers of cells for biochemical analysis. An additional reason for wanting to grow cells more rapidly is an economic one. Each refeeding of the cultures that can be eliminated reduces both the cost of the labor involved in caring for the cells and the cost of the medium, particularly the serum, in which the cells are grown.

II.   Shortening the Time between Amniocentesis and Analysis

Two approaches to shortening the time between amniocentesis and analysis have been suggested. One is miniaturization of the system so that analysis can be performed on fewer cells (see chapter by Galjaard, this volume). This approach has been particularly useful for the diagnosis of biochemical disorders, but unfortunately the microanalytic techniques required are not readily available or applicable to all situations. The other approach, which is the subject of this article, has been to stimulate the cells to proliferate more rapidly by the use of exogenous growth-promoting substances, the so-called growth factors. At the present time neither approach is in vogue, and the vast majority of cytogenetic and biochemical analyses are coupled with standard mass-culture techniques or, in some laboratories, with clonal culture techniques and conventional cytogenetic methods (see chapter by Hoehn and Salk in this volume).

If the objective is to obtain a certain number of cells more rapidly, then two aspects of the growth of amniotic fluid cells are potential sites of attack. One is the original attachment and outgrowth of the cells. Despite the relatively ample number of cells initially placed into culture, the number of cells that actually attach and form colonies is quite low, of the order of 10 in a conventional plate or flask. Therefore, any approach that would improve the plating efficiency of the cells could bring about the desired outcome. However, this increase in plating efficiency would have to be several fold (at least 3–4) in magnitude to produce a meaningful shortening of the time required to obtain the necessary number of cells. To date, no systematic investigation of means of improving plating efficiency has been reported, but it can be visualized that the proper choice of culture vessel (type of glass or plastic), the application of a special substrate (for example, collagen, gelatin, fibronectin), alteration of the medium, or even the use of nonproliferating feeder layers (when only cytogenetic analysis is to be undertaken), could produce the desired enhancement (see, for example, Reidy and Chen, 1979).

The other potential point of intervention in an attempt to decrease the time required for cell culture is the cell cycle itself. If the length of the cycle could be reduced, for example, by half, then only half as much total culture time would be required to obtain the same number of cells. This would mean that a culture period of 14 days could be shortened to about 8 to 10 days. The shortening is not strictly proportional to the reduction in cell cycle length because of the lag period of several days before net cell proliferation actually occurs. However, even a 25% reduction in the length of the cell cycle could shorten a 14-day culture period to 10–12 days. More significantly, it could reduce a 28-day period, such as is sometimes encountered when amniotic fluid cell cultures are being expanded for biochemical analysis, by close to a week.

III.   Growth Factors

A variety of growth factors have been used in an attempt to achieve a significant shortening of the length of the cell cycle. The general area of growth factors, particularly their identities, effects, and modes of action, has been the scene of considerable activity during the past decade, and the state of work in the area has been well summarized by Gospodarowicz and Moran (1976) and by Papaconstantinou and Rutter (1978). Growth factors have been assigned to several categories on the basis of their sites of origin or the material from which they are isolated. These categories include factors from the bloodstream (serum, plasma, platelets), from tissues (submaxillary gland, pituitary, brain, cartilage, mesenchyme), and from the media of cells cultured *in vitro*. Some of these factors are highly specific in their actions (e.g., erythropoietin, which stimulates proerythroblasts, and nerve growth factor, which sustains the growth of the sympathetic nervous system), whereas others are much more general and act on several cell types. Hormones, such as insulin and steroids, also function as growth factors, and many of the other factors are polypeptides or small proteins of relatively low molecular weight, between 7000 and 22,500.

The effects of three nonhormonal growth factors on the proliferation of amniotic fluid cells have been investigated. These include the fibroblast, epidermal, and cartilage growth factors. In addition, limited work with insulin and dexamethasone has also been reported. In considering the results of these studies it is necessary to distinguish between effects produced on primary cell cultures established directly from amniotic fluid and on secondary cultures derived from already existing amniotic fluid cell cultures. The former are relevant to the general situation obtaining when cytogenetic analysis is the objective, whereas the latter are more applicable to circumstances, such as biochemical determinations, in which large numbers of cells are required.

IV. Effects of Growth Factors on Primary Amniotic Fluid Cell Cultures

Two studies of the effects of fibroblast growth factor (FGF) on the proliferation of primary human amniotic fluid cell cultures have been reported. Gospodarowicz and collaborators (1977) found that 100 mg/ml of FGF, a saturating amount, added 1 day after initiation of the culture to an optimal medium containing Dulbecco's modified Eagle's medium (DME) with 20% fetal calf serum, increased the number of cells obtained after 15–18 days of culture by 2- to 280-fold, the median enhancement being approximately 5.5-fold (Table I). Of 10 sets of treated and control cultures, 6 pairs showed a statistically significant difference (at $p \leq 0.05$) in favor of the FGF-treated cells. In examining these data, it is apparent that the wide range of enhancement observed is a function primarily of the tremendous variation in the growth of the control cultures (from 0.01 to 6.4×10^5 cells per 60-mm dish). Similar experiments were also carried out with bovine amniotic fluid cells, and enhancements ranging from 2.4- to 108-(median 12.5) fold were observed.

Chettur et al. (1978) also looked at the effects of FGF on primary human amniotic fluid cells, again grown in DME with 20% fetal calf serum. Rather than directly determining cell numbers, they measured the incorporation of [^{3}H]thymidine into DNA (Table I). In their hands, a concentration of FGF of 200 ng/ml was necessary for maximal effect and resulted in about a doubling of the rate of [^{3}H]thymidine incorporation. However, when insulin and dexamethasone were also present, at concentrations of 100 ng/ml each, the rate of [^{3}H]thymidine incorporation was increased 6-fold over the control and 3-fold over FGF alone. To evaluate the potential practical usefulness of the growth enhancement produced by FGF, insulin, and dexamethasone, a study was carried out of the time between initiation and harvesting the cultures. With standard DME with 20% fetal calf serum, the time required was 15.2 ± 0.88 (SD) days, whereas with the supplemented medium it was 11.0 ± 0.86 days, a difference of 4.2 ± 0.75 days. These data are somewhat difficult to evaluate because there is no evidence that the experiments were performed blindly, an experimental condition necessary to ensure an unbiased interpretation of the status of the cultures.

Gospodarowicz and co-workers (1977) also studied the effects of epidermal growth factor (EGF) on primary human and bovine amniotic fluid cell cultures. At a saturating concentration of 100 ng/ml, EGF enhanced the growth of the human cells by 1.3- to 5-(median between 1.5 and 2.0) fold (Table I) and of bovine cells by 0.009- to 8.8-(median between 1.8 and 3.4) fold, but none of the differences were significant at $p \leq 0.05$.

Rüdiger et al. (1974) investigated the effects of a "human growth factor" prepared by concentrating the proteins of MW $\geq 20,000$ in human urine. It is possible that this material is related to EGF or urogastrone, which is present in

TABLE I

The Effect of Growth Factors on the Growth of Cultured Human Amniotic Fluid Cells

Factor	Primary cultures		Secondary cultures			References
	Concentration of factor	Numbers of cells: factor/control	Concentration of factor	Doubling time: factor/control	Numbers of cells: factor/control	
Fibroblast	100 ng/ml	5.5 (2–280) [15–18][a]	100 ng/ml	0.25	200 [8][b]	Gospodarowicz et al. (1977)
	200 ng/ml	1.8 [12][b,c]				Chettur et al. (1978)
	200 ng/ml + insulin[d] + dexamethasone	4.4 [12][b,c]				
Epidermal	100 ng/ml	1.8 (1.3–5.0) [15–18][a]	100 ng/ml	0.5	2.5 [8][b]	Gospodarowicz et al. (1977)
					4.0 [12][b]	
"Human" (urinary)	5% (v/v) of concentrate	(72% versus 46% of cultures positive)[e]				Rüdiger et al. (1974)
Cartilage	200 μg/ml	1.7 [16][b]	500 μg/ml		2.0 [11][b]	Golbus et al. (1980)
					2.6 [15][b]	

[a] Median (range) [time in days]
[b] Mean [time in days]
[c] Relative cell numbers based on [³H]thymidine incorporation.
[d] Insulin and dexamethasone added at concentrations of 100 ng/ml each.
[e] Data expressed as proportion of microwell cultures showing growth.

human urine, although the latter has been reported to have a molecular weight of less than 6000. When added to human amniotic fluid cells cultured with DME containing 20% fetal calf serum, the ability of cells to grow in the wells of microtiter plates was increased, and the proportion of wells not showing growth after 6 days decreased from 54% to 28%. Although comparison of these results with those obtained with mass-culture techniques is not possible, they do suggest that the urine factor does improve cell growth, either by direct stimulation or by increasing plating efficiency. Even a small increase in the latter would be likely to have a significant effect on the proportion of positive cultures observed in what is essentially a cloning method of culture initiation.

The one other growth factor that has been examined with primary human amniotic fluid cells is cartilage growth factor (CGF) obtained from bovine cartilage (Klagsbrun *et al.*, 1977). When added at a concentration of 200 μg/ml in minimal essential medium supplemented with 20% fetal calf serum, an increase of cell numbers of 1.8-fold was observed after 16 days in culture (Golbus *et al.*, 1980). However, when the effect of CGF on the time necessary for the cultures to reach a density sufficient for chromosome analysis was assessed blindly, a significant difference between CGF (13.8 $\pm$ 2.4 SD days) and control cultures (15 $\pm$ 1.5 SD days) was not observed.

Taken together, the data on FFG, EGF, and CGF suggest that these growth factors can enhance the proliferation of primary human amniotic fluid cells. Of the factors tested to date, the results with FGF have been the most impressive. However, it is not at all certain that these factors can significantly reduce the time between initiation of the culture and their reaching a density appropriate for cytogenetic analysis.

V.   Effects of Growth Factors on Secondary Amniotic Fluid Cell Cultures

When large numbers of amniotic fluid cells are required, the primary cultures are harvested and replated as secondary cultures. These cultures are no longer maintained under clonal conditions, and the cells are already adapted to proliferation *in vitro*. The effects of FGF, EGF, and CGF have been tested on such secondary cultures, and in each instance a stimulating effect has been noted. The results of these studies are summarized in Table I. FGF and EGF, at concentrations of 100 ng/ml, produced 4- and 2-fold stimulations, respectively, in the rate of proliferation of "fibroblastic" human amniotic fluid cells plated under sparse conditions (3000 cells per 60-mm dish) (Gospodarowicz *et al.*, 1977). FGF significantly shortened the lag time between plating and the onset of log-phase growth, and beneficial effects were also obtained with epithelioid amniotic fluid cells. Similarly, CGF, at a concentration of 500 μg/ml, produced a 2.6-fold increase in the proliferation of secondary cell cultures plated at a density of 1000 cells per T25 flask (Golbus et al, 1980).

It appears, therefore, that both FGF and CGF can significantly enhance the rate of cell division in secondary cultures. Given a doubling time of about 3 days (Gospodarowicz et al., 1977), this increase in the rate of proliferation could shorten by as much as a week the time required to grow cells in amounts of the order of $1-2 \times 10^6$ per dish.

VI.   Potential Deleterious Effects of Addition of Growth Factors

Because of concern about altering the biochemical or chromosomal properties of the cells by addition of growth factors, the chromosomes and some enzymes of stimulated cell cultures have been examined. Neither FGF (Chettur et al., 1978) nor CGF (Golbus et al., 1980) caused any untoward cytogenetic effects, and CGF did not alter the specific activities of the medically important enzymes, arylsulfatase A, β-galactosidase, hexosaminidase A, and total hexosaminidase (Golbus et al., 1980). The latter results are of particular importance because of the need to carry out enzyme assays of amniotic fluid cells under carefully controlled conditions and with the appropriate normal reference cells.

VII.   Future Uses of Growth Factors in Prenatal Diagnosis

As has already been mentioned, growth factors, despite their apparent usefulness in potentiating the growth of amniotic fluid cells, particularly in secondary culture, are not in general use. The reasons for this are several. In addition to lack of knowledge about their effects, these factors are not generally available and, as the paucity of literature referred to in this chapter testifies to, they have been little studied. Furthermore, except in the special instance of obtaining large numbers of cells, which represents but a small fraction of the total load of a laboratory culturing cells for prenatal diagnosis—for example, only 1.4% of cases in a large series from a general prenatal diagnosis service (Golbus et al., 1979)—it is still to be proven that the enhancing effect of the growth factors, at least under the conditions examined to date, is sufficient to warrant a change in existing procedures.

However, it is also clear that more investigation is still in order. This point is brought home particularly by the results of Chettur et al. (1978), in which the addition of insulin and dexamethasone greatly increased the enhancing effect of

FGF. Unfortunately, the effects of these hormones alone, without FGF, have not been studied, and neither have the potential synergistic effects of these hormones with the other growth factors. Although there must be a limit to the rate of proliferation of amniotic fluid cells that can ultimately be achieved, it is quite possible that this limit has not been reached by any of the culture regimens tested so far.

Ironically, it may turn out that the decision to use growth factors in the culture of amniotic fluid cells may not rest on considerations of time but on the more mundane question of the availability of fetal calf serum. All of the culture media now in use are made up with substantial quantities of this serum. This commodity, in addition to rapidly becoming more expensive, is gradually becoming difficult to obtain at any price. Therefore, it may eventually become necessary to use substitutes for fetal calf serum, and one such may be a growth factor or combination of factors. Evidence that this might be feasible is presented by Rüdiger et al. (1974), who showed that addition of their human (urinary) growth factor to cultured diploid fibroblasts could restore the rate of cell growth to normal when the fetal calf serum concentration was lowered to 2%. In this case, the growth factor did not lead to a growth performance better than was obtained with fetal calf serum, but it could at least lead to one that was as good. A less dramatic but still significant effect was obtained by Chettur et al. (1978) with primary human amniotic fluid cell cultures. In this case, fetal calf serum could be reduced to 10% and 5% with decreases in the rates of [^{3}H]thymidine incorporation of about 25% and 50%, respectively.

It appears, therefore, that exogenous growth-promoting substances may have an important role to play as long as the growth of cells is required for prenatal diagnosis, and further investigation is certainly warranted.

REFERENCES

Chettur, L., Christensen, E., and Phillip, J. (1978). *Clin. Genet.* **14**, 223–228.
Golbus, M., Loughman, W. D., Epstein, C. J., Halbasch, G., Stephens, J. D., and Hall, B. D. (1979). *N. Engl. J. Med.* **300**, 157–163.
Golbus, M., Djalali, M., Klagsbrun, M., Kaback, M. M., Levenson, R. M., and Epstein, C. J. (1980). *Am. J. Med. Genet.* **6**, 107–111.
Gospodarowicz, D., and Moran, J. S. (1976). *Ann. Rev. Biochem.* **45**, 531–557.
Gospodarowicz, D., Moran, J. S., and Owashi, N. D. (1977). *J. Clin. Endocrinol. Metab.* **44**, 651–659.
Klagsbrun, M., Langer, R., Levenson, R., Smith, S., and Lillehei, C. (1977). *Exp. Cell Res.* **105**, 99–108.
Papaconstantinou, J., and Rutter, W. J., eds. (1978). "Molecular Control of Proliferation and Differentiation." Academic Press, New York.
Reidy, J. A., and Chen, A. T. L. (1979). *Am. J. Hum. Genet.* **31**, 31A.
Rüdiger, H. W., Wolff, R., Wendel, V., and Passarge, E. (1974). *Humangenetik* **22**, 81–84.

Chapter 10

Fetal Cells from Maternal Blood: Their Selection and Prospects for Use in Prenatal Diagnosis[1]

DAVID R. PARKS[2] AND LEONARD A. HERZENBERG

Department of Genetics
Stanford University School of Medicine
Stanford, California

[1]This work was supported in part by grants from the National Institutes of Health (GM-17367 and HD-13025).
[2]Recipient of a Senior Fellowship, American Cancer Society, California Division.

I. Introduction

We are attempting to improve methods for obtaining fetal cells from samples of maternal blood early in pregnancy using a fluorescence-activated cell sorter (FACS). Our goal is to use these cells for prenatal diagnosis of chromosome abnormalities and other genetic disorders.

It would be very desirable to have a minimally invasive technique for prenatal diagnosis of genetic defects that could be applied to all pregnancies. The low but significant risks of amniocentesis restrict its use to pregnancies in which the risk of fetal defects is relatively high. Prenatal diagnosis from a maternal blood sample would not only decrease the risks in cases where amniocentesis is now recommended but would also allow testing in low-risk pregnancies, which because of their greater number actually result in the birth of the majority of infants with trisomy 21 and other chromosome abnormalities (Holmes, 1978).

In addition, such a technique might allow prenatal diagnosis results to be obtained at an earlier stage in the pregnancy than is possible with amniocentesis. This could result if fetal cells are present in maternal circulation early in pregnancy or if the cells could be cultured to yield karyotypable mitoses in a few days rather than the few weeks required for culture of amniotic fluid cells.

Our approach has been to label differentially maternal and fetal cells[3] with fluorescein-tagged antibodies to cell-surface antigens such as paternal histocompatibility (HLA) antigens. Cells with appropriate labeling are isolated from the bulk of the maternal cells using the FACS. Our verification procedure is to stain the selected cells with quinacrine mustard (QM) and examine them for the presence of Y-chromatin spots (Y-bodies), indicative of their origin from a male fetus. We hope to be able to culture the still-viable sorted cells to obtain fetal karyotype information and possibly use them to test for biochemical defects.

II. Previous Studies—Detection of Fetal Cells without Enrichment

There have been a number of reports of the detection of (male) fetal cells in maternal blood during pregnancy. The results were based on identification of XY mitoses following mitogen stimulation of cells from maternal blood (Walknowska et al., 1969; de Grouchy and Trebuchet, 1971; Schindler et al.,

---

[3]In this article the term fetal cells refers to the fetal cells found in maternal blood unless otherwise specified. Abbreviations used include FACS, for fluorescence-activated cell sorter and QM for quinacrine mustard.

1972) or on identification of Y-chromatin-positive interphase cells with or without mitogen stimulation (Schröder and de la Chapelle, 1972; Grosset et al., 1974; Schröder et al., 1974; Siebers et al., 1975; Zilliacus et al., 1975). The identification of rare XY mitoses by the conventional techniques used in the earlier studies (Walknowska et al., 1969; de Grouchy and Trebuchet, 1971; Schindler et al., 1972) is open to question (Schröder, 1975), and a later attempt to find such mitoses using quinacrine staining yielded zero XY mitoses out of 112,000 mitoses studied (Zilliacus et al., 1975).

The studies on interphase cells used quinacrine or quinacrine mustard staining to reveal Y-chromatin. In each study Y-chromatin-positive cells were found primarily but not exclusively in blood samples from women who subsequently delivered boys (Schröder and de la Chapelle, 1972; Grosset et al., 1974; Schröder et al., 1974; Siebers et al., 1975; Zilliacus et al., 1975). The average observed frequencies of such cells range from less than 0.2% (Schröder and de la Chapelle, 1972; Schröder et al., 1974; Zilliacus et al., 1975) to almost 4% (Siebers et al., 1975). The time of earliest appearance of Y-chromatin-positive cells is also different in different studies. The discrepancies among the studies and the sources of incorrect diagnoses have been discussed (Schröder, 1975; Schröder and Herzenberg, 1980), but none of the data would support the use of this technique for accurate fetal sex determination.

Our results are consistent with the lowest frequency estimates, because unenriched control slides usually yield no Y-chromatin-positive cells among 1000–2000 cells examined.

The tissue of origin of the fetal cells found in maternal blood during pregnancy is unknown. Those identified by quinacrine or quinacrine mustard staining usually show a morphology like lymphocytes, often with larger nuclei than the smallest lymphocytes. However, they seem to be unresponsive to phytohemagglutinin (Zilliacus et al., 1975) and may in fact be precursor cells to erythrocytes or lymphocytes, and so on; or they may be of placental, perhaps trophoblast, origin.

III. Fetal Cell Project Design and Published Results

Our research program has been designed to (1) verify the presence of nucleated fetal cells in maternal blood, (2) obtain cell fractions enriched with such fetal cells in selected maternal–fetal pairs, (3) generalize the enrichment techniques to be applicable to all pregnancies, (4) improve the purity of the fetal cell-enriched fractions, and (5) find culture conditions and stimulants that will induce the fetal cells to enter mitosis so that fetal karyotypes can be analyzed. Each aspect of the work both draws on and contributes to our understanding of the characteristics and possible origins of the fetal cells. This characterization is particularly necessary in finding appropriate culture conditions, but it is important for all aspects of the work.

The first two objectives have been achieved through fetal cell labeling for paternally derived HLA-A2 antigen, FACS sorting of the labeled cells, and identification of the fetal cells by examination for QM-stained Y-chromatin (Herzenberg et al., 1979; Iverson et al., 1981). Table I shows the data on Y-body observations in relation to typing of the informative male babies with the anti-HLA-A2 serum. The impressive correlation clearly demonstrates that Y-chromatin-positive cells of fetal origin were present in the maternal blood and that they were selectively enriched by sorting for the HLA-A2 marker. In five of the eight cases with HLA-A2-positive male infants, two or three maternal blood samples were tested beginning at 15 weeks gestation. Y-chromatin-positive cells were found in each sample. Finding such cells in all samples where they would have been expected a posteriori is the most convincing evidence that they are usually present as early as 15 weeks and that they continue to be present through midpregnancy. The data do not allow a firm estimate of the fraction of fetal cells in maternal blood, but the assumption that the fetal cells stain for paternal HLA like cord blood lymphocytes do and that they show a comparable frequency of visible Y-chromatin leads to estimates of 1/800 to 1/60,000 with a mode between 1/1000 and 1/5000 (Iverson et al., 1981).

The one case in which Y-chromatin-positive cells were observed but the baby's cells were not stained by the antiserum may have been due to an unusually high number of fetal cells in the mother's blood, allowing them to be detected without enrichment. Among the 19 cases in which sorting of fetal cells was attempted and the baby turned out to be a girl, Y-chromatin-positive cells were

TABLE I

ENRICHMENT OF Y-CHROMATIN-POSITIVE CELLS IN RELATION TO THE
HLA TYPE OF MALE BABIES[a]

Y-Chromatin-positive cells found in samples sorted from maternal blood	Cord blood typing with sorting serum (no. of cases)	
	HLA-A2+	HLA-A2−
Yes	8	1
No	0	17

[a] The probability of obtaining such results by random association is 5.8×10^{-6} (Fisher Exact Test).

found in only one sample. Later samples from the same woman did not yield Y-chromatin-positive cells. The unusual result remains unexplained and was probably due to some technical error.

The procedures used in obtaining the data just summarized have been published (Herzenberg *et al.*, 1979; Iverson *et al.*, 1981), so they will be explained only briefly here. Mononuclear cell suspensions were prepared from maternal blood samples drawn between the fifteenth and thirtieth week of pregnancy. The cells were stained with a rabbit antiserum to HLA-A2 kindly provided by Dr. J Strominger, Harvard University (Robb *et al.*, 1975), followed by a second step of goat anti-rabbit immunoglobulin. Both antisera were absorbed to obtain specific staining. If the bulk of the maternal cells were not stained by this procedure, the brightest cells having light-scatter properties like small lymphocytes were sorted with the FACS (usually the brightest 0.1 to 1% were selected). The sorted cell samples were QM-stained to reveal Y-chromatin. The reading for Y-chromatin-positive cells was carried out blindly in that neither the fetal sex nor HLA reactivity was known. When the babies were born, their sex was noted and their cord blood mononuclear cells were tested for reactivity with the selecting antiserum.

The ability of the FACS to examine several thousand cells per second and to isolate cell fractions as pure as the specificity of the fluorescent-staining reagent allows has made it possible to obtain fetal cell-enriched fractions from maternal blood. However, the low frequency of fetal cells and the great variety of cell types in maternal blood make it difficult to achieve stains that mark only the fetal cells. In the cases just quoted the Y-chromatin-positive cells averaged less than 0.4% of the total in the appropriate enriched samples. Thus even enriched fractions contained predominantly maternal cells, and the QM Y-chromatin technique was required to confirm the enrichment of fetal cells.

When sorts for fetal cells were divided into several subsamples with different fluorescence ranges, Y-chromatin-positive cells were often found in the lower fluorescence range just above unstained maternal cells and well below most positive control staining of adult lymphocytes. Thus the fetal cells seem to stain less brightly for paternal HLA than ordinary adult lymphocytes do. This may be part of the reason for the limited enrichments observed.

In the next sections we will discuss (1) the basic operation and capabilities of the FACS and modifications that have been made to facilitate fetal cell sorting; (2) the QM Y-chromatin technique for identification of male cells; and (3) work in progress toward improving fetal cell selection, including the use of monoclonal antibodies to HLA polymorphisms, monoclonal antibodies to trophoblast cells, and use of double-labeling techniques. Following that we will describe FACS-based investigations of fetal–maternal transfer of erythrocytes in humans and in a rhesus monkey model.

IV.   Basic Flow Cytometry

Flow-cytometry systems have been described in a number of places (Hulett *et al.*, 1973; Herzenberg *et al.*, 1976; Herzenberg and Herzenberg, 1978), so we will present a brief overview, outline the capabilities and limitations of such systems, and then discuss the specific modifications we have made to facilitate selection of fetal cells.

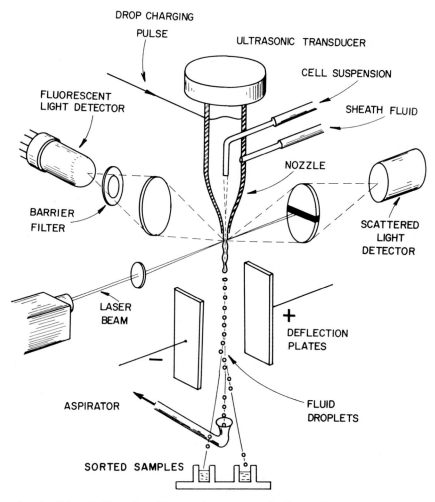

FIG. 1.   Schematic illustration of the central components of a flow analysis and sorting system. The functions of the various components are described in the text.

A. Equipment and Operation

Figure 1 is a sketch of a flow analysis and sorting system. The focal point of the system is the intersection of a laser beam with a liquid jet from a small nozzle. This jet consists mostly of cell-free sheath fluid and has a diameter of 50 to 100 μm. The suspension of fluorescent-labeled cells is injected at the center of the nozzle and forms a small central core in the jet. As a cell passes through the laser beam, fluorescent molecules it carries are excited and emit fluorescent light, which is collected by a lens, filtered to block out scattered laser light, and converted to an electrical signal by a photomultiplier detector. In addition, laser light scattered by the cell in the forward direction is measured by another detector. This gives information on cell size and for some cell types allows discrimination of live and dead cells. Electronic signals proportional to the amount of light scatter and fluorescence from each cell are amplified in linear or logarithmic fashion, processed, and digitized for computer analysis or pulse height analyzer display. We have recently built high-speed logarithmic amplifiers that work over a signal ratio range of about 10,000 to 1. They are used for almost all fluorescence work because the range is enough to cover all usual fluorescence signals, making amplifier gain changes unnecessary. In addition, we have found that the logarithmic presentation makes the relevant features of immunofluorescent distributions more visible and easier to interpret than linear presentation does.

For cell sorting the nozzle is vibrated at a frequency of 20 to 40 kHz by a piezoelectric transducer. This results in breakup of the jet into extremely uniform droplets. When a cell is detected that fulfills present conditions in scatter and fluorescence, droplets containing that cell are electrically charged. The drops fall through an electric field, produced by two statically charged plates, which draws charged droplets out of the stream of uncharged ones so that they can be collected as sorted samples.

B. FACS Capabilities and Limitations

The capabilities and limitations of flow-cytometric measurements and sorting with FACS-type instrumentation are outlined in the following points:

1. Flow-cytometric techniques can be applied to any type of cell that can be obtained in single-cell suspension. For good measurements and sorting the nozzle orifice diameter should be at lease five times the cell diameter.

2. The fluorescent label may be any dye associated with the surface or interior of the cell whose fluorescence can be excited by the laser light. The commonly used argon-ion laser has a number of available emissions from 350 nm in the near UV to 514 nm in the green. For longer wavelengths a krypton-ion laser operating at 568 nm or a tunable dye laser excited with an argon-ion laser (with emission range determined by the dye used) may be suitable.

3. The FACS makes a quantitative measurement of the fluorescence of each cell. Using appropriate standards, this measurement may be calibrated in terms of the actual number of dye molecules per cell.

4. The sensitivity of the measurements depends on the properties of the dye and on how well its excitation efficiency is matched to the available laser wavelengths, but for the best dyes such as fluorescein, lymphocytes with only 10,000–20,000 dye molecules can be clearly distinguished from a population of unstained cells. The limit is set by the background fluorescence of the unstained cells. The number of labeled sites (such as surface-antigen molecules) required to yield adequate staining may be quite small if dye labeling is amplified by coupling the labeling reagent to fluorescent microspheres or a multiple dye molecule tail.

5. Any characteristics that allow cells to be discriminated on the basis of light scattering and/or fluorescence can be used for sorting.

6. Sorting is normally carried out at a total cell-flow rate of 2000–3000 cells per second (7–10 million cells per hour). Losses due to the appearance of cells too close together to be separated in the deflected drops increase in relative frequency as the cell-flow rate is increased.

7. The ability of FACS systems to select rare cells is limited only by the specificity of the labeling technique in distinguishing wanted from unwanted cells and by the time required to run enough cells to find the required number of the rare type.

8. The viability and functional capacities of most types of cells are not affected by passage through the FACS.

9. Sterile sorting can be carried out routinely so that sorted cell fractions are suitable for either short- or long-term tissue culture.

C.   Sorter Modifications and Developments for Fetal Cell Selection

Sorts for fetal cells typically select 0.1–1% of the cells run. This presents significant problems in recovering and handling the small number of cells. Sorted cells are collected in small wells containing culture medium mounted on microscope slides. The wells are produced by attaching short lengths of 5-mm internal diameter glass tubing to the slides with wax. In sorting, the stream of undeflected droplets is intercepted and aspirated away at a point above the collecting wells (see Fig. 1).

To ensure that the trajectories of the deflected drops remain constant it is necessary to monitor the deflections during the sorting. However, observation of the deflected drops is difficult when only a few cells are being sorted per second, so we devised a variable-delay strobe-light system triggered by the drop charging pulse. The delay is set so that the flash occurs when the deflected drops are about to enter the collection vessel. The drops of each deflection event can be seen and sorting conditions adjusted to ensure that each deflected cell is collected.

The assurance of collecting each deflected cell has also been increased by shortening the path from the FACS nozzle to the collector and by grounding the collection vessel to prevent static charge buildup, which can cause the charged drops to be repelled out of the well.

V. Quinacrine Y-Chromatin—Background and Techniques

Either quinacrine or quinacrine mustard can be used to reveal Y-chromatin in interphase cells. The results are similar, but QM is probably better because it is used at a lower concentration for staining, it binds more strongly (even covalently) to DNA, and its fluorescence is more resistant to fading under illumination (Caspersson and Zech, 1970). They are intercalating dyes that bind relatively uniformly to DNA with little preference for particular local nucleotide base compositions (Latt et al., 1974). However, the fluorescence quantum efficiency shows a strong maximum in an A-T rich environment (Latt et al., 1974). The distal half of the long arm of the human Y-chromosome contains A-T-rich heterochromatin, and that area shows bright fluorescence when stained with QM. The Y-chromosome fluorescence is the brightest area in metaphase chromosome spreads from most males. Other chromosomes may show relatively bright areas particularly at the centromere (Caspersson et al., 1972).

A QM bright spot (Y-body), identifiable with the relatively condensed Y-chromatin, is visible in interphase nuclei of many male cells (Pearson et al., 1970; Mukjerjee et al., 1972). The fraction of cells exhibiting a Y-body varies from one cell type to another and from person to person. Fibroblast cells have been reported to show a Y-body frequency of 71–81% (Mukjerjee et al., 1972), whereas blood lymphocytes are commonly in the 35–66% range (Schröder and de la Chapelle, 1972). In lymphocytes the Y-body appears as a small bright spot often near the margin of the nucleus. The treatment used for QM staining makes it difficult to distinguish different cell types, but in our experience the Y-body-positive cells found in maternal blood generally have round nuclei and look more or less like small or medium lymphocytes.

Use of the Y-body technique for identification of male cells is limited by the fact that not all male cells show a Y-body and by the appearance of fluorescent spots in cells for reasons other than the presence of Y-chromatin. In particular, a small fraction of interphase cells from people who have bright fluorescent spots on one or more autosomes may show a spot bright enough to be taken for a Y-body. Staining artifacts also occur that may occasionally be difficult to distinguish from Y-bodies. Often examination of such a cell by white light will expose the artifact because Y-bodies are essentially invisible without fluorescence (Holbrook and Tishler, 1980).

The other major limitation on the technique is that the reading is subjective. Obtaining reliable results depends on the training and consistency of the reader as well as on careful experimental design to include adequate controls and to assure that the reading is "blind."

VI.   Broadening Fetal Cell-Selection Capability and Reagent Evaluation

In order to improve the enrichment of fetal cells and devise fetal cell-selection techniques applicable to most or all pregnancies, we are exploring several types of labeling reagents and different selection strategies. The reagents include monoclonal antibodies to HLA types and to trophoblast antigens. Selection strategies have been expanded to include selection with two independent fluorescent labels.

A.   Monoclonal Antibodies for HLA Polymorphisms

There were three problems with the rabbit anti-HLA-A2 serum used in our earlier enrichment of fetal cells: (1) it was available in limited quantity; (2) even after extensive absorptions to make it specific, most sorted cells were of maternal origin; and (3) as an HLA-type reagent it was usable only when the mother and fetus differed in that particular HLA type. Monoclonal antibodies to HLA-A2 and HLA-B7 (named PA2.1 and BB7.1, respectively) were obtained as mouse ascites fluids from Dr. Peter Parham (Brodsky *et al.*, 1979). Both are of the IgG1 isotype and are available in large quantities. They require only minimal processing, such as ammonium sulfate precipitation and ion-exchange chromatography, to give almost pure antibody. By binding assays on cells of known HLA type and inhibition of binding by purified HLA antigens, the two monoclonal antibodies show the same pattern of reactivities as the HLA-A2 and HLA-B7 types defined by conventional serology.

Our previous work was limited to HLA-A2-incompatible pregnancies in which the mother was HLA-A2 negative, partly because of the need to conserve the antiserum. With the monoclonals this limitation is removed, and it is reasonable to sort for unlabeled fetal cells in a sample of maternal mononuclear cells that stain with the antibody. This doubles the fraction of mother–fetus pairs that are appropriate for fetal cell selection. With an HLA-A2 gene frequency of about 25%, fetal cell selection based on an HLA-A2 difference should be possible in about 28% of pregnancies.[4] For HLA-B7 with a gene frequency of about 8% the sortable fraction is 14%. A battery of perhaps 5 or 10 of such reagents would make it possible to select for fetal cells in most (but not all) pregnancies.

We have compared several two-step staining procedures with these reagents, including the use of fluorescein-conjugated whole goat anti-mouse-IgG1 and F(ab')2 of this as second steps. We have also used biotin-conjugated forms of the monoclonal anti-HLAs with fluorescein-conjugated avidin as a second step (Bayer and Wilchek, 1978). For our purposes it is not staining brightness or staining specificity per se that is important, but rather the ability to discriminate a few (fetal) cells of one type from a large heterogeneous population of another. To test the staining reagents, each was titrated for staining of cells of the appropriate type and of cells that should be negative. Fluorescence histograms for each sample were collected on the FACS and analyzed by positive–negative pairs with the same reagents and concentrations.

To optimize the titrations and compare one reagent to another, we used computer analysis of the histograms to ask, "If a few of this kind of cell had been mixed with a large number of that kind of cell and the mixture sorted for cells in a particular fluorescence range, what fraction of the few cells would we expect to recover, and what enrichment of these cells would we expect in the sorted fraction compared to the original mixture?" A single optimizing measure or Figure of Merit was obtained by weighting the factors of fractional recovery and enrichment equally. Sample results are shown in Fig. 2 for a biotin–avidin stain and a goat anti-mouse immunoglobulin second-step stain. The optimum in each case occurs with the "sort" fraction, including a little less than 1% of the nondesired cells, but the Figure of Merit is four times higher for the biotin–avidin stain. The set of such analyses showed that the biotin–avidin system was superior to the anti-mouse Ig second steps tested, even though its staining brightness was not as great as with some of the second-step antisera. In these tests the anti-HLA-A2 performed better than the anti-HLA-B7 because background staining levels were comparable, whereas the anti-HLA-A2 staining brightness was more than twice that of the anti-HLA-B7. This may reflect a real difference in average antigen density or may be due to differences in the monoclonal antibody affinities.

The reagent analysis was extended by sorting from actual mixtures of adult blood mononuclear cells at ratios of one to several thousand. In order to minimize postsorting variables, the "rare" cells were prelabeled with the UV-excited DNA-labeling dye Hoechst 33342 (Arndt-Jovin and Jovin, 1977). This is a viable cell dye and is totally invisible under the 488-nm laser illumination used to excite fluorescein in the FACS. These cells were then mixed with unlabeled

---

[4]Assuming random assortment, the relationship between gene frequency (f) and total sortable cases is: fraction sortable $= 2f(1 - f)^2$.

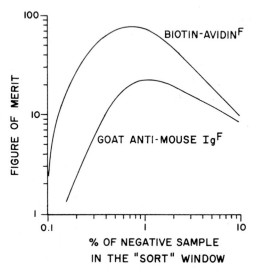

FIG. 2.   Comparison of the quality of two-step stains for fetal cell enrichment. Adult blood mononuclear cell populations positive and negative for HLA-A2 were stained by different two-step procedures, using the monoclonal anti-HLA-A2 first step. Each cell sample was analyzed on the FACS to yield a computerized data set of cell frequencies versus cell fluorescence. For various simulated sorting ranges in fluorescence, the fraction of the HLA-A2$^-$ cell population (fNeg) and the fraction of the HLA-A2$^+$ population (fPos) that would have been sorted were calculated. The Figure of Merit for the expected quality of a sorting of rare HLA-A2$^+$ cells from a mixture of the two is as follows:

Figure of Merit = (Estimated enrichment factor for rare cells) × (Fraction of the rare cells
in the sort window)
= (fPos)^2/fNeg

The figure plots the Figure of Merit as a function of fNeg.

cells with an appropriate HLA difference, and the mixture was stained with the appropriate anti-HLA reagent at the optimal concentration indicated by the previous testing. Mixtures in which the "rare" cells should be stained and those in which the "rare" cells should be unstained and the majority stained were both tested. Cells with the appropriate fluorescence for "rare" cells were sorted with the FACS and collected into small wells mounted on microscope coverglasses. An inverted fluorescence microscope with appropriate excitation and emission filters was used to count Hoechst 33342-labeled cells and other cells in each well. In the course of such experiments each prelabeled cell retains most of its Hoechst 33342, and no other cell absorbs enough of what is released to cause any confusion. Data taken with biotin–avidin staining are shown in Table II.

The biotin–avidin system gave better results than other two-step stains. Such tests also indicated that sorting for unstained fetal cells should be as good as

TABLE II

Results of Sorts from Mixtures of HLA-A2[+] and HLA-A2[−] Cells

	Mixture HLA-A2[+]/HLA-A2[−] (cells:cells)	Recovery[a]	Purity[b]	Figure of Merit[c]
Sort for bright cells	1:2900	33%	63%	600
Sort for unstained cells	4500:1	58%	24%	625

[a] Percentage of the "rare" cells run that were recovered in the sorted fraction.
[b] Percentage of sorted cells that were of the "rare" type, i.e., labeled with Hoechst 33342.
[c] Equals the product of the enrichment factor (e.g., 2900 × 0.63) and the recovery factor (e.g., 0.33).

sorting for stained fetal cells. In fact, we have now selected Y-body-positive cells from the blood of pregnant women by sorting unstained cells when the woman was HLA-A2 positive.

So far, however, the frequency of fetal cells in enriched fractions sorted with the monoclonal reagents has been similar to that found with the rabbit anti-HLA-A2. Tests using blood samples from nonpregnant persons have shown a number of stained (or unstained) cells comparable to that found with our pregnant subjects. Sorting and FACS reanalysis of such cells has demonstrated that most of them are in fact being measured correctly by the FACS. Fluorescence microscopy on such "improperly stained" cells shows some artifacts, but the staining pattern of a large fraction of the cells looks like that of properly stained cells. The sources of this limitation on staining specificity are under investigation. It is even possible that individuals express histocompatibility antigens different from their nominal HLA types on a small fraction of cells as a result of genetic variation.

B. Antitrophoblast Monoclonal Antibodies

The ideal way to select fetal cells would be with antibody to a fetal antigen not found on any adult blood mononuclear cells. We are exploring the possibility that the fetal cells in maternal blood include trophoblast cells. Monoclonal antibodies were produced by immunizing BALB/cN mice with human choriocarcinoma cells of the BeWo line and fusing their spleen cells with the mouse myeloma line NS-1 (Lipinski et al., 1981). Culture fluid from each of many subcultures was tested by radioimmunoassay for antibody reacting with BeWo cells. Those that showed such activity were tested by two-step immunofluorescent staining and FACS analysis for antibody binding to human red and white blood cells and platelets. Hybridoma cells from interesting subcultures, particularly those that had antibody activity to BeWo cells but not to blood cells, were cloned with the

FACS. In this application the FACS deposits single viable cells (with or without selection for fluorescent markers) in the wells of microculture plates containing "feeder" cells. This is a rapid and efficient cloning method (Parks *et al.*, 1979). This work has now yielded two trophoblast-specific monoclonal antibodies (Lipinski *et al.*, 1981).

We have begun to test several of the antibodies as immunofluorescent-staining reagents on samples of blood mononuclear cells from pregnant women. Sorting labeled cells and examining the sorted fraction for enrichment of Y-body-positive cells will show whether these antibodies selectively mark the fetal cells. Although significant results are not as yet available, these trophoblast-specific monoclonal antibodies will be useful in establishing whether fetal cells in maternal blood include cells from this tissue and should allow their routine sorting if they are there.

The other obvious possibility for obtaining fetal cell-specific antibodies is to immunize mice with human fetal blood cells and attempt to obtain monoclonal antibodies that react with fetal but not adult blood cells. Specific fetal leukocyte-differentiation antigens have not yet been described in humans, but it is worth a serious attempt with monoclonal antibody techniques. Yet another possibility for general fetal cell selection with male fetuses would be a good anti-H-Y-staining antibody. Although monoclonal antibodies to H-Y do exist (Koo and Hammerling, personal communication), so far they do not seem to be sufficiently selective of male cells for our purposes.

C. Better Fetal Cell Characterization

Increasing our knowledge of the characteristics of the fetal cells is difficult because the processing for QM Y-body analysis results in identified fetal cells that are not only dead but are even unsuitable for ordinary morphological observation. More information about their surface markers is needed for designing efficient selection procedures, and further, successful culturing to obtain karyotypes will be helped by knowledge of the exact origin of the fetal cells.

To investigate the surface antigens of the fetal cells while continuing to rely on the Y-body-identification technique, we plan to carry out FACS selection based on pairs of different fluorescent stains. One will be a proven selective stain such as antibody to paternal HLA, and the other will mark an antigen whose presence on the fetal cells we want to assess. Using different fluorescent dyes for the two stains a fetal cell-enriched fraction defined with reference to paternal HLA staining can be subdivided on the basis of staining for the second antigen. The staining pattern of the fetal cells for the second marker is then indicated by which sorted subfraction(s) yield Y-chromatin-positive cells on subsequent examination. Comparison of these results with analyses of fetal tissues such as blood and placenta stained with the same characterizing antibodies will help to identify the origin of the fetal cells. The fetal cell-characterization data will also be used to devise efficient two-reagent selection procedures to give higher purity fetal cell-enriched fractions.

Double-staining experiments are possible with our present FACS system in which both fluorescein and tetramethylrhodamine dyes can be excited by mixed laser light at 488 nm and 514.5 nm. The two fluorochromes are measured separately by a combination of optical filtering and electronic manipulation of the signals from two detectors (Loken et al., 1977). However, the compromises and signal losses required for such measurements are a problem. This is especially true when monoclonal antibody reagents are used, because their monospecific binding tends to give clean but not bright staining.

To avoid such difficulties we are adding a tunable dye laser (Arndt-Jovin et al., 1980) to our FACS system. It will be used together with the usual argon-ion laser to excite two dyes separately and optimally, thus allowing better measurements on doubly stained cells. With this we expect to retain the normal enrichment efficiency of the regular selective stain while using the second independent stain for defining subfractions.

VII.   Fetal Red Blood Cell Transfer

A.   Human Rh D-Antigen Labeling

We have been associated with Drs. Paul Hensleigh and Arnold Medearis, Department of Gynecology/Obstetrics, Stanford University, in a project assessing the frequency and amount of fetal–maternal hemorrhage during pregnancy and investigating the effect of procedures such as amniocentesis (Medearis et al., 1980). The concern arises from the risk of maternal or fetal isoimmunization, particularly for Rh D, through such hemorrhage. The experimental objective is to do accurate quantitation of transferred cells when they occur at frequencies as low as 1:100,000 by differentially labeling maternal and fetal cells for erythrocyte-expressed polymorphisms and using the FACS to analyze the staining and to sort rare labeled cells (Jan and Herzenberg, 1973).

To date the work has focused on the Rh D (rhesus) antigen. The procedure is to stain erythrocytes from an Rh D⁻ woman with a commercial high-titer human anti-D serum followed by a fluoresceinated goat anti-human immunoglobulin second step. The sample is run on the FACS and examined for the presence of stained erythrocytes. The second-step antiserum will label B-lymphocytes and monocytes in the sample, but they can be excluded from the analysis because they give larger light-scatter signals than erythrocytes.

Under optimal staining conditions a population of only a few in 100,000 can be seen and counted as a definable stained population after several million cells have been analyzed (Jan and Herzenberg, 1973). The count of labeled erythrocytes can be verified and extended to lower frequencies by sorting the cells that give appropriate light-scatter and fluorescence signals into a small medium-filled well mounted on a microscope coverglass. Gentle centrifugation to bring the cells to the coverglass and examination with an inverted fluorescence microscope make it possible to distinguish between properly labeled erythrocytes and artifacts, because the vast majority of artifacts are not erythrocytes at all and/or do not show the correct staining pattern on the cell.

In the initial survey, samples from Rh D^- women were drawn near term and examined for the presence of Rh D^+ red cells. They were found in all 11 patients who delivered Rh D^+ babies; the frequencies ranged from 1:4000 to 1:80,000 with an average of about 1:25,000 when the baby was ABO compatible with the mother (10 cases). The average frequency corresponds to a transfer of about 200 μl of fetal blood to the mother's circulation (taking the average maternal blood volume to be about 5 liters).

The sensitivity and accuracy of this technique will make it possible to monitor for effects of clinical procedures such as amniocentesis and to follow the decline of fetal erythrocyte frequency after delivery.

B.   Rhesus Monkey Model

We have carried out several experiments to measure the amount and kinetics of the transfer of fetal erythrocytes into maternal circulation in a monkey model. The work has been carried out in collaboration with Drs. Arthur Malley and Miles J. Novy of the Oregon Regional Primate Center, Beaverton, Oregon. The surgical preparations were initiated for experimental work requiring measurement of hormone levels in maternal and fetal blood. The experiments were performed on rhesus monkeys (*Macaca mulatta*) pregnant 120–135 days (term is 167 days). Our work was started only after the animals were stabilized and we could be confident that no fetal–maternal blood contact was resulting from the surgical procedure.

After the surgery to chronically catheterize the maternal and fetal circulations, a fetal blood sample amounting to about 3% of the blood supply was drawn. The cells were labeled with fluorescein isothiocyanate (FITC) and returned to the fetus. Small samples of fetal blood were withdrawn periodically to measure the fraction of labeled cells and to confirm that it was relatively constant. We expected that fetal cells entering the maternal circulation would not be cleared rapidly because labeled fetal cells injected into unrelated adults circulated with little loss for at least 3 days. Samples of maternal blood were drawn periodically and analyzed for the presence of labeled fetal cells.

Before running maternal samples on the FACS we measured the fluorescence of the labeled cells in the fetal samples in order to select the correct brightness range for sorting from the maternal samples. Having access to two FACS machines, we avoided any risk of contamination of the maternal samples with leftover fetal cells by running the fetal samples on one machine and the maternal

TABLE III

TRANSFER OF LABELED FETAL ERYTHROCYTES TO MATERNAL CIRCULATION

Experiment no.	Time after return of labeled cells		
	0–3 hours	24 hours	3–4 days
1	0/6[a]	5/134	
2	0/75	1–4[b]/75	32/75
3	0/100	3/100	4/100
4	0/200	0/200	1/200

[a] Number of labeled cells observed/millions of maternal cells examined.

[b] Due to the low brightness of labeling in this experiment, three fluorescent cells were found whose fluorescence could not be confirmed as being the same color as that of the fluorescein label.

samples on the other. The maternal samples were run at about 30,000 cells per second (10^8 cells per hour), with the analysis circuitry threshold set to process only the few hundred most fluorescent objects per second. Those objects with fluorescence and light-scatter characteristics comparable to the labeled fetal cells were sorted into small wells filled with medium mounted on microscope coverglasses. After gentle centrifugation the sorted cells were examined with an inverted fluorescence microscope to identify erythrocytes with the uniform green fluorescence characteristic of the FITC-labeled cells.

The results of four experiments are summarized in Table III. Maternal blood samples were drawn (1) before or shortly after the return of the labeled fetal cells, (2) at about 24 hours, and (3) at 3 to 4 days. Labeled fetal cells were found in very small numbers in most of the maternal samples taken 1 to 4 days after the return of labeled cells to the fetus. Correction for cell losses in the sorting and confirmation process might double the observed frequencies.

Although the numbers of labeled fetal cells observed have been small, they indicate the magnitude of the blood transfer from the fetal to maternal circulation. Calculating back from the above data and the approximate 5000-ml maternal blood volume gives transfer rates in the range from 0 to 2 μl/day. The low but usually detectable rate of transfer implies that the placental barrier is only slightly compromised by direct blood flow.

VIII. Summary

We have demonstrated that fetal cells can be selected from maternal blood using appropriate reagents and the FACS. However, in the nucleated cell work the original techniques lacked generality and yielded sorted fractions in which the fetal cells were still a small minority. We are approaching this problem from several directions, including the use of monoclonal antibodies and improved staining procedures for paternal HLA, development of monoclonal antibodies to human trophoblast antigens, and use of double-staining techniques.

Besides improving the selection of fetal cells from maternal blood, this work will help to characterize such cells so that appropriate culture conditions can be chosen and information suitable for prenatal diagnosis obtained. We hope such techniques will be developed into a form suitable for prenatal diagnosis on a routine clinical basis.

In addition, FACS-based techniques are proving to be useful in investigations of fetal–maternal transfer of erythrocytes.

ACKNOWLEDGMENTS

In addition to the authors of Herzenberg et al. (1979) and Lipinski et al. (1981), work on the project as a whole has included Dr. Paul Hensleigh, Dr. Roman Malvehy, Ms. Jenny Scott, Ms. Virginia Bryan, Mrs. Jennifer Royce, Dr. Carol Greene, and Mr. Eugene Filson.

REFERENCES

Arndt-Jovin, D. J., and Jovin, T. M. (1977). *J. Histochem. Cytochem.* **25**, 585–589.
Arndt-Jovin, D. J., Grimwade, B. G., and Jovin, T. M. (1980). *Cytometry* **1**, 127–131.
Bayer, E., and Wilchek, M. (1978). *Trends in Biochem. Sci.* **3**, N257–N259.
Brodsky, F. M., Parham, P., Barnstable, C. J., Crumpton, M. J., and Bodmer, W. F. (1979). *Immunol. Rev.* **47**, 3–61.
Caspersson, T., and Zech, L. (1970). *Science* **170**, 762.
Caspersson, T., Lindsten, J., Lomakka, G., Moller, A., and Zech, L. (1972). *Int. Rev. Exp. Pathol.* **11**, 1–72.
de Grouchy, J., and Trebuchet, C. (1971). *Ann. Genet.* **14**, 133–137.
Grosset, L., Barrelet, V., Odartchenko, N. (1974). *Am. J. Obstet. Gynecol.* **120**, 60–63.
Herzenberg, L. A., and Herzenberg, L. A. (1978). *In* "Handbook of Experimental Immunology" 3rd Edition (D. M. Weir, ed.), pp. 22.1–22.21 Blackwell, Oxford.
Herzenberg, L. A., Sweet, R. G., and Herzenberg, L. A. (1976). *Sci. Am.* **234**, 108–117.
Herzenberg, L. A., Bianchi, D. W., Schröder, J., Cann, H. M., and Iverson, G. M. (1979). *Proc. Natl. Acad. Sci. U.S.A.* **76**, 1453–1455.
Holbrook, D. A., and Tishler, P. V. (1980). *Cytogenet. Cell Genet.* **26**, 59–60.
Holmes, L. B. (1978). *N. Engl. J. Med.* **298**, 1419–1421.
Hulett, H. R., Bonner, W. A., Sweet, R. G., and Herzenberg, L. A. (1973). *Clin. Chem.* **19**, 813–816.
Iverson, G. M., Bianchi, D. W., Cann, H. M., and Herzenberg, L. A. (1981). *J. Prenatal Diagnosis* **1**, 61–73.
Jan, W. H., and Herzenberg, L. A. (1973). Presentation at SAMA-UTMB National Student Research Forum, Galveston, Texas, April 24–28.
Latt, S. A., Brodie, S., and Munroe, S. H. (1974). *Chromosoma* **49**, 17–40.

Lipinski, M., Parks, D. R., Rouse, R. V., and Herzenberg, L. A. (1981). *Proc. Natl. Acad. Sci. U.S.A.* **78**, 5147-5150.

Loken, M. R., Parks, D. R., and Herzenberg, L. A. (1977). *J. Histochem. Cytochem.* **25**, 899-907.

Medearis, A. L., Hensleigh, P. A., and Herzenberg, L. A. (1980). Presentation at 27th Annual Meeting, Society for Gynecologic Investigation, Denver.

Mukjerjee, A. B., Moser, G. C., and Nitowsky, H. M. (1972). *Cytogenetics* **11**, 216-227.

Parks, D. R., Bryan, V. M., Oi, V. T., and Herzenberg, L. A. (1979) *Proc. Natl. Acad. Sci. U.S.A.* **76**, 1962-1966.

Pearson, P. L., Bobrow, M., and Vosa, C. G. (1970). *Nature* **226**, 78-80.

Robb, R. J., Humphreys, R. E., Strominger, J. L., Fuller, T. C., and Mann, D. L. (1975). *Transplantation* **19**, 445-447.

Schindler, A. M., Graf, E., and Martin-du-Pan, R. (1972). *Obstet. Gynecol.* **40**, 340-346.

Schröder, J. (1975), *J. Med. Genet.* **12**, 230-242.

Schröder, J., and de la Chapelle, A. (1972). *J. Hematol.* **39**, 153-162.

Schröder, J. P., and Herzenberg, L. A. (1980). *In* "Genetic Disorders of the Fetus: Diagnosis, Prevention and Treatment" (A. Milunsky, ed.), pp. 541-555. Plenum, New York.

Schröder, J., Tiilikainen, A., and de la Chapelle, A. (1974). *Transplantation* **17**, 346-360.

Siebers, J. W., Knauf, I., and Hillemanns, H. G. (1975). *Humangenetik* **28**, 273-280.

Walknowska, J., Conte, F. A., and Grumbach, M. M. (1969). *Lancet* **1**, 1119-1122.

Zilliacus, R., de la Chapelle, A., Schröder, J., Tiilikainen, A., Kohne, E., and Kleihauer, E. (1975). *Scand. J. Haematol.* **15**, 333-338.

Chapter 11

Application of Cell-Fusion Techniques to Induce Amniotic Fluid Cells to Express Special Functions and for Complementation Analysis

GRETCHEN J. DARLINGTON

Division of Human Genetics
Department of Medicine
Cornell University Medical College
New York, New York

I. Introduction

Amniotic fluid cells obtained from second-trimester pregnancies have been used to diagnose chromosomal abnormalities, inherited enzyme defects, and hemoglobin abnormalities. Most diseases that may be diagnosed prenatally are those whose gene products are expressed ubiquitously in cells of the body including amniotic fluid cells. In general, tissue-specific genes have not been accessible for examination because these loci are not active in amniocytes. Globin is one

297

tissue-specific gene that can be assessed. In this case the DNA-sequence coding for this erythrocyte protein is examined directly (see Chap. 12).

Another approach to examining specialized genes and their products in amniotic fluid cells utilizes the technique of somatic cell hybridization. Several investigators have reported the expression of tissue-specific genes in hybrids between a differentiated rodent tumor line and a cell type of a different histogenetic origin (cf. Davidson, 1974; Darlington and Ruddle, 1975; Bernhard, 1976). For example, Peterson and Weiss (1972) demonstrated the production of mouse albumin in hybrids between a line of rat hepatoma cells and mouse fibroblasts. The rat line expressed rat albumin in the unfused state but the murine cells did not produce mouse albumin. This phenomenon of expression of the homologous specialized gene product from the ''undifferentiated'' parental genome was termed activation.

Several other studies have suggested that activation is frequently observed in both intra- and interspecific cell hybrids. In an intraspecific fusion, the γ-globin of mouse teratocarcinoma origin was expressed by hybrids between this germ cell tumor line and Friend erythroleukemia cells (McBurney et al., 1978). Mouse albumin was produced by mouse lymphoid cell $\times$ rat hepatoma crosses (Malawista and Weiss, 1974), and mouse tyrosine aminotransferase and aldolase B, two other liver-specific loci, were activated in these same hybrids (Brown and Weiss, 1975). From these studies, the array of genes activated in cell hybrids would seem to be broad.

In addition to rodent $\times$ rodent hybrids, rodent $\times$ human crosses have been studied. The expression of human albumin in mouse hepatoma human leukocyte hybrids was reported in 1974 (Darlington et al., 1974). The rodent parent expressed a number of liver-specific functions in vitro (Darlington et al., 1980). These included mouse serum albumin, transferrin, alpha-fetoprotein, ceruloplasmin, and alpha-1-antitrypsin (alpha-1-AT). The human parental cell was a diploid peripheral lymphocyte. Subsequently, we have examined many cell types and have found that fibroblasts, amniocytes, lymphoblastoid cells, and fetal hepatocytes all express human hepato-specific genes following hybridization to mouse hepatoma cells. Furthermore, several human proteins (albumin, transferrin, ceruloplasmin, and alpha-1-AT) were produced by hybrids from human amniocytes (Rankin and Darlington, 1979). The frequency and type of activated hybrids is shown in Table I. The fact that human amniotic fluid cells can express these genes following cell fusion suggests the usefulness of hybridization as a tool for prenatal diagnosis of defects in hepato-specific loci.

Other specialized human gene products have also been observed in hybrids, although in these studies fibroblasts or leukocytes rather than amniotic fluid cells have been used as the human parent. Willing et al. (1979) have described the production of human γ-globin in hybrids between the Friend erythroleukemic line and human fibroblasts. Interestingly, these interspecific hybrids did not

TABLE I

Frequency of Activated Mouse Hepatoma × Human
Amniocyte Hybrids[a,b]

Protein secreted	No. of colonies
Colonies secreting	
no human proteins	26
Albumin	17
Alpha-1-AT	6
Transferrin	3
Ceruloplasmin	7
Haptoglobin	0

[a] From Rankin and Darlington (1979).

[b] The total number of hybrids examined was 55. Twenty-nine expressed one or more human serum proteins. Four clones secreted two human products.

produce γ-globin, the form of globin expressed during gestation. Schwaber and Cohen (1973) also observed the expression of a differentiated human gene product, the kappa chain of immunoglobulin and the γ-heavy chain. The rodent tumor line was a mouse myeloma, whereas the human parent cells were peripheral leukocytes. It is unclear whether or not this study is an example of activation as the human cell may well have had the capacity to synthesize immunoglobulin.

From published work, it seems likely that activation of a variety of genes that ordinarily are not expressed in amniocytes may occur in hybrid cells. The extent of genes subject to activation is unknown. However, some loci appear to be refractile to activation, for example the γ-locus of globin (Willing *et al.*, 1979) and alpha-fetoprotein (Darlington *et al.*, 1982b). Both of these genes are expressed during fetal development but decline in synthetic activity, reaching low levels shortly after birth. These findings suggest that temporally expressed genes may fall under a different mode of regulation, one that does not permit turn-on in the hybrid cell.

Although several systems would appear amenable for use in prenatal testing, to date I know of no example of a disorder diagnosed using this approach. My own interests have centered on the diagnosis of alpha-1-AT deficiency and I will discuss the methodology that we are devising to test for this and other hepatic disorders as an example of the usefulness of this system. Clearly other genes expressed by other tissues and organs may well require different assays and different culture conditions than those described here.

A second goal of this article is to enumerate the disorders in which complementation analysis has been performed. Complementation between cells from

individuals with inherited diseases has been used to define the genetic
heterogeneity of conditions that present a clinically similar picture. Cell fusion is
used for these studies as well as for gene activation, and it is the technology that
links the two topics in this article.

II.   Methodologic Approaches to Prenatal Testing Using Cell Hybrids

A.   Development of Differentiated Rodent Cell Lines

There exists in the cell culture laboratories of the world a host of established
rodent cell lines, which continue to express tissue-specific products *in vitro*. The
compilation of Naval Biosciences Laboratory[1] and the Linscotts' catalog[2] citing
cell lines of different species are helpful manuals. The reason for choosing a
rodent parental line as opposed to another one of human origin is that the gene
products can be distinguished from one another due to speciation. Established
human lines might also be acceptable provided the gene products in question
differ between the amniocyte and the immortal human parent. Nonsenescing or
established lines are also likely to be most successful because the hybrid may
require several generations of proliferation before analysis. We have used a
murine hepatoma in our laboratory that was adapted to *in vitro* growth following
the procedure of Buonassisi and co-workers (1962), which called for alternate *in
vivo/in vitro* passage of the tumor cells. This procedure appears to work well for
tumors that grow rapidly in the animal but may not be useful for tumors that
proliferate slowly *in vivo*.

Important characteristics of the rodent tumor line include the following:

1. The stable retention of the expression of differentiated phenotypes. The
importance of this trait might seem to be obvious to the reader. In actuality, it has
not been established that the expression of a particular gene in the rodent parent is
essential for its expression by the hybrid. In fact, McMorris and Ruddle (1974)
described the appearance of choline acetyltransferase activity in hybrids between
mouse neuroblastoma cells and human fibroblasts, neither of which had activity
for this enzyme in the unfused state. Evidence that activation is dependent on
expression by one parental cell type is circumstantial. Considering a large
number of studies together, the vast majority of the specialized products pro-

---

[1]"Catalog of Human and Other Animal Cell Cultures," Naval BioSciences Laboratory, Naval
Supply Center, Oakland, California 94625.
[2]Linscott, W. D., and Linscott, N. "Linscotts' Catalog of Immunologic Reagents," 40 Glen
Drive, Mill Valley, California 94941.

duced by hybrids were also expressed by the rodent tumor line. However, few other traits were examined in the hybrids. For example, globin was not assayed in the hepatoma hybrids we studied, and it is probable that the serum proteins were not examined in the mouse erythroleukemia fusion products. However, it would seem logical to assume that the expression of a tissue-specific gene in the rodent cell would ensure that all the appropriate mechanisms for processing, secretion, and so forth would be functional, thus increasing the likelihood of the human product being observed in the hybrid.

2. The parental line should be karyotypically stable and not generate hybrids with rapid loss or rearrangement of the human genome. Mouse × human hybrids lose human chromosomes preferentially. The trait of a stable karyotype is a highly desirable one, but one that cannot be predicted or manipulated. One potential cause of chromosome instability is mycoplasma infection (Fogh and Fogh, 1965; Aula and Nichols, 1967); this can be identified and, with precautions, avoided. The problem created by rapid chromosome loss and/or rearrangement is simply that the human gene of interest will be present in only a few hybrid cells unless either there is a syntenic marker for which selection can be applied, or the hybrids retain a large subset of the human genome with slow random loss of human chromosomes.

3. The rodent line should be hyperdiploid. This trait may not be essential to the activation of the human genome; however, considerable evidence from studies of the FU-5 rat hepatoma suggests that gene dosage influences the frequency of this phenomenon. For example when Malawista and Weiss (1974) compared a stem cell line of the rat hepatoma ($2S$ Faza; S stands for stem cell chromosome number) that had a hypertetraploid number of chromosomes to the $1S$ line, the frequency of activated clones was considerably greater for the $2S$ derivatives. Furthermore, when the gene-dosage relationships favored the differentiated rat hepatoma parent, the expression of rat hepatic enzymes (tyrosine aminotransferase, aldolase B, and alcohol dehydrogenase) and the activation of the mouse form of these enzymes were found.

4. The line should contain an enzyme deficiency or genetic marker that permits selection. Following fusion of the rodent line with human amniocytes it is necessary to select the true hybrid from the population of unfused parental cells. The most commonly used selection protocol calls for the introduction of an enzyme deficiency in the rodent parent line. Deficiencies for hypoxanthine phosphoribosyltransferase, thymidine kinase (Littlefield, 1964), and adenosine phosphoribosyltransferase (Kusano and Green, 1971) have been most universally employed.

The isolation of the mutant enzyme-deficient line is accomplished by treating a mass population of cells with a cytotoxic analog of the enzyme substrate. Cells lacking the enzyme do not incorporate the analog and proliferate in its presence. Several other selectable markers have proven useful in Chinese hamster ovary cells (Puck, 1976), and are generated in a different fashion. Human amniocytes are cultured prior to fusion in order to generate a population with a high percentage of viable cells.

B.   Generation of Hybrid Cells

The scheme for the production of hybrids is shown in Fig. 1.

Cell lines vary considerably in their sensitivity to both Sendai virus and polyethylene glycol (PEG), two agents that have been used extensively for cell fusion. We have employed PEG almost exclusively in recent years, but testing the differentiated parent for the degree of fusion and toxicity with both agents is recommended, varying time of exposure and concentration of the fusogen. A

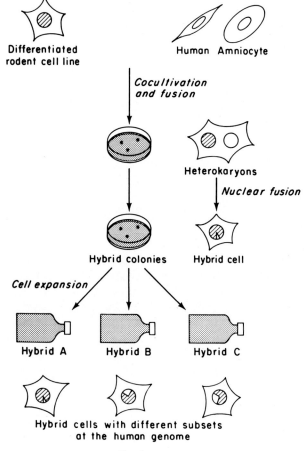

Fig. 1

detailed account of the preparation and use of Sendai virus is given by Giles and Ruddle (1973), and the description of Davidson and Gerald (1976) and Davidson et al. (1976) for the use of PEG is informative.

Following fusion, the mixture of human cells and hybrids is placed in selective medium. Unfused parental rodent cells are eliminated by nutritional deprivation of purines or pyrimidines (see Littlefield, 1964; Kusano and Green, 1971), and the human cells may be selectively killed by the addition of $10^{-6} M$ ouabain (Baker et al, 1974). Rodent cells are inherently resistant to ouabain at the 10^{-4} to $10^{-5} M$ level, and this resistance is a dominant trait. Hybrids survive by receiving normal enzyme activity from the human parent and resistance to ouabain from the mouse.

C.   Selection or Screen for Hybrids Producing the Specialized Gene Product of Interest

Once hybrid colonies arise in the culture dish, it is possible to isolate, expand, and examine them for the production of human gene products. It is this step of clonal isolation and cell proliferation that is time-consuming, labor-intensive, and expensive.

It would be preferable to have either an efficient screening system for small numbers of cells or the ability to select for the phenotype of interest. One example of each type has been considered by us and will be described.

A screen for secreted proteins has been developed for murine albumin (Sammons et al., 1980). We are presently trying to adapt this procedure to the detection of human proteins, especially alpha-1-AT. In general the human proteins are secreted at lower levels (1–10%) than the mouse products. The protocol for screening colonies for secreted protein is shown in Fig. 2. The principle is that hybrid colonies secreting human alpha-1-AT will be identified at the 300- to 500-cell stage by overlaying the colonies with 1% agarose containing anti-human alpha-1-AT. The antibody in the agarose and the antigen secreted by the cells form a precipitin complex above the colony. We have established that there is no cross-reactivity between the anti-human alpha-1-AT (Kallestad, Chaska, Minn.) and any proteins secreted by the mouse cells. Colonies that do not secrete human alpha-1-AT will not have an immunologic reaction in the agar. The ability to unequivocally distinguish the human gene product from that of the mouse is essential. The agar patty is removed, washed, and stained with a protein stain to identify the protein–antibody complexes, thereby identifying clones that secrete alpha-1-AT. These hybrid colonies can be isolated and examined by Pi typing (Fagerhol and Laurell, 1970) or two-dimensional electrophoresis for the isozymic form of alpha-1-AT in order to discriminate the abnormal ZZ variant from the normal M isozyme.

This theoretical protocol has several technical problems that need to be ad-

IMMUNO-OVERLAY PROCEDURE FOR HYBRID
CELLS SECRETING HUMAN PROTEINS

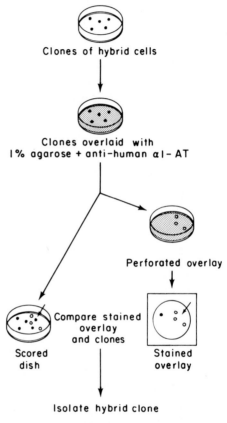

FIG. 2

dressed before actual testing can begin. The first is the sensitivity of the overlay procedure for identifying secreting clones. It should be possible to increase the sensitivity of the overlay by an additional step employing ^{125}I-labeled protein A from *Staphylococcus aureus* or second antibody. A second problem is whether or not the ZZ protein would be secreted by the cells at all. There is evidence that in the hepatocytes of ZZ alpha-1-AT deficient individuals, alpha-1-AT accumulates (Eriksson and Larsson, 1975). The low level of alpha-1-AT in serum may be due to a failure of the protein to be secreted. We are examining this question by studying hybrids formed from the lymphocytes of a ZZ patient. To date, two clones that contain chromosome 14, to which alpha-1-AT has been assigned

(Darlington *et al.*, 1982a; Croce *et al.*, 1979), do not secrete human alpha-1-AT. Intracellular levels are being examined.

Another gene of potential interest for prenatal diagnosis is phenylalanine hydroxylase. A deficiency of this liver-specific enzyme is associated with phenylketonuria (PKU), an autosomal recessive disorder that leads to severe mental retardation unless treated soon after birth by dietary restriction of phenylalanine. Although the importance of identifying PKU individuals may be debated because there is a mechanism for neonatal screening in most states and a treatment for the disease, it is offered as an example of a selectable enzyme defect.

Hepatocytes have activity for phenylalanine hydroxylase as do some hepatoma lines (Haggerty *et al.*, 1975; Choo *et al.*, 1980), although many, including the Hepa mouse hepatoma, do not (D. F. Haggerty, personal communication). This enzyme converts phenylalanine to tyrosine, an essential amino acid for cell growth. Medium containing phenylalanine but lacking tyrosine should permit the growth of only those cells containing the liver enzyme. By selecting a hepatoma line that does not itself produce phenylalanine hydroxylase, it may be possible to obtain activated hybrids expressing the human form of the enzyme. The major question that must be addressed in this theoretical protocol is whether or not this enzyme will be activated or expressed in the hybrids if the differentiated parent does not produce it.

Comparing screening procedures for assay of gene products with selection systems, the immuno-overlay technique has perhaps greater potential because many proteins can be used to generate specific antisera. The number of selectable genes is limited. Even intracellular production of the product may be detected by mixing the clones and using immunofluorescent techniques. Replicate plating of hybrid clones would permit the retention of a viable hybrid population for expansion when the detection assay kills the cells. Monoclonal antibodies may have sufficient specificity to discriminate the normal from the abnormal protein in some disorders where cross-reacting material is present.

Controls for the detection of activated proteins would of course include hybrids with normal amniocytes assayed simultaneously. In the instance where selection is applied for activated enzymes, a failure to observe growth of hybrids could be due to either a defective enzyme or a technical failure to obtain hybrids. It is consequently important to include positive controls in the assay.

III. Potential Problems with Using Cell Hybrids for Prenatal Diagnosis

Some of the specific problems to be faced when considering the use of cell hybrids for antenatal diagnosis have already been mentioned. More general difficulties will be mentioned now.

Perhaps the major drawback in this system is the length of time the assay requires. A minimum of 6 weeks is required for the test, if one allows 10 days for amniocyte expansion plus 2 weeks for hybrid colonies to form and an additional 2 weeks for hybrid cell expansion and analysis.

Some possibilities can be explored for reducing this time period, including using amniotic fluid cells without an *in vitro* expansion period. This may require a larger volume of fluid than is presently used for karyotypic analysis. It may also be possible to analyze hybrid colonies at the 500- to 1000-cell stage without further expansion. The development of microassays for specific proteins would be important in this regard. Another approach is the use of heterokaryons (multinucleate cells generated by cytoplasmic fusion) as opposed to hybrids. The examination of the heterokaryon can be done within a short time after fusion, eliminating the time required for growth of hybrid cells. Relatively few studies of differentiated gene expression have been done using heterokaryons (see Ringertz and Savage, 1976), and the effects of gene dosage have not been examined. Gene-dosage relationships are likely to be quite important in heterokaryons where chromosomal segregation does not occur and entire genomes remain intact in the cell.

A second concern for the use of somatic cell hybrids as a diagnostic tool is the possibility that the genes in question will not be turned on at a high frequency. Our own findings suggest that whereas albumin is found in 31% of amniocyte hybrids, only 5% expressed transferrin. Given a limited number of amniocytes and a low frequency of hybrid cell formation, a small number of hybrid colonies might not give informative data.

In addition to the problem of having a low frequency of activated hybrid clones, one may face the problem of low levels of human protein in the hybrids that are activated. Although the levels vary from clone to clone, we have found that on the average the hybrids express the human product at a level less than 10% of the amount of mouse protein. Low levels of expression will require highly sensitive and specific assays.

The use of immunoassays for human proteins may work well when no protein product is formed from the defective gene. However, any cross-reacting material would give a positive result and would require expansion of the cells for analysis of function or other physical properties.

Finally, it is important to know the basis of the the defect under study. The possibility exists that the mouse parental cell can "correct" the human defect. For example, a defect in processing or secretion of a protein might be compensated for by the appropriate rodent enzymes and cell structures. In this case immunoassay might show immunologically reactive human protein product leading to an incorrect assumption of normality.

IV.   Complementation Analysis

Complementation analysis provides information about the degree of genetic heterogeneity of a disease state and gives an estimate of the number of genes that may be responsible for producing a clinical phenotype. Although complementation analysis has not been used to diagnose any disorders prenatally, many diseases have been examined and their genetic and/or biochemical bases elucidated.

Complementation studies may be done with either mononucleate hybrid cells or heterokaryons. Most reports in the literature have used heterokaryons formed between two human diploid cell lines. Many of the techniques for cell fusion are similar to those already described.

One of the first reports of complementation was described by de Weerd-Kastelein et al. (1972). These investigators studied heterokaryons made between fibroblasts from patients with xeroderma pigmentosum. This disorder is due to defects in enzymes that repair thymine dimers. The patients are sensitive to the ultraviolet spectrum from sunlight, and their cells in culture fail to incorporate thymidine after treatment with UV light. Fusion of normal fibroblasts with those from an XP individual resulted in the correction of the repair defect as determined by the incorporation of tritiated thymidine into XP nuclei in heterokaryons; XP homokaryons did not incorporate the labeled pyrimidine. Furthermore, heterokaryons formed between different patients could result in the complementation of each disorder, giving normal repair capacity (de Weerd-Kastelein et al., 1973). These experiments established the multigenic nature of XP. Some seven complementation groups have now been described (Bootsma and Galjaard, 1979).

Tay-Sachs disease and Sandhoff disease have been similarly studied by analyzing the A and B isozymes of hexosaminidase in heterokaryons (Galjaard et al., 1974; Gravel et al., 1979b). Maple-syrup urine disease is a third disorder for which evidence of multiple genes has been acquired via complementation in heterokaryons (Lyons et al., 1973). GM_2-gangliosidosis (Thomas and Taylor, 1974; Rattazzi et al., 1976; Wood, 1978), methylmalonicacidemia (Gravel et al., 1975; Willard et al., 1978), and propionic acidemia (Gravel et al., 1977; Wolf et al., 1978; Saunders et al., 1979) have also been shown to be heterogeneous disorders by this procedure—making a total of six.

One of the difficulties faced in the analysis of heterokaryons is the necessity of single-cell assays or a good fusion index, resulting in a high proportion of multinucleate cells. In disorders where the defect results in complete absence of an enzyme or phenotype, small numbers of heterokaryons may give sufficient activity above background to indicate complementation. However, in conditions where the activity is present at low levels, it becomes difficult to demonstrate complementation if only a few cells are involved in fusion.

Gravel (1979a) has suggested an approach to the analysis of heterokaryons by mechanically selecting multinucleate cells, thus enriching the population for heterokaryons. By isolating multinucleate cells from the fusion of two different propionic acidemia lines with five or more nuclei, the increase in enzyme activity was 7- to 12-fold above background.

At least two reports describe complementation between the cytoplasm of one cell type and whole cells from a second. Cytoplasts from enucleated infantile Type 1 GM_1-gangliosidosis fibroblasts complemented adult Type 4 fibroblasts (de Wit-Verbeck *et al.*, 1978), and "I-cell" fibroblasts were corrected or complemented by each of the following types of cytoplasts: GM_1-gangliosidosis, Sandhoff disease, and mannosidosis (D'Azzo *et al.*, 1980).

Mononucleate, proliferating cell hybrids, either interspecies or intraspecies, can also potentially be used for complementation analysis. For example, Patterson *et al.*, (1974; Patterson, 1975) have isolated mutant Chinese hamster ovary cells that require adenine for growth. These mutants fall into several different complementation groups. Each class of mutant (most of which are well defined biochemically) could serve as fusion partner for cells obtained from patients with defects of any one of the enzymes involved. Failure to grow in the absence of adenine would suggest a common deficiency. In this case, direct biochemical analysis for the enzyme in question would be preferable to complementation analysis. However, it is conceivable that in instances where the biochemical basis for the mutations have not been well defined, hybrid cells using auxotrophic mutants may discriminate between human disease genes.

V.   Summary

This speculative discussion of the use of cell hybridization as a tool in prenatal diagnosis has, I hope, pointed out the potential of the system and some of the problems to be faced when considering its application.

The greatest advantage of the cell hybrid system is that it permits an examination of genes expressed in specialized tissues using amniotic fluid cells rather than cells taken directly from the organ or tissue. Despite the technical difficulties yet to be faced in the utilization of this system, the potential would seem to be great. The variety of differentiated rodent cell lines to be used as parental cells would suggest that a considerable number of specialized human gene products might be studied in activated cell hybrids.

References

Aula, P., and Nichols, W. W. (1967). *J. Cell Physiol.* **70**(3), 281–289.

Baker, R. M., Brunette, D. M., Mankovitz, R., Thompson, L. H., Whitmore, G. F., Siminovitch, L., and Till, J. E. (1974). *Cell* **1**, 9–21.

Bernhard, H. P. (1976). *Int. Rev. Cytol.* **47**, 289–325.

Bootsma, D., and Galjaard, H. (1979). *In* "Models for the Study of Inborn Errors of Metabolism" (F. A. Hommes, ed.). Elsevier-North Holland, Amsterdam.

Brown, J. E., and Weiss, M. C. (1975). *Cell* **6**, 481–494.

Buonassisi, V., Sato, G., and Cohen, A. I. (1962). *Proc. Natl. Acad. Sci U.S.A.* **48**, 1184–1190.

Choo, K. H., Cotton, R. G. H., Jennings, I. G., Fowler, K., and Damks, D. M. (1980). *Biochem. Genet.* **18**, 955–968.

Croce, C. M., Shander, M., Martinis, J., Cicurel, L., D'Ancona G. G., Dolby, T. H., and Koprowski, H. (1979). *Proc. Natl. Acad. Sci. U.S.A.* **76**, 3416–3419.

Darlington, G. J., and Ruddle, F. H. (1975). *In* "Modern Trends in Human Genetics" (A. E. H. Emery, ed.), Vol. 2, pp. 111–137. Butterworth, London.

Darlington, G. J., Bernhard, H. P., and Ruddle, R. H. (1974). *Science* **185**, 859–862.

Darlington, G. J., Bernhard, H. P., Miller, R. A., and Ruddle, F. H. (1980). *J. Natl. Cancer Inst.* **64**, 809–819.

Darlington, G. J., Astrin, K. H., Muirhead, S. P., Desnick, R. J., and Smith, M. (1982a). *Proc. Natl. Acad. Sci. U.S.A.* **79**, 870–873.

Darlington, G. J., Rankin, J. K., and Schlanger, G. S. (1982b). *Somatic Cell Genet.* (in press).

Davidson, R. L. (1974). *Ann. Rev. Genet.* **8**, 195–218.

Davidson, R. L., and Gerald, P. S. (1976). *Somatic Cell Genet.* **2**, 165.

Davidson, R. L., O'Malley, K. A., and Wheeler, T. B. (1976). *Somatic Cell Genet.* **2**, 271–280.

D'Azzo, A., Konings, A., Verkerk, A., Jongkind, J. F., and Galjaard, H. (1980). *Exp. Cell Res.* **127**, 484–487.

de Weerd-Kastelein, E. A., Keijzer, W., and Bootsma, D. (1972). *Nature* **238**, 80–83.

de Weerd-Kastelein, E. A., Kleijer, W. J., Sluyter, M. L., Keijzer, W. (1973). *Mutat. Res.* **19**, 237–243.

deWit-Verbeek, A., Hoogeveen, A., and Galjaard, H. (1978). *Exp. Cell Res.* **113**, 215–218.

Eriksson, S., and Larsson, C. (1975). *Hum. Hered.* **10**, 354–359.

Fagerhol, M. K., and Laurell, C. B. (1970). *Prog. Med. Genet.* **7**, 96–111.

Fogh, J., and Fogh, H. (1965). *Proc. Soc. Exp. Biol. Med.* **119**, 233–238.

Galjaard, H., Hoogeveen, A., deWit-Verbeek, A., Reuser, A. J. J., Keijzer, W., Westerveld, A., and Bootsma, D. (1974). *Exp. Cell Res.* **87**, 444–448.

Giles, R. E., and Ruddle, F. H. (1973). *In Vitro* **9**, 103–107.

Gravel, R. A., Mahoney, M. J., Ruddle, F. H., and Rosenberg, L. E. (1975). *Proc. Natl. Acad. Sci. U.S.A.* **72**, 3181–3185.

Gravel, R. A., Lam, K. F., Scully, K. J., and Hsia, Y. E. (1977). *Am. J. Hum. Genet.* **29**, 378–388.

Gravel, R., Leung, A., Saunders, M., and Hosli, P. (1979a) *Proc. Natl. Acad. Sci. U.S.A.* **76**, 6520–6524.

Gravel, R., Lowden, J. A., Callahan, J. W., Wolfe, L. S., and Ng Yin Kin, N. M. K. (1979b). *Am. J. Hum. Genet.* **31**, 669–679.

Haggerty, D. F., Young, P. L., and Bruse, J. V. (1975). *Dev. Biol.* **44**, 158–168.

Kusano, T., Long, C., and Green, H. (1971). *Proc. Natl. Acad. Sci. U.S.A.* **68**, 82–86.

Littlefield, J. W. (1964). *Science* **145**, 709–710.

Lyons, L. B., Cox, R. P., and Dancis, J. (1973). *Nature* **243**, 533–535.

Malawista, S. E. and Weiss, M. C. (1974). *Proc. Natl. Acad. Sci. U.S.A.* **71,** 927–931.

McBurney, M. W., Featherstone, M., and Kaplan, H. (1978). *Cell* **15,** 1323–1330.

McMorris, A. F., and Ruddle, F. H. (1974). *Dev. Biol.* **39,** 226.

Patterson, D. (1975) *Somatic Cell Genet.* **1,** 91–110.

Patterson, D., Kao, F. T., and Puck, T. J. (1974). *Proc. Natl. Acad. Sci. U.S.A.* **71,** 2057–2061.

Peterson, J. A., and Weiss, M. C. (1972). *Proc. Natl. Acad. Sci. U.S.A.* **69,** 198–201.

Puck, T. T. (1976). *Adv. Pathobiol.* **3,** 72–80.

Rankin, J. K., and Darlington, G. J. (1979). *Somatic Cell Genet.* **1,** 1–10.

Rattazzi, M. C., Brown, J. A., Davidson, R. G., and Shows, T. B. (1976). *Am. J. Hum. Genet.* **28,** 143–154.

Ringertz, N., and Savage, E. (1976). "Cell Hybrids." Academic Press, New York.

Sammons, D. W., Sanchez, E., and Darlington, D. J. (1980). *In Vitro* **16,** 918–924.

Saunders, M., Sweetman, L., Robinson, B., Roth, K., Cohn, R., and Gravel R. A. (1979). *J. Clin. Invest.* **64,** 1695–1702.

Schwaber, J., and Cohen, E. (1973). *Nature* **244,** 444–447.

Thomas, G. H., and Taylor, H. A. Jr. (1974). *Nature* **250,** 580–582.

Willard, H. F., Mellman, I. S., and Rosenberg, L. E. (1978). *Am. J. Hum. Genet.* **30,** 1–13.

Willing, M. C., Nienhuis, A. H., and Anderson, W. F. (1979). *Nature* **277,** 534–538.

Wolf, B., Hsia, Y. E., and Rosenberg, L. E. (1978). *Am. J. Hum. Genet.* **30,** 455–464.

Wood, S. (1978). *Hum. Genet.* **41,** 325–329.

Chapter 12

Prenatal Analysis of Human DNA-Sequence Variation

DAVID KURNIT

Division of Clinical Genetics
Children's Hospital Medical Center
and
Division of Genetics (Obstetrics and Gynecology)
Brigham and Women's Hospital
Boston, Massachusetts

STUART ORKIN

Division of Hematology–Oncology
Children's Hospital Medical Center
Boston, Massachusetts

AND

RAY WHITE

Department of Microbiology
University of Massachusetts Medical School
Worcester, Massachusetts

METHODS IN CELL BIOLOGY, VOL. 26

Until recently, human genetic diagnosis has been, of necessity, indirect. Genetic alterations have been analyzable only by the ascertainment of secondary changes (e.g., abnormal gene products or phenotypes) resulting from the primary mutation (or permutation) of DNA sequence. The complexity of the human genome, consisting of over 3 billion base pairs per haploid chromosome set (Bachmann, 1972), is responsible primarily for previous difficulties in making straightforward genetic diagnoses at the DNA-sequence level. This review will summarize the techniques and concepts that underlie the remarkable advances in molecular biology that have overcome such difficulties and allowed for the first successful prenatal diagnoses at the nucleic acid level. These techniques can be expected to have broad applicability and wide usage because they are highly accurate, have the potential of spanning the entire genome, and require only nucleated cells readily obtainable by routine amniocentesis, venipuncture, or biopsy.

I. Techniques

In the last decade, the "3 Rs" have become available to molecular biologists: restriction enzymes, recombinant-DNA technology, and readout of DNA sequences. Taken together with the previously established ability to separate DNA chains and allow them to reassociate with their complementary chain (Schildkraut *et al.*, 1961), a process termed "hybridization," these techniques have resulted in increasingly sophisticated mapping and characterization of normal and abnormal genes and genetic processes.

Restriction enzymes are endonucleases that recognize and incise DNA strands at precisely defined short nucleotide sequences. These enzymes are purified from a variety of microorganisms in which they serve as a barrier against the intrusion of foreign DNAs; a directory of these enzymes can be found in Roberts (1980). A most successful stratagem for the detection of specific DNA segments has been to cleave a complex DNA preparation of interest with an appropriate restriction endonuclease, separate the resultant DNA fragments by size using gel-electrophoretic techniques (Southern, 1975), and transfer the fragments to a solid matrix (e.g., nitrocellulose paper) in a manner that maintains the spatial orientation of the fragments from the original gel. The immobilized DNA is then hybridized *in situ* with a radioactive probe yielding a correlation between the specific probe and the size of the specific DNA fragments on which it (the probe) lies in the complex preparation of DNA of interest. Named after its inventor, this technique is termed a "Southern transfer." Protocols for restriction-enzyme digestions and Southern transfers are provided in the Appendix, Section IV.

Restriction-enzyme/Southern-transfer technology has already been successfully adapted to prenatal diagnosis (Orkin *et al.*, 1978). The key to the success of this method is that total cellular DNA can be utilized as the substrate for the analysis; thus fetal amniotic fluid cells can be processed immediately (Kan and Dozy, 1978) or after a few weeks of cellular proliferation *in vitro,* permitting diagnosis in a clinically suitable time frame. In addition, the resources of manpower and equipment required are not dissimilar from those required for prenatal karyotyping.

In contrast with the above technologies that have been demonstrated to be directly applicable to rapid and economical prenatal diagnosis, DNA-sequencing techniques are more likely to be used in an ancillary way to support the aforementioned diagnostic methodology than to be used directly for prenatal diagnosis. Although rapid DNA-sequencing techniques have been developed (Maxam and Gilbert, 1977; Sanger *et al.*, 1977), even at the rate of 1000 bases per week it would still require nearly 60,000 years to sequence a human haploid genome end to end. On paper, it would be feasible to isolate fetal cellular DNA, prepare an appropriate "library" of cloned DNA fragments (Blattner *et al.*, 1978; Maniatis *et al.*, 1978), select a clone containing the gene of interest, and obtain the DNA sequence of that gene. Although the technology to perform such a *tour-de-force* exists, the time constraints of prenatal diagnosis, the equipment and manpower needs, and the necessity to be sure that both alleles of a diploid fetus have been examined make it unlikely that such a strategy will have widespread clinical utility in the near future. However, recombinant-DNA and DNA-sequencing technology will remain important for obtaining probes and for guiding the appropriate choice of restriction enzymes to look for specific mutations. In summary, current DNA technology will not allow for wholesale determination of fetal genomic DNA sequences but does allow for the detection of a variety of sequence and organization changes that can be discerned following cleavage with restriction enzymes. The remainder of the review consists of a discussion of the various ways in which such changes have been or could be used for prenatal diagnosis.

II. Applications

A. Quantitative Variation

The existence of quantitative variation reflects the existence in eukaryotic genomes of sequences that are present in multiple copies. The first successful prenatal diagnosis using DNA technology was, in fact, a gene-counting experiment in which hybridization of a labeled probe complementary to α-globin messenger RNA was used to titrate the α-globin gene content of a fetus at risk for deletion of the α-globin genes (Kan *et al.*, 1976). Although this method for analyzing this number of copies of genes present in a few copies per haploid genome may be useful in a limited number of specific cases, other methods to be described are more likely to be used in cases of gene deletion because the titration method is tedious and less accurate. Variation of more highly repeated sequences—for example, tandem repeats of genes coding for histones, ribosomal RNA, transfer RNA, and 5S RNA; interspersed repetitive sequences (Houck *et al.*, 1979), which may include translocatable elements (Cohen and Shapiro, 1980); satellite (simple sequence) DNAs, which comprise constitutive heterochromatin (John and Miklos, 1979; Kurnit, 1979a)—can also be quantitated in fetal DNA. The lack of known deleterious effects that result from such variations among highly repeated DNA sequences (Young *et al.*, 1976; Kurnit, 1979a) limits the clinical indications for such studies. However, such variations are most useful for purposes of prenatal cytogenetic analysis in which cytologically apparent heteromorphisms (Jacobs, 1977), which result from quantitative variation of highly repeated DNA sequences (Kurnit, 1979a), can furnish useful information about the parental identity of individual chromosome homologues (for review, see Kurnit and Hoehn, 1979).

B. Qualitative Variation

1. DIRECT METHOD

Restriction enzymes are sufficiently specific to permit direct detection of single nucleotide changes in DNA. For example, mutant hemoglobin chains can at times be identified by such DNA analysis (Little *et al.*, 1980a). An example of this approach is the identification of the hemoglobin 0 Arab mutation within the β-globin gene (5'-GAATTC-3' is mutated to 5'-AAATTC-3'). The pattern of β-globin-specific EcoRI-DNA fragments is altered due to obliteration of an intragenic EcoRI site normally present. Detection of this fragment has resulted in antenatal diagnosis of an 0 Arab allele (Phillips *et al.*, 1979) that in association with a β-sickle allele leads to a severe sickle syndrome. (The experimental design corresponds to part A of Fig. 1.) Of greater importance, the sickle globin mutation can also be recognized in this direct manner. Using the enzyme DdeI, Geever *et al.* (1981) were able to distinguish the sickle and wild type β-globin alleles. However, the small size of β-globin-specific DNA fragments generated by DdeI presents technical problems. More recently, Orkin *et al.* (1982) have used MstII, which generated larger β-globin-specific DNA fragments, to distinguish these alleles. Mst II recognizes the sequence 5'-CCTNAGG-3' (in which N represents any nucleotide). The sickle globin mutant results in loss of the MstII-recognized wild type sequence 5'-CCTGAGG-3' to the altered sequence 5'-CCTGTGG-3'.

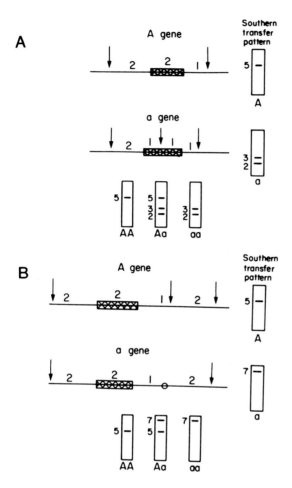

FIG. 1. Detection of genetic variation at the DNA level. (A) Changes of endonuclease-recognition sites within genes. The restriction-endonuclease map of a putative wild-type (*A*) gene is shown. Endonuclease-recognition sites are designated by arrows. Arabic numbers give distances in kilobases (kb), where a kilobase is 1000 bases. The *A* gene, which is 2 kb long, has no endonuclease-recognition sites within the gene, and is flanked by endonuclease-recognition sites 2 kb upstream from the left side of the gene and 1 kb downstream from the right side of the gene. After restriction-endonuclease digestion, the gene will lie on a single fragment 5 kb long, which would appear as a single band following Southern transfer and *in situ* hybridization with a radioactive probe specific for the gene.

A mutant allele (a gene), resulting from a mutation within the gene that caused the creation of a new endonuclease-recognition site, would alter the restriction map as shown. Following restriction-endonuclease digestion, two fragments containing the gene would be detected following Southern transfer: a 3-kb and a 2-kb piece. Thus the Southern transfer pattern from a wild-type homozygote (*AA*) would show only a 5-kb fragment; from a heterozygote (*Aa*), 5-kb, 3-kb, and 2-kb fragments; and from an affected homozygote (*aa*), only 3-kb and 2-kb fragments.

(B) Changes of recognition sites in flanking sequences. An expanded restriction map of the *A* gene

This methodology should become the preferred analysis for prenatal diagnosis of the sickle globin mutation. In theory, utilization of a battery of restriction enzymes currently available should be capable of detecting approximately half of the 135 known single amino acid substitution variants of human α-globin chains (Roberts, 1980; Wilson *et al.*, 1980). However, the point remains that many point mutations do not create or delete enzyme recognition sites readily amenable to direct analysis with this method.

In contrast with the case for point mutations where the direct method will not detect most mutants, rearrangements involving deletions, insertions, and/or inversions can be analyzed. In fact, the first reported use of the restriction-enzyme/Southern-transfer method for prenatal diagnosis involved ascertainment of thalassemias caused by globin-gene deletion (Orkin *et al.*, 1978). In the case of the α-globin gene family, deletion of all four α-globin genes, which results in hydrops fetalis, can be readily detected by the total absence of any fragments available to hybridize with the characteristic pattern and specificity of genomic α-globin DNA. Deletions with the human $\gamma\delta\beta$-globin gene complex are associated with rare thalassemias. In these disorders in which the production of more than one β-like globin chain is not produced ($\delta\beta$-thalassemia, HPFH (hereditary persistence of fetal hemoglobin), and $\gamma\delta\beta$-thalassemia), various deletions have been identified by direct analysis (Orkin and Nathan, 1980). These conditions constitute a minority of thalassemias and are rare or nonexistent (e.g., $\gamma\delta\beta$-thalassemia) in the homozygous state. Thus, β-thalassemias are the only clinical entities with this class of potential significance. However, detailed mapping of the deletions identifiable in the $\gamma\delta\beta$-complex may help define regions involved in controlling hemoglobin switching (Fritsch *et al.*, 1979; Orkin and Nathan, 1980). In general, standard application of restriction mapping to the analysis of classical β-thalassemias (in which only β-globin synthesis is impaired) is unrewarding (Flavell *et al.*, 1979; Orkin *et al.*, 1979). Both β^0- and β^+-thalassemias are generally associated with normal appearing β-globin structural loci. Nevertheless, a partial deletion of the structural gene seen in three Asian Indians (Flavell *et al.*, 1979; Orkin *et al.*, 1979, 1980) suggests that some de-

---

is shown, which demonstrates an additional endonuclease-restriction site 2 kb downstream from the site located 1 kb from the right end of the gene. In this case, the mutant *a* gene does not result in the creation of a new recognition site within the gene. However, the mutation is closely linked to a DNA sequence change 1 kb downstream from the right end of the gene, resulting in an altered sequence that no longer functions as a recognition site. As before, endonuclease digestion of DNA containing the *A* gene followed by Southern transfer will result in detection of a 5-kb fragment. However, digestion of DNA containing the *a* gene will result in a longer 7-kb fragment. Again, this will allow for distinction between the *AA* (5 kb only), *Aa* (5 kb and 7kb), and *aa* (7 kb only) genotypes. Reproduced with permission from the *Annual Review of Genetics*, Volume 13. © 1979 by Annual Reviews Inc.

letions may be "private," that is, specific for a given racial group or pedigree. Study of the molecular basis of thalassemia in many families may ultimately permit tailoring direct detection of abnormal genes to the family at risk.

Genic probes are required for utilization of the direct method. This requirement has restricted the clinical applicability of the method to diagnosis of hemoglobin variants. As DNA probes for human genes other than globin become increasingly available, it is anticipated that this method will be applied to analysis of other genetic disorders. In summary, the direct method has the advantage of examining the primary DNA-sequence change responsible for a given genetic lesion. However, the applicability is limited by the requirements for specific gene probes and (in the case of point mutations) by limitations in the number of restriction endonuclease-recognition sequences.

2. INDIRECT APPROACH

In order to obviate the limitations of the direct method just described, an alternative strategy has been devised that relies on the utilization of linkage between a gene of interest and nearby restriction endonuclease-recognition sites. Variations in restriction sites (given the acronym RFLPs to represent restriction-fragment length polymorphisms) can be utilized as mendelian co-dominant markers to follow the inheritance pattern of cis-linked genes (Botstein *et al.*, 1980). Given that the diploid human genome of roughly 6×10^9 base pairs undergoes about 6×10^1 crossovers per meiotic event, an average of 1 meiotic crossover per 10^8 base pairs per generation can be expected (i.e., 1 morgan $\approx 10^8$ base pairs and 1 centimorgan $\approx 10^6$ base pairs in humans). Thus RFLPs resulting from changes in restriction endonuclease-recognition sites as far away as 10^7 base pairs from a given gene are of potential utility for following the inheritance of that gene.

The potential to utilize RFLPs for purposes of human genetic analysis is analogous in theory to previous linkage studies using protein and chromosomal polymorphisms. Nonrandom familial segregation of a chromosomal heteromorphism of chromosome 1 with the blood-group marker Duffy was used to make the first human autosomal gene assignment (Donahue *et al.*, 1968). A number of such protein polymorphisms have been used clinically, including linkage between HLA and the 21-hydroxylase (Dupont *et al.*, 1977) and hemochromatosis loci (Krayitz *et al.*, 1979); secretor antigen and myotonic dystrophy (Schrott *et al.*, 1973); ABO blood group and nail patella syndrome (Renwick and Lawler, 1955); and glucose-6-phosphate dehydrogenase and hemophilia (Boyer and Graham, 1965). The known human markers are, however, insufficient in number; thus most disease loci are not known to be linked to useful markers. Further, in order to be useful, a marker must be sufficiently polymorphic as well as closely linked to a gene of interest. Quantitative estimates of the degree of polymorphism, denoted as PIC (polymorphism information content), have been considered by Botstein *et al.* (1980). From these considerations, it is apparent that there are only a handful of co-dominant protein polymorphisms with PIC values sufficient to be useful clinically. Therefore, although protein polymorphisms have been applied in a few clinical situations to discern segregation of alleles with nearby genes of medical significance, it is clear that the quantity and diversity of such polymorphisms will permit this analysis only in a small number of cases. In contrast, both theoretical expectations and preliminary experiments (Kan and Dozy, 1978; Jeffreys, 1979; Wyman and White, 1980) indicate that DNA polymorphisms should be more suitable than protein polymorphisms, both in number and in PIC.

Successful prenatal diagnosis using DNA technology to detect linkage between a RFLP and the $\gamma\delta\beta$-globin locus has already been performed. Kan and Dozy (1978) detected a change in a recognition site for the endonuclease Hpa I located 5000 bases downstream from the β-globin locus. The alteration they detected at this site was highly associated with the presence of the sickle mutation at the β-globin locus. Kan and Dozy utilized this association to ascertain which restriction variants of Hpa I and hence which β-globin alleles were present in fetal DNA following hybridization with a radioactive probe from β-globin. (The experimental design corresponds to Fig. 1B). In the population Kan and Dozy studied (i.e., the U.S. blacks in California), the degree of linkage disequilibrium was sufficient so that accurate and sensitive diagnosis was possible in the majority of couples at risk by knowing only fetal and parental Hpa I-restriction patterns following Southern blotting (Southern, 1975) with a β-globin probe (for calculations, see Appendix of Kurnit and Hoehn, 1979).

In the study of Kan and Dozy (1978), there are two main sources of error inherent in the diagnostic protocol. First, as in any linkage study, recombination leads to diagnostic error; this error should be very small, because the chance of meiotic recombination between the β-globin locus and the Hpa I site should be roughly

$$\frac{5000 \text{ base pairs separating } \beta\text{-globin locus and the Hpa I site}}{10^8 \text{ base pairs/recombinational event/generation}} =$$

1/20,000 per parent (Kurnit, 1979b). The ability to obtain such close linkage is one of the major advantages of using DNA technology for linkage studies. Second, a larger error comes from the assumption that the linkage phase in an individual can be predicted from the linkage disequilibrium seen in the population. In the case of the high degree of linkage disequilibrium seen by Kan and Dozy, this error remains small (1% false-positive and false-negative rates; for calculations, see Appendix of Kurnit and Hoehn, 1979); however, subsequent studies of U.S. blacks on the East Coast have shown a lower degree of linkage disequilibrium (Feldenzer *et al.*, 1979; Phillips *et al.*, 1980) than that seen by Kan and Dozy

(1978). This decrement in the degree of disequilibrium results in a markedly larger error rate expected from using population date to deduce the linkage phase in a given individual; specifically, the error rate of 1% calculated in Kurnit and Hoehn (1979) would increase to 10% using the population data in Phillips *et al.* (1980). The implication of this higher error rate is that family studies will be required to establish the actual linkage phase of the β-globin alleles and Hpa I RFLPs in prospective parents at risk for offspring with sickle cell anemia. Because most RFLPs will be unlikely to demonstrate the high degree of linkage disequilibrium seen between β-globin genes and adjacent loci, it will be necessary to perform such extended family studies in virtually all prenatal studies using linkage between genes and RFLPs. Two other examples of the indirect strategy in genotyping are the use of a Bam HI polymorphism 3' to the β-locus to exclude β-thalassemia in Sardinians (Kan *et al.*, 1980), and of Hind III polymorphisms within the γ-globin genes to identify thalassemia and β^s-chromosomes (Little *et al.*, 1980b; Phillips *et al.*, 1980b). The studies using linkage between β-globin variants and closely linked RFLPs illustrate the potential of this concept for prenatal diagnosis. However, these studies still require a probe either at or closely linked to the gene of interest. Botstein *et al.* (1980) have suggested a more general approach with the potential to obtain a genetic map of numerous RFLP markers spanning the human genome. They conclude that a very large number of DNA-sequencing polymorphisms should exist in the human population. With the identification of several hundred RFLPs at arbitrary sites, most disease loci would be closely linked (i.e., within about 10 centimorgans).

There are several potential approaches to obtaining RFLP loci from diverse locations about the human genome. One approach is to screen a clone library of large genomic DNA segments (15,000–20,000 base pairs long) (Blattner *et al.*, 1978; maniatis *et al.*, 1978) with a probe containing intermediate-repetitive human DNA (Gusella *et al.*, 1980). Although most such clones contain such repetitive DNA sequences (and hence cannot be utilized to define unique loci), a few percent of the genomic clones lack these repeats and are suitable as probes. The first such locus to be characterized in detail (Wyman and White, 1980) will likely be useful because more than 8 alleles were obseved in a sample of 50 individuals, yielding a high PIC. Most families and matings should be informative with this marker. Further, stable mendelian segregation was observed through several generations. A large number of such probes exist and we estimate that a significant fraction should contain RFLPs with a useful PIC. The polymorphic locus examined by Wyman and White resulted from DNA-rearrangement events. In principle, it should be feasible to screen directly for analogous polymorphic loci by probing larger fragments with smaller probes generated by the same restriction enzymes. Another likely source of useful probes will be arbitrary human genic cDNA clones (Kurnit *et al.*, in preparation).

In summary, the protocol of Botstein *et al.* (1980), which requires several hundred highly polymorphic loci scattered about the human genome, appears to be feasible with current DNA technology. Another likely source of useful probes will be to hybridize with arbitrary human genic cDNA clones (Kurnit *et al.*, 1982).

III.   Potential Pitfalls

Recent findings concerning the plasticity of the eukaryotic genome are germane to a discussion of the detection of rearrangements in fetal DNA. It is clear that insertions and deletions of DNA are more common than the earlier dogma of an "invariant genome" predicted previously. In particular, unequal crossovers among units of tandemly repeated sequences (Smith, 1976; John and Miklos, 1979; Kurnit, 1979a; Petes, 1980; Szostak and Wu, 1980; Zimmer *et al.*, 1980), movement of interspersed repetitive sequences, and/or translocatable elements (Cameron *et al.*, 1979; Strobel *et al.*, 1979; Young, 1979; Cohen and Shapiro, 1980), and specific rearrangement and deletion events involved in antibody formation (Brack *et al.*, 1978; Seidman *et al.*, 1978) all underscore that normal variability of complex eukaryotic genomes exist. Most of these rearrangements are associated with mitotic DNA replication (Kurnit, 1979a; John and Miklos, 1979), although some—for example, some ribosomal DNA unequal crossovers (Petes, 1980)—occur in early meiosis before chiasma formation as well. Fortunately, in spite of the potential for this variability to interfere with attempts to distinguish genic pathology from normal genome rearrangements, no such interference has been encountered to date in attempts to perform prenatal diagnosis using DNA technology. This lack of difficulty is in accord with a study that demonstrated that the bulk of DNA in *Drosophila* does not undergo such rearrangements (Potter and Thomas, 1977). Further, other potential tissue-specific modifications (e.g., methylation) that could interfere with restriction-enzyme analysis of fetal DNA (Singer *et al.*, 1979) have not posed problems so far with prenatal analyses. DNA rearrangements may be responsible for a significant proportion of the burden of genetic disease in humans (34), and for a significant number of useful RFLPs (Neel, 1978). Therefore, it will be mandatory to ensure that the variations that will be observed are, in fact, reflective of pathology rather than representing normal human variation. Family studies before attempting prenatal diagnosis will be most helpful in this regard, to ensure that stable mendelian inheritance is maintained for the polymorphism being scrutinized. In addition, pilot studies to monitor the expression of a given RFLP in amniotic fluid cells will be required. In the case of RFLPs within and adjacent to globin genes, initial studies have shown that these RFLPs retain their parental type of organization and can be used to follow segregation of parental globin alleles. As discussed previously, family studies will also be required in most cases to ascertain the linkage phase between RFLPs and adjacent genes.

In summary, the following sources of error can be anticipated using both the direct and indirect methods:

1. Experimental error
2. Errors in knowledge of linkage phase from inaccuracies (e.g., paternity errors) or lack of appropriate pedigree data
3. *De novo* rearrangements of fetal DNA
4. Recombination

We are optimistic that all these sources of error can be minimized so that DNA technology can be utilized to provide highly efficacious prenatal diagnosis for a large proportion, if not the entire, human genome. In particular, the methodology (see Appendix, Section IV) is reliable and can be run at sufficiently low cost even when including the required family study. *De novo* rearrangements should be rare (Potter and Thomas, 1977). Recombination can be minimized once an RFLP–gene association has been established by using locus expansion to obtain further RFLPs even closer to the gene in question. Thus, given accurate pedigree data (which is necessary for any attempt to perform antenatal genetic analysis), DNA technology should result in accurate and reliable prenatal diagnoses of human genetic disorders.

IV.   Appendix: Useful Procedures for Obtaining, Labeling, and Hybridizing DNA Probes for Restriction-Fragment Analyses

A.   DNA Preparation from Amniotic Fluid Cells

1. Wash cell pellet; may be frozen at this stage.
2. Add roughly 20 volumes of lysing solution:
   10 mM Tris (pH 8)
   10 mM NaCl
   10 mM EDTA
   0.5% sodium dodecyl sulfate (SDS)
   100–200 μg/ml Proteinase K
Incubate at 50–55°C for 2 hours.
3. Phenol-extract once; chloroform: isoamyl alcohol (24:1) extract twice; ethanol precipitate.
4. Resuspend DNA in small volume of 0.5 mM EDTA, pH 8 (use about half the volume in step 2).

From buffer stocks, bring solution to following concentrations:

50 m*M* Tris (pH 8)

10 m*M* NaCl

10 m*M* EDTA

RNase A to 50 μg/ml

Incubate at 37°C for 4 hours.

5. Add SDS to 0.5%; Proteinase K to 100–200 μg/ml. Incubate 2 hours at 50–55°C. Repeat step 3.

6. Resuspend DNA in small amount of appropriate buffer.

B. Isolation of DNA from White Blood Cells

1. CELL LYSIS

1. Transfer thawed white blood cell pack from Pro-Vial to 15-ml plastic Corning (orange or blue cap) tube. Break up clump of cells by pipetting several times using a pasteur pipet and shaking vigorously.

2. Add sufficient lysis buffer (0.01 *M* Tris–0.1 *M* NaCl–0.001 *M* EDTA, to pH 7.8 with HCl) to bring volume to 10 ml. Shake vigorously to ensure homogeneous distribution of cells.

3. Place 10 ml of lysis buffer and 1% SDS and 0.4 mg/ml Proteinase K (Boehringer) into each of a siliconized 125- to 250-ml Erlenmeyer flask with screw cap. Add dropwise while swirling the white cell–lysis buffer mix from the plastic tube. Allow to swirl 2 hours at room temperature.

2. CRUDE EXTRACTIONS

4. Phenol extraction (two times): Add 20 ml of equilibrated (pH 7.5) liquid phenol. Shake vigorously to form emulsion, then let swirl 1 hour. Pour into 40-ml polyallomer centrifuge tubes and spin at 5000 rpm for 5 minutes at 4°C. Discard lower (phenol) phase, including white material at the interface.

5. Chloroform–isoamylalcohol extraction (two times): Use 20 ml of a 24:1 mixture of chloroform–isoamylalcohol to extract phenol as in step 4. Phase separation by gravity occurs readily so spinning is not necessary.

3. DNA RECOVERY

6. Isopropanol precipitation: Add 50 ml isopropanol (assuming extracted aqueous phase is 20 ml in volume) to a 150- to 250-ml siliconized beaker. Pour in aqueous phase containing DNA. Pour solution back and forth

between containers just until a ball of DNA appears (about three pours). Hook DNA from the solution by means of a curved pasteur pipet tip and transfer immediately to 20 ml ultracentrifuge density-gradient solution less CsCl and ethidium bromide [50 mM Tris-HCl (pH 8)–200 mM NaCl–1 mM EDTA–6.0 g (w/v) sucrose] in siliconized 50-ml Erlenmeyer flasks with screw tops. Parafilm tops and allow to swirl 24 hours or until DNA is completely in solution, at room temperature.

4.   PURIFICATION

7. Cesium chloride density-gradient ultracentrifugation: From the white blood cell pack from 50 ml of blood, DNA yields were between 305 and 1127 μg, which can be further purified on a CsCl density gradient using the Sorvall TV-850 rotor.
   a. Tube loading: Measure volume of dissolved DNA sample using plastic Dispo pipet into 25 × 89-mm polyallomer tubes (Sorvall/Dupont). Add sufficient CsCl to bring final concentration to 0.88 g/ml and sufficient ethidium bromide to bring concentration to 300 μg/ml. Bring total volume in tube to 32 ml using gradient solution [50 mM Tris-HCl (pH 8.0)–200 mM NaCl–1 mM EDTA–6 g/ml (w/v) sucrose–300 μg/ml ethidium bromide–0.88 g/ml CsCl]. Balance tubes and pair.
   b. Rotor assembly: Be sure rotor chambers and threads are clean and dry prior to assembly. Seat a chambered ring (fat edge down) on the lip of each chamber just below the threads. Insert tube. Place white cap on top of tube so beveled edge fits partially into tube. Grease an "O" ring lightly with vacuum grease and seat in groove on top of white cap. Grease the threads of red screw cap lightly with Versilube-Plus. Seat on top of chamber opening. Using only the two-pin headpiece of the torque wrench, rotate the red cap counterclockwise until beginning of thread catch can be felt. Carefully rotate cap clockwise as long as correct threading can be felt. If cap jams, it is probably cross-threaded. Back off cap and begin again. When correctly threaded cap is tightened as much as possible by hand, then apply a torque of 160 inch-pounds to complete sealing of chamber.
   c. The run: Load rotor into Sorvall Ultracentrifuge. Run at 42,000 rpm at 20°C. First make speed and temperature settings. With time control on "off," press "start" button. Turn time control to "hold." When rotor velocity reaches 5000 rpm or more, press "reogradprogram" button. Equilibrium is reached in 24 hours.
   d. Taking down gradient: Stop rotor by turning time control to "off." Remove caps from tube and place in a 1:5 dilution of Beckman rotor-cleaning solution. Remove tubes from chambers using a syringe needle

to push tube side away from chamber surface and gripping with a pair of hemostats. Pull tube slowly and continuously from its chamber. Visualize band under long-wave UV light. Insert a 16-gauge hypodermic needle using a 6-cc syringe into side of tube just slightly below band and angled up at band. Insert needle carefully, making sure not to puncture opposite side of tube. Collect band by slow but continuous suction of the syringe.

e. Isopropanol extraction: Place band in a Corning plastic screw-cap tube and extract with two volumes of isopropanol until no more ethidium bromide can be visualized under long-wave UV light. Phases separate by gravity and isopropanol is the top phase. It usually takes three extractions to completely remove the ethidium bromide from the aqueous phase. Use for extraction isopropanol that has been equilibrated against an equal volume of 0.88 g/ml aqueous CsCl; isopropanol is the top phase.

f. Dialysis: Dialyze extracted samples for at least 12 hours at room temperature against 5mM Tris–0.1 mM EDTA (TE^{-4}) and 0.5 M NaCl. Then dialyze twice against TE^{-4} and 0.3 M sodium acetate at 4°C for at least 12 hours each.

g. Ethanol precipitation: Precipitate dialyzed samples with two and one half volumes of ethanol in siliconized Corex tubes.

C.   Nick Translation of DNA

Buffers and Solutions

DNase: 1 mg/ml in 0.01 N HCl, store in 50-μl aliquots frozen at -20°C
DNase Buffer: 10 mM Tris-HCl (pH 7.5)–5 mM MgCl–1 mg/ml BSA
Nick translation (NT) buffer (5×): 0.25 M Tris-HCl (pH 7.4)–25 mM MgCl$_2$
100 mM β-Mercaptoethanol: 7 μl β-ME to 1.0 ml
Sephadex G-50 in TE^{-4}–0.1 M NaCl–0.5% SDS
4 N NaOH
2 M Tris-HCl (pH 7.0)
150 μM dGTP in TE^{-4}

1. Dry   50 μl of 1 mCi/ml: [^{32}P]dATP
        50 μl of 1 mCi/ml: [^{32}P]dCTP
        50 μl of 1 mCi/ml: [^{32}P]TTP
        2 μl of 150 μM: dGTP

2. *DNase activations*
   Add 450 μl DNase buffer to an aliquot of DNase. Thaw for 2 hours on ice. Dilute to the proper concentration with 1 × NT buffer.

3. *Nick translation*
   Take up in a 10-μl final reaction volume, in order:
   2 μl 5 × NT buffer

2 μl 100 mM β-ME
   0.5 g DNA
1 μl DNase (this can be varied by altering dilution)
2 μl NEN-100 DNA Polymerase I (8 units)
   dd H_2O to 10 μl.

Mix well and incubate at 15°C for 90 minutes. The labeled DNA may now be dealt with in one of two ways: Denatured and passed a G-50 column or precipitated several times and run on a gel.

4. *Sephadex G-50 purification*

Add 5 μl 4 N NaOH to reaction and incubate for at least 30 minutes at 37°C. Add 10 μl 2 M Tris-HCl (pH 7.0). Pass the DNA–triphosphates mixture over a Sephadex G-50 column of about 17 cm equilibrated with TE^4–0.1 M NaCl–0.5% SDS. Elute the DNA with TE^{-4}–0.1 M NaCl–0.5% SDS. It is in the exclusion volume while the triphosphates are in the inclusion volume. Collect 15-drop fractions and the DNA peak will be in fractions 13–20 (usually 15–18); the triphosphates will come off the column later (fractions 23–35). The ^{32}P-labeled DNA is usually in a volume of 325–350 μl. A 5-μl aliquot of the final pooled peak should be TCA precipitated. (The specific activity is based on this number.) Store the material frozen at −20°C.

5. *Purification by precipitation*

Add 200 μl of 3.3 M NH_4Ac–20 mM EDTA and 20 μg of tRNA to the reaction mixture. Add 440 μl 95% EtOH: and place in a dry ice–ethanol bath. Spin for 4 minutes and wash the pellet two times with 70% EtOH–0.5 M NH_4Ac and once with 95% EtOH. Resuspend.

D.   Nick Translation of DNA (Alternate Protocol)

For reaction containing ≥ 100 ng of DNA:

1. Prepare 2× reaction mix from following stock solutions:
   0.1 ml of 1 M Tris-HCl (pH 7.5)
   0.01 ml of 1 M $MgCl_2$
   0.0015 ml of β-mercaptoethanol
Bring volume to 1 ml with water.

2. In a small microcentrifuge tube, lyophilize DNA to be nick translated with 25 μCi each of dATP, dCTP, dTTP, and dGTP (each radioactive nucleotide is from a stock at 400 Ci/mmol)

3. Add 10 μl H_2O and resuspend DNA and nucleotides.
Add 10 μl of 2× reaction mix.
Add 2–5 units of DNA Polymerase I (Boehringer-Mannheim).
Keep at room temperature for 2–4 hours.

4. Stop reaction by adding EDTA to final concentration of 10 mM

5. Recovery excluded material from Sephadex G-50 or G-100 column in 5 mM Tris (pH 7.4)–0.1 mM EDTA.
6. Boil probe 5 minutes and quick-cool before use.

E. Transfer of DNA from Agarose Gel to Nitrocellulose Paper (Southern, 1975)

1. Prepare and run standard agarose gel (0.7–1.2%).
2. Stain gel with ethidium bromide (0.5 μg/ml) and photograph.
3. Place gel for 40–60 minutes in 1 N NaOH.
4. Neutralize for 60–75 minutes in 3 M NaCl–1 M Tris (pH 7.5).
5. Place gel in 6× SSC (1× SSC is 0.15 M NaCl–0.015 M sodium citrate, pH 7) for 20–30 minutes and wet nitrocellulose paper at this time by floating paper onto liquid surface.
6. Wet sponge pad in large tray containing 6× SSC.
7. Lay wet Whatman 1 paper on sponge.
   Lay gel on paper avoiding air bubbles.
   Place glass plates on left and right of gel for support of top papers.
   Lay nitrocellulose paper on gel without bubbles.
   Lay 1 sheet Whatman 1 wetted on nitrocellulose and then multiple sheets of Whatman 1 and paper towels.
   Change towels when wet.
   Transfer for 24 hours.
8. Peel off paper and soak nitrocellulose paper in 2XSSC rinsing off surface to remove agarose bits.
9. Bake for 2 hours at 75–80°C under vacuum.

Hybridization
10. Prehybridize blot in tray at 65–68°C containing:
    6× SSC
    0.5% SDS
    10× Denhardt's solution
    10 mM sodium phosphate (pH 7.0)
    1 mM EDTA
    25 μg/ml heat-denatured salmon sperm DNA
    25 μg/ml poly A
    Optional: add dextran sulfate to 10% w/v to accelerate hybridization.
    Preincubate for 1 hour or more.
11. Squeeze out prehybridization buffer and add probe in small volume (usually 1–2 ml) of same buffer; the specific activity of the probe should be at least 10^8 cpm (Cerenkov)/μg and 200,000–1,000,000 cpm are usually added per milliliter of hybridization buffer. Incubate at 68°C for 18 hours.

12. Wash filter in tray at 68°C in following solutions:

2× SSC–10 mM sodium phosphate (pH 7)–0.5% SDS–1 mM EDTA for 1 hour

1× SSC–10 mM sodium phosphate (pH 7)–0.5% SDS–1 mM EDTA for 1 hour

0.5× SSC–10mM sodium phosphate (pH 7)–0.5% SDS–1 mM EDTA for 1 hour

0.2× SSC–10 mM sodium phosphate (pH 7)–0.5% SDS–1 mM EDTA for 1 hour

0.1× SSC–10 mM sodium phosphate (pH 7)–0.5% SDS–1 mM EDTA for 1 hour

13. Dry and expose with intensifying screen.

F.   Transfer of DNA from Agarose Gel to DBM Paper (Alwine *et al.*, 1979)

1. After gel running, photograph entire gel under short-wave UV light.
2. Place gel in wash tray with gel restrainer. Gently slide gel on its bottom surface just enough to break adhesion between it and the plastic surface so solution contact can be made from the bottom surface as well as the top surface.
3. Pour 0.25 N HCl into gel-wash tray to a depth of 0.5 cm above top gel surface. Begin gentle agitation on orbital shaker. This initial acid wash should be continued until the bromphenol blue dye band has been completely converted to a yellow color. (This can be most accurately assessed by viewing the dye band from the side gel box wall.) For a 400-ml, 0.5% agarose gel this takes about 15 minutes. After complete dye color change has occurred, immediately change wash solutions and wash for 15 minutes again with 0.25 N HCl.
4. Immediately change wash solutions after the second acid wash to a solution of 0.5 N NaOH and 1 M NaCl. Continue this first basic wash until bromphenol blue has reverted completely to its former color. For a 0.5%, 400-ml agarose gel this takes 20–25 minutes. Change wash solutions and wash in same solution again for 15 minutes.
5. Empty basic wash solution, and add 1 M sodium acetate buffer (pH 4.0). Wash for 30 minutes. Repeat this wash once again.
6. Begin diazotization of NBM paper immediately after first buffer wash of gel has begun. Have NBM paper cut to desired size and have a 60°C, constant-temperature water bath preheated. Place NBM paper in the bottom of a flat-bottomed tray, not much larger than the paper area itself. For each 100-cm^2 of paper, add 40 ml of freshly prepared 20% (w/v) sodium dithionite in H_2O, agitate, and squeeze out any bubbles from underneath

paper. Cover tray with Saran Wrap to prevent evaporation and place a weight on the tray to keep it level. Allow this incubation to proceed for 30 minutes with occasional agitation of the tray.

7. After 30 minutes of incubation in the sodium dithionite, wash paper in tray many times with distilled water to remove as much of the H_2S odor as possible. This may require 10 or more rinses. Then wash paper for about 3 minutes in 1.2 N HCl.

8. Place paper in tray on ice and for each 100 cm² of paper add 30 ml of ice-cold 1.2 N HCl and 0.8 ml of a 10 mg/ml sodium nitrite solution. Add the sodium nitrite solution (after the HCl) dropwise, using a pipet while agitating the tray. Place this assemblage in the cold (4°C) to incubate for 30 minutes with occasional agitation.

9. Before $NaNO_2$ incubation of the paper is complete, the second gel-buffer wash should be done. Remove gel box with gel from wash tray. Cut gel, if desired, and cut off a small piece from the upper left-hand corner to preserve the orientation of the lanes. Have sponges large enough to accommodate gel surface in trays, and soaked with 1 M sodium acetate buffer (pH 4.0), with about 2 cm excess buffer in the tray. Place a piece of Whatman 3-mm paper soaked in the acetate buffer about 1 cm larger on all sides than gel on top surface of gel. Place a Plexiglas plate over paper and invert gel. Slide gel box (now on top) off gel and then slide 3-mm paper (gel on top of paper) onto sponge so that gel is completely on sponge. Keep top surface of gel constantly soaked with the acetate buffer to prevent its drying out. Border all sides of gel with 3- to 4-cm wide strips of parafilm. *Keep gel surface moist!*

10. When $NaNO_2$ incubation of paper is complete, rinse paper two times for about 30 seconds each with ice-cold distilled water. (During the second rinse, the paper should begin to assume a faint to prominent yellow color.) The rinse two times for 30 seconds each with ice-cold 0.02 M sodium acetate buffer (pH 4.0).

11. Immediately position DBM paper on *wet* gel surface so that the area of gel to be transferred is completely covered. Quickly place a piece of 3-mm paper (soaked in the acetate buffer) that is identical in size to DBM paper on top, so it covers DBM paper completely. Place four to five more "perfect fit" dry sheets of 3-mm paper on top of this and then add a 3-in. stack of flat paper towels cut to size. Place a light weight (such as a glass plate) on top and allow transfer to proceed for 4 hours. Be sure none of the wicking material comes in contact with the sponge or the solution in the tray during the transfer.

12. When transfer time is complete, remove all wicking material. By this time, the DBM paper should have a deep orange color. Wash filter in distilled water for a few minutes, then two times for a few minutes each in

0.2 *M* Tris-HCl buffer (pH 8.0). Filter is now ready for prehybridization or storage at 4°C.

Note: Be sure complete contact between DBM paper and gel is made (i.e., no trapped air bubbles) when laying down the DBM paper before blotting. Likewise with the first sheet of 3-mm paper placed on top of the DBM paper.

References

Alwine, J. C., Kemp, D. J., Parker, B. A., Reiser, J., Renart, J., Stark, G. R., and Whal, G. M. (1979). *In* "Methods in Enzymology" (Wu, R., ed.), Vol. 68, pp. 220–242.

Bachmann, K. (1972). *Chromosoma* **37**, 85–93.

Blattner, F. R., Blechl, A. E., Denniston-Thompson, D., Faber, H. E., Richards, J. E., Slightom, J. L., Tucker, P. W., and Smithies, O. (1978). *Science* **202**, 1279–1284.

Botstein, D., White, R. L., Skolnick, M., and Davis, R. W. (1980). *Am. J. Hum. Genet.* **32**, 314–331.

Boyer, S. H., IV, and Graham, J. B. (1965). *Am. J. Hum. Genet.* **17**, 320–324.

Brack, C., Hirama, M., Lenhard-Schuller, R., and Tonegawa, S. (1978). *Cell* **15**, 1–14.

Cameron, J. R., Loh, E. H., and Davis, R. W. (1979). *Cell* **16**, 739–751.

Cohen, S. N., and Shapiro, J. A. (1980). *Sci. Am.* **75**, 40–49.

Donahue, R. P., Bias, W. B., Renwick, J. H., and McKusick, V. A. (1968). *Proc. Natl. Acad. Sci. U.S.A.* **61**, 949–955.

Dupont, B., Oberfield, S. E., Smithwick, E. M., Lee, T. D., and Levine, L. S. (1977). *Lancet* **2**, 1309–1312.

Feldenezer, J., Mears, J. G., Burns, A. L., Natta, C., and Bank, A. (1979). *J. Clin. Invest.* **64**, 751–755.

Flavell, R. A., Bernards, R., Kooter, J. M., DeBoer, E., Little, P. F. R., Annison, G., and Williamson, R. (1979). *Nucleic Acids Res.* **6**, 2749–2760.

Fritsch, E. F., Lawn, R. M., and Maniatis, T. (1979). *Nature* **279**, 598–603.

Geever, R. F., Wilson, L. B., Nallaseth, F. S., Milner, P. F., Bittner, M., and Wilson, J. T. (1981). *Proc. Natl. Acad. Sci. U.S.A.* **78**, 5081–5085.

Gusella, J. F., Keys, C., Varsanyi-Breiner, A., Kao, F.-T., Jones, C., Puck, T. T., and Housman, D. (1980). *Proc. Natl. Acad. Sci. U.S.A.* **77**, 2829–2833.

Houck, C. M., Rinehart, F. P., and Schmid, C. W. (1979). *J. Mol. Biol.* **132**, 289–306.

Jacobs, P. A. (1977). *Prog. Med. Genet.* **2**, 251–274.

Jeffreys, A. (1979). *Cell* **18**, 1–10.

John, B., and Miklos, G. L. G. (1979). *Int. Rev. Cytol.* **58**, 1–114.

Kan, Y. W., and Dozy, A. M. (1978). *Lancet* **2**, 910–911.

Kan, Y. W., Golbus, M. S., and Dozy, A. M. (1976). *N. Engl. J. Med.* **295**, 1165–1167.

Kan, Y. W., Lee, K. Y., Furbetta, M., Angius, A., and Cao, A. (1980). *N. Engl. J. Med.* **302**, 185–188.

Kravitz, K., Skolnick, M., Cannings, C., Carmelli, D., Baty, B., Amos, B., Johnson, A., Mendell, N., Edwards, C., and Cartwright, G. (1979). *Am. J. Hum. Genet.* **31**, 601–619.

Kurnit, D. M. (1979a). *Hum. Genet.* **47**, 169–186.

Kurnit, D. M. (1979b). *Lancet* **1**, 104.

Kurnit, D. M., and Hoehn, H. (1979). *Ann. Rev. Genet.* **13**, 235–258.

Kurnit, D. M., Wentworth, B. M., de Long, L., and Villa-Komaroff, L. (1982). *Cytogenet. Cell Genet.* (in press).

Little, P. F. R., Whitelaw, E., Annison, G., Williamson, R., Kooter, J. M., Flavell, R. A., Goosens, M., Sergeant, G. R., and Montgomery, D. (1980a). *Blood* **55,** 1060–1062.

Little, P. F. R., Annison, G., Darling, S., Cleamson, R. W., Camba, L., and Modell, B. (1980b). *Nature* **285,** 144–147.

Maniatis, T., Hardison, R. C., Lacy, E., Lauer, J., O'Connell, C., Quon, D., Sim, G. K., and Efstratiadis, A. (1978). *Cell* **15,** 687–701.

Maxam, A. M., and Gilbert, W. (1977). *Proc. Natl. Acad. Sci. U.S.A.* **74,** 560–564.

Mears, J. G., Ramirez, G., Leibowitz, D., and Bank, A. (1978). *N. Engl. J. Med.* **299,** 1258.

Neel, J. V. (1978). *Can. J. Genet. Cytol.* **20,** 295–306.

Orkin, S. H. (1978). *N. Engl. J. Med.* **299,** 1258.

Orkin, S. H., and Nathan, D. G. (1980). *Adv. Hum. Genet.* **11,** 233–280.

Orkin, S. H., Alter, B. P., Altay, C., Mahoney, M. J., Lazarus, H., Hobbins, J. C., and Nathan, D. G. (1978). *N. Engl. J.Med.* **299,** 166–172.

Orkin, S. H., Old, J. M., Weatherall, D. J., and Nathan, D. G. (1979). *Proc. Natl. Acad. Sci. U.S.A.* **76,** 2400–2404.

Orkin, S. H., Kolodner, R., Michelson, A., and Husson, R. (1980). *Proc. Natl. Acad. Sci. U.S.A.* **77,** 3558–3562.

Orkin, S. H., Little, P. F. R., Kazazian, H. H., Jr., and Boehm, C. D. (1982). Submitted for publication.

Petes, T. D. (1980). *Cell* **19,** 765–774.

Phillips, J. A., III, Scott, A. F., Kazazian, H. H., Jr., Smith, K. D., Stetten, G., and Thomas, G. H. (1979). *Johns Hopkins Med. J.* **145,** 57–60.

Phillips, J. A., III, Panny, S. R., Kazazian, H. H., Jr., Boehm, C. D., Scott, A. F., and Smith, K. D. (1980). *Proc. Natl. Acad. Sci. U.S.A.* **77,** 2853–2856.

Potter, S. S., and Thomas, C. A., Jr. (1977). *Cold Spring Harbor Symp. Quant. Biol.* **42,** 1023–1031.

Renwick, J. H., and Lawler, S. D. (1955). *Ann. Hum. Genet.* **19,** 312–331.

Roberts, R. (1980). *Nucleic Acids Res.* **8,** r63–r80.

Sanger, F., Nicklen, S., and Coulson, A. R. (1977). *Proc. Natl. Acad. Sci. U.S.A.* **74,** 5463–5467.

Schildkraut, C. L., Marmur, J., and Doty, P. (1961). *J. Mol. Biol.* **3,** 595–617.

Schrott, H. G., Karp, L., and Omenn, G. S. (1973). *Clin. Genet.* **4,** 38–45.

Seidman, J. G., Leder, A., Nau, M., Norman, B., and Leder, P. (1978). *Science* **202,** 11–17.

Singer, J., Roberts-Ems, J., Luthardt, F. W., and Riggs, A. D. (1979). *Nucleic Acids Res.* **7,** 2369–2389.

Smith, G. P. (1976). *Science* **191,** 528–535.

Southern, E. M. (1975). *J. Mol. Biol.* **98,** 503–517.

Strobel, E., Dunsmuir, P., and Rubin, G. M. (1979). *Cell* **17,** 429–439.

Szostak, J. W., and Wu, R. (1980). *Nature* **284,** 426–430.

Wilson, J. T., Wilson, L. B., Reddy, V. B., Cavallesco, C., Ghosh, P. K., deReil, J. K., Forget, B. G., and Weissman, S. M. (1980). *J. Biol. Chem.* **255,** 2807–2815.

Wyman, A., and White, R. L. (1980). *Proc. Natl. Acad. Sci. U.S.A.* **77,** 6754–6758.

Young, B. D., Hell, A., Birnie, G. D. (1976). *Biochim. Biophys. Acta* **454,** 539–548.

Young, M. W. (1979). *Proc. Natl. Acad. Sci. U.S.A.* **76,** 6274–6278.

Zimmer, E. A., Martin, S. L., Beverley, S. M., Kan, Y. W., and Wilson, A. C. (1980). *Proc. Natl. Acad. Sci. U.S.A.* **77,** 2158–2162.

Index

CONTENTS OF RECENT VOLUMES

(Volumes I–XX edited by David M. Prescott)

Volume X

Volume XIII

Volume XV

Volume XVI

Volume XVII

Chromatin and Chromosomal Protein Research. II

Volume XVIII

Chromatin and Chromosomal Protein Research. III

Volume XIX

Chromatin and Chromosomal Protein Research. IV

Volume XX

Volume 21A

Volume 21B

*Normal Human Tissue and Cell Culture B. Endo-
crine, Urogenital, and Gastrointestinal Systems*

Volume 22

Three-Dimensional Ultrastructure in Biology

Volume 24

The Cytoskeleton.

Part A. *Cytoskeletal Proteins, Isolation and
Characterization*

Volume 25

The Cytoskeleton

Part B. *Biological Systems and in Vitro Models*